The Whartons'
BACK BOOK

End back pain with this simple
revolutionary programme

JIM & PHIL WHARTON
WITH BEV BROWNING

RODALE

This edition first published in 2004 by
Rodale International Ltd
7-10 Chandos Street
London W1G 9AD
www.rodale.co.uk

Printed and bound in China
1 3 5 7 9 8 6 4 2

A CIP record for this book is available from the British Library
1-4050-3285-5

This paperback edition distributed to the book trade by Pan Macmillan Ltd

Produced for Rodale Books International by
studio cactus ©
Design: Laura Watson and Dawn Terrey
Editorial: Jake Woodward and Clare Wallis
Commissioned Exercise Photography: Gary Ombler
Illustration: Claire Moore

Notice
This book is intended as a reference volume only, not as a medical manual. The information given
here is designed to help you make informed decisions about your health. It is not intended as a substitute
for any treatment that may have been prescribed by your doctor. If you suspect that you have a medical
problem, we urge you to seek competent medical help.

Mention of specific companies, organisations or authorities in this book does not imply endorsement by
the publisher, nor does mention of specific companies, organisations or authorities imply that they endorse this
book. Internet addresses and telephone numbers given in this book were accurate at the time it went to press.

To Robert R. Glass

CONTENTS

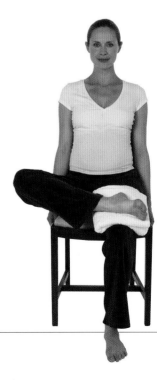

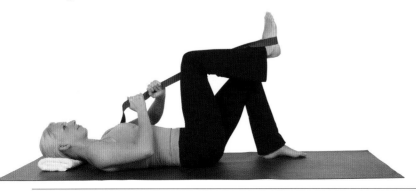

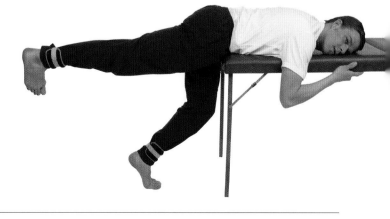

INTRODUCTION

When your back isn't working right, nothing in your life works right. Trying to understand what has gone wrong and how to correct it has led you to this book and a unique opportunity to explore injury not as a patient, but as an athlete.

'Athlete?' you're thinking. 'I'm not an athlete.'

Yes, you are! We are all athletes. If you're living in a body and using it every day to create your life and your work, you're an athlete in need of optimal health, strength, flexibility, balance and more.

Seeing yourself as an athlete affords you a unique perspective. You view yourself not as a helpless victim, but as a person on a mission to take control. You approach getting well with energy that comes into focus only when you reach for the best in yourself. Use this book, and you'll not only relieve and prevent pain – you'll find yourself stronger and more fit than when your back problems began, secure in the knowledge that they won't happen again. Together, we'll get you there.

WE'VE BEEN WHERE YOU ARE TODAY

Are you in pain? Struggling with a chronic injury? Or do you just want to relieve stiffness, a lack of mobility, or a surprising twinge that comes and goes, taking your breath and your confidence with it?

We can help.

Your success is personal to us because we began our careers trying to solve a back problem. When Phil developed scoliosis, we learned what would become the Active-Isolated Stretching and Strengthening programme. Using this method not only relieved his pain but entirely reversed his condition, preventing the need for surgery or an immobilising brace. Today, we are a father-and-son training team that travels the world, helping relieve the back pain of hundreds of high-profile athletes, performers and other luminaries. Now, we want to help you, too!

We started our practice nearly 20 years ago, out of a small office in New York City. Our practice grew by whispers, behind the scenes of some of the largest arenas and venues in the world. Soon, we were training and rehabilitating professional athletes, Broadway dancers, famous musicians and Hollywood actors with roles that were physically challenging. We were especially delighted when, during the 1992 Olympic Games in Barcelona, Spain, the athletes with whom we worked brought home 13 gold medals. (If we were our own country, we would have been placed third in the world!)

Quietly, discreetly, our reputations as 'The Mechanics' spread, on account of our reported ability to fine-tune a high-performance body or 'fix' one when things go wrong. All this, with nothing more than a flat surface, an exercise strap or length of rope and the Active-Isolated method.

What's our secret? Well, over the years, we've certainly learned a lot about physiology and the inherent talents and changing moods of the human body. We can tell you what is the best move to do, when and why, and we can help you coax your body into position. But the truth is, while we may be helpful, we're not miracle workers – but the Active-Isolated method is. We've seen, beyond a doubt, that the same training method that unlocks and relieves the pain of Olympic medalists, hulking American football players and delicate ballerinas can and will work for everyone who's ready to take control. And that means you!

REVOLUTIONARY TRAINING AND REHABILITATION

With this book, we tailor our trademark Active-Isolated method to help prevent and cure back pain. You'll learn a quick, easy method that can help get you out of pain immediately and strengthen your back so that pain will be a thing of the past. In the process, you'll also enjoy better circulation and mobility, enriched sleep, lowered stress and increased energy. You'll do more and hurt less. By giving your back new life, you'll get your own life back.

First, we want to help you understand the anatomy of your back. Ever notice how when your knee goes out, your back acts up two days later? We'll trace those seemingly mystical links and explain how your back is really the epicentre of all sensation in your body.

From medical and biomechanical standpoints, we'll review some of the things that can go wrong with your back, and why. Then we'll advise you on professional care available for diagnosis, treatment and rehabilitation, and the results you can expect.

The core of the book is a training programme of your own. With your doctor's permission and using our signature systems of Active-Isolated Stretching and Strengthening, you can improve your back and your entire fitness level.

Later in the book, we cover some of the situations and conditions that can lead to back pain, and we'll give you complete strategies for preventing and relieving pain in those key moments – exactly when and how you need them.

At the back of the book, we've included easy-reference illustrations of the body's key muscle sets and details for some of the national organisations you may wish to contact regarding conventional or complementary therapies.

Throughout the book, you'll read about the experiences of some of our favourite clients – all of whom have found relief with this very same programme. (Please note: we've changed some of our clients' names and personal details to protect their privacy.)

With the Active-Isolated method, even the smallest efforts will yield surprising, even revolutionary, results. You'll feel better from the very first time you try these exercises. Your healthy back – flexible, strong and pain-free – is waiting for you, athlete. Let's get started!

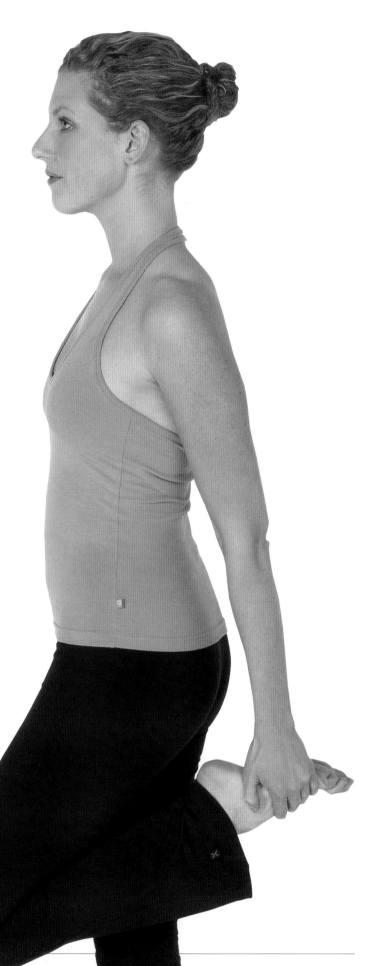

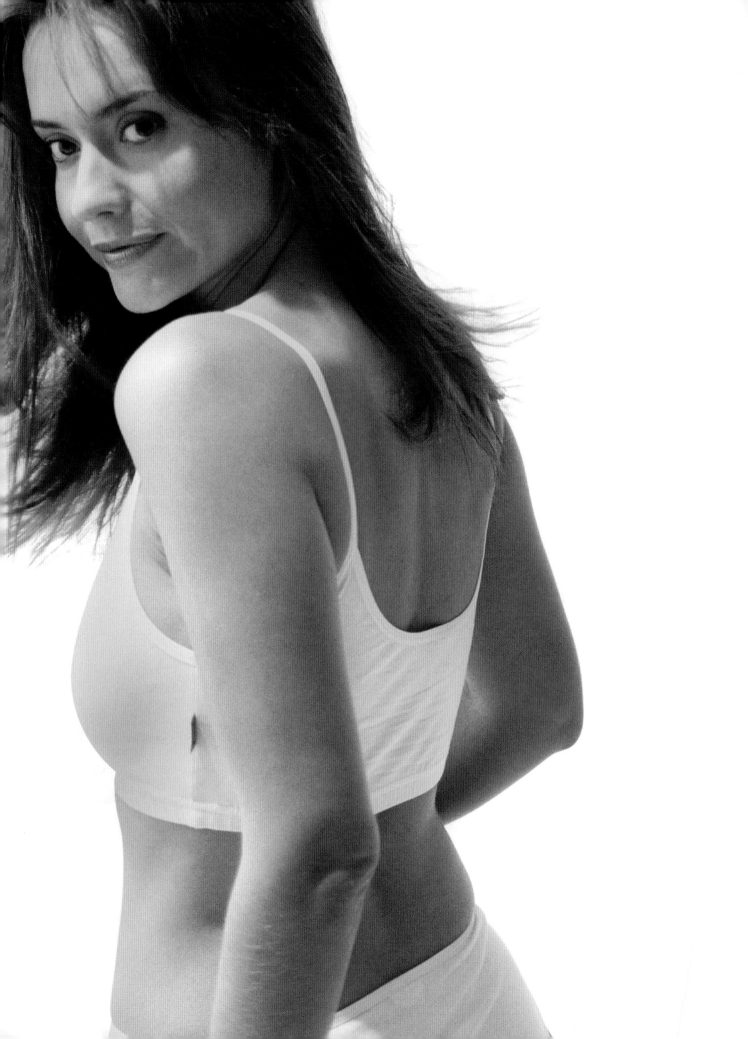

1

THE PAIN-FREE BACK

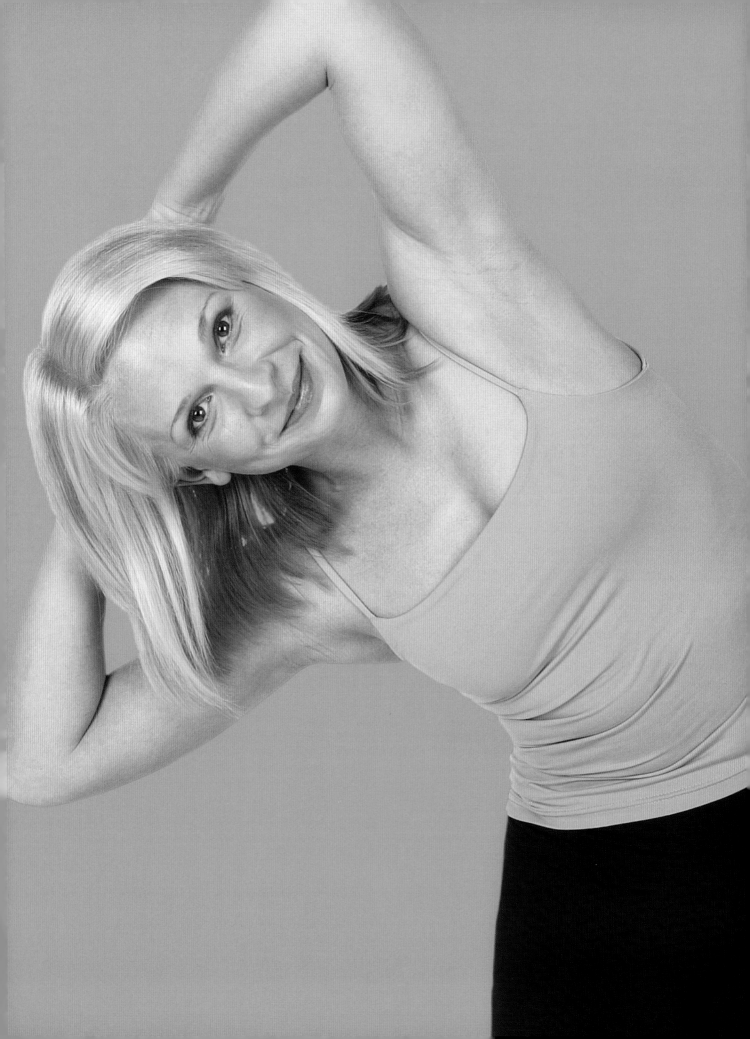

CHAPTER 1

A NEW WAY TO THINK ABOUT YOUR BACK

If you are unfortunate enough to suffer with back *pain, you aren't alone. It is estimated that between 60 and 80 per cent of people will experience back pain at some time in their lives, particularly in the lower-back region. Three working days per employee are lost annually due to backache, and there has been a three-fold increase in sick leave due to backache over the last 20 years.*

As sympathetic as we are, we're also convinced that most of these problems are absolutely preventable. And once they manifest, they can be easily treated in their early stages, before they become debilitating and expensive. Even when they become extreme, surgery might not be the only answer.

Sound crazy? Believe it. We've seen the proof, hundreds of times. And we're going to show you how a simple, do-it-yourself method has helped hundreds of our clients prevent, diminish or completely obliterate their back pain, quickly, easily and often forever.

What it will take is a shift in your thinking. We know that when your back isn't working right, nothing in your life works right. Your attempts to understand what's happening and to control your pain have led you to us. Now we're here to help you seize this opportunity to, as we said earlier, explore your injury not as a *patient*, but as an *athlete*.

We think it's very interesting that our elite athletes never think of back injury as 'injury'. Although almost all are very knowledgeable in anatomy and biomechanics and are certainly well-informed about every aspect of the pain they're suffering, they never define the injury at all. They see it merely as a mistake in training or performance. Perhaps it's even a wake-up call.

Well, here is your wake-up call. You can control your own pain. You can rehabilitate your body. You can even learn to 'PREhabilitate' your back, to prevent pain from striking again. Just listen to the stories of your fellow athletes.

BANISHING PAIN ON STAGE AND ON THE COURT

Take this case, for instance: the actress, Lauren Bacall, had just completed an arduous run on Broadway when she consulted us about back pain that had resulted from the demands made on her by the performances. Rather than succumb to the pain and retreat to bed, she was already working out at La Palestra, one of the best gyms in New York City, to try to bring her body back into alignment. We examined her and realised that a knee irritation, which she had had for some time, was causing her to favour her other leg. Because she was compensating, she had thrown her back into imbalance; pain and weakness followed.

We pointed out to Lauren that performing on stage is no different from performing in an Olympic arena. Both are athletic and require the same training and preparation. She smiled. She already knew. We were on the same wavelength. We worked out with her and taught her the same techniques that we'll show you in chapter 4. We got her out of pain very quickly.

The point is that this graceful actress knew that her body is her gift and her responsibility. When her back was in pain, she didn't cave in. She headed straight for the gym and eventually to us. She didn't fixate on the injury. She used it as a wake-up call. As a result, she's doing better than ever: still active and energetic, and still very beautiful.

We'll give you another example. A leading American basketball team, the New York Knicks, invited us to their pre-season training to teach the players short routines to prepare and recover quickly. The Knicks were facing an 81-game season, and there was concern about keeping everyone healthy and on the basketball court.

Over a series of visits to their training centre, we got to know the players pretty well. They're great people who responded appreciatively to our care. But one player was particularly interested: Patrick Ewing.

Patrick admitted that he'd been suffering with back pain for a couple of years. We suspected that it had stemmed from a slight knee injury (just like Lauren), so we designed an intensive personal programme for him. We started first with flexibility and strengthening, concentrating on his knee. When we straightened that problem out, Patrick reported that his back stopped hurting. He was willing to do the work, even when he couldn't quite make the direct connection between the imbalances caused by his knee and the pain in his back.

He didn't give up. He's not about injury – he's about winning. He used the work to become a better athlete. He used the opportunity to take performance to the next level.

New Attitude, New You

As we've discussed, athletes view injuries as mistakes and opportunities; their bodies have pointed out mistakes and have given them the chance to make corrections and rocket their performances to the next level.

Non-athletes, on the other hand, sometimes fixate on injuries. In an effort to avoid further pain, they may allow the injury to limit their activity, sometimes to the point that life itself winds down to nearly nothing. Sadly, the approaches between athlete and non-athlete are 180 degrees off each other. But they shouldn't be.

We want you to think like an athlete. We want you to see a back problem as an opportunity. Suffering and surgery might be prevented if you are willing to switch your mindset. You *are* an athlete. You might not play in a basketball team or dance in musicals but if you use your body to live, work, play and love, then you are an athlete. You deserve to be flexible, strong, fit, healthy... and pain-free. You deserve to reclaim your life.

Our Story

Your success is personal to us because we began our careers trying to solve a back problem. Let us tell you the story of how an injury turned out to be the opportunity of a lifetime.

In high school, Phil was an up-and-coming track athlete who averaged 35 miles (55km) of running per week and took summers off to rest and recover from the pounding his body took during the school year. The hard work paid off when Phil was accepted to the University of Florida to run with the prestigious Florida Track Team.

Phil had ramped up his running to 80 miles (130km) per week and all but eliminated the rest cycle when things suddenly started going very wrong. At first, he felt a twinge in his hip. Then he felt an ache in his back. Day by day, 'discomfort' – at first easily explained and even ignored – turned uglier. It wasn't long before every step that he ran fired a jolting, searing pain up his spine.

His whole life started to unravel. Like most people trying to solve back problems, Phil and his coaches tried every therapy they thought might bring relief, from massage and rest to chiropractics and medications. The team doctors at the University of Florida finally diagnosed him with scoliosis, curvature of the spine, and suggested implanting rods on either side of his spine to straighten it. They also informed him that if he didn't stop running, they could practically guarantee that his disability was going to get considerably worse. He might even suffer permanent nerve damage or paralysis.

Implanting the rods would mean that his running career would be over anyway, which the surgeons thought would be a small price to pay for the relief he would get. But the surgeons didn't understand the heart of a runner. Running was Phil's life. Period. There had to be another way.

The Breakthrough

Randy Brower, a trainer who worked with the Florida Track Team, had one more suggestion, even though it was a long shot. He directed Phil to Aaron Mattes, a well-respected

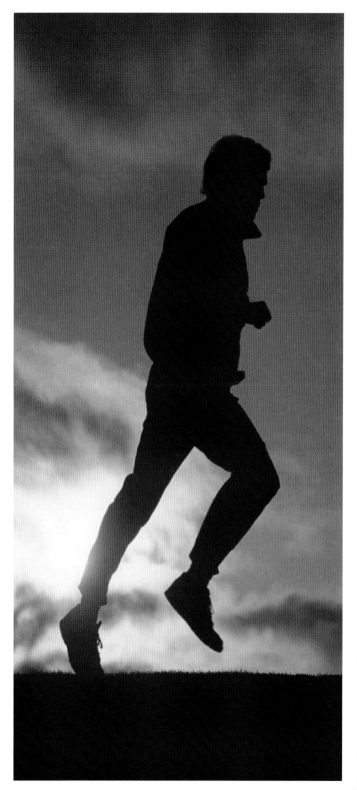

▲ Back on track

Phil Wharton's running career seemed over when he was diagnosed with curvature of the spine, but Active-Isolated training provided a non-surgical remedy to this debilitating condition.

kinesiologist with a clinic only a few hours away in Sarasota. Aaron conducted a muscle-by-muscle evaluation of Phil's body and matter-of-factly pointed out areas that were weak and imbalanced.

Weak and imbalanced?! Heresy! Impossible! Phil was a front-runner for the mighty Florida Track Team. Aaron wasn't impressed at all. He flatly informed us that he thought the scoliosis had nothing to do with any deformity of Phil's spine. It had everything to do with Phil's being out of balance on one side and drawing his spine out of alignment and into curvature. In fact, *he* was causing the problem.

Before Phil could catapult from initial shock into righteous indignation and outrage, Aaron told us that he thought he could help. And he did. After one session with Aaron, Phil felt measurable relief. Against overwhelming odds, we had found the answer. We were believers.

We both were intrigued by Aaron's approach, for it combined all that we understood about physics with our knowledge of the biomechanics of running. Everything Aaron said made a lot of sense. Besides, we had nothing to lose and everything to gain by following his advice.

Together, we embarked on a year of hard work to get Phil out of pain and back onto the track. Phil worked with Active-Isolated Stretching and Strengthening exercises six days a week for a full year; he was a man on a mission. Once a week, the two of us would travel to Aaron's clinic in Sarasota for an evaluation to check progress and finely tune the workouts.

Here's the happy ending: Phil corrected the imbalances and strengthened the weaknesses. His spine straightened, and his pain disappeared. He returned to running – this time 100 miles (160km) per week – with no problem.

Today, 20 years later, he trains every day without injury and competes on the world-class level in the 26.2-mile (42km) marathon. Not only did we find a solution to Phil's back problem that would actually improve his performance, but we also became students of Aaron Mattes. It meant starting all over again and going back to school for both of us, but the sacrifices of an abrupt about-face would be worth the effort.

We embarked on a long, long journey that would change the course of our lives and the world of sports forever. Today, we train and rehabilitate athletes all over the world. Our clinic in New York City is a small, unassuming haven on the Upper West Side just off Central Park in Manhattan. But don't let 'small, unassuming' fool you. Our clinic looks like a public relations junket for the finest athletes and entertainers in the world. Among unrecognisable faces are those of NBA basketball players, Kenyan runners, Italian football players, and Olympic swimmers chatting with famous actors and Broadway dancers. All are there for one of two reasons: either they are injured and need fast, effective rehab, or they are preparing to do something that will make unfamiliar demands on their bodies, and they need to be properly trained to achieve the next level.

We want you to have those same opportunities. We want to open the doors of our clinic to you through the pages of this book. We want to get you to stop thinking like a patient with a bad back and start thinking like an athlete who needs rehabilitation or requires training to take performance to the next level.

HOW TO USE THIS BOOK

This book is divided into the following six parts:

1. The Pain-free Back
2. Try PREhab, Not Rehab
3. Stopping the Pain
4. Protecting Your Back as Your Body Changes
5. Stress and Slumber
6. Pain-free Solutions for Everyday Situations

How you use the book depends on why you're reading it. If you want to prevent back problems, you'll be particularly interested in training like an athlete to become as strong and flexible as you can. You'll benefit from the general information in part one and the PREhab programme in part 2.

PREhab (as opposed to rehab) is a term we coined when we found our early practice dominated by rehabilitating athletes who had made basic biomechanical mistakes with catastrophic consequences. After treating the thousandth injury, we decided to step into athletes' lives earlier – *before* they got hurt. Now we design PREhabilitation programmes, so we have to do less rehabilitation.

We'd rather work this way, of course, but it's not always possible. If you're reading the book because you're already suffering with back pain, in part 3 we'll help you design your own at-home rehab programme. We call it your Get-Out-of-Pain-Free-Plan. If that doesn't do the trick, we'll help you make decisions about the right professional help. After you're well, and with your doctor's blessing, you can continue with training to make sure you'll stay out of trouble for a lifetime.

We understand that no back exists in a perfect, unstrained world, so in parts 4, 5 and 6, we'll advise you on how to avoid, and also cope with, a number of situations in which you may become injured, feel pain or aggravate old injuries.

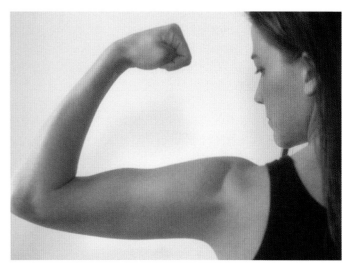

▲ Flexing and relaxing for fitness
The basic principle of Active-Isolated training is that all muscles work in opposite pairs. An obvious example of this is when your triceps muscle relaxes to allow your biceps to contract.

You'll discover the best way to prepare for these situations, and you'll learn 'quick-release' moves to help relieve you from those painful seize-ups that can instantly immobilise you, those moments that can make you want to lie down on the floor and never get up. We've been there, and we're here to help.

ACTIVE-ISOLATED? WHAT DOES THAT MEAN?

When we say that our method is called 'Active-Isolated', what does that mean, exactly? We'll explain more later, but, essentially, you'll be encouraging your muscles to function in the way nature intended.

Muscles work in opposite pairs. Every time one contracts, a companion muscle must relax.

Why not try it yourself: make a fist and flex your elbow to bend your arm up. Your biceps, the muscle on the front side of your upper arm, contracts to bring your fist up. At that very same moment, your triceps muscle, the one at the back side of your upper arm, is completely relaxed. It needed to let go and elongate so that your biceps could then shorten.

This simple principle underlies all of the Active-Isolated work. You isolate a specific muscle or group of muscles and activate, or 'fire', them one at a time in a prescribed sequence. As you do this, the opposite muscles will relax for a good stretch, allowing a greater range of motion and a fuller, more complete workout of the muscle fibres from one end to the other. The same principle applies during an Active-Isolated Strengthening move, except this time you'll relax one muscle so that the opposite muscle can then fire for the lift.

How is this different from conventional methods? Well, Mother Nature designed the muscles in the body to be helpful to each other. When one is weak, fatigued, cramped or struggling, your body automatically recruits volunteers – other muscles that can kick in to get the job done. So let's imagine that you are trying to do a sit-up, but your abdominal muscles aren't very strong. What happens? Your body recruits other volunteer muscles to assist – probably ones in your hip – and those weaker ab muscles get shut out, remain weak, and get progressively weaker as time goes on.

What if the goal had been to strengthen that weak muscle, instead of just doing the sit-up? What if the goal had been to stretch a weak muscle, instead of getting your nose to your knee? This is exactly what Active-Isolated work is all about.

The goal of your Whartons' workout is to isolate a muscle or a muscle group, so your body will not be able to recruit others against your wishes. You activate the targeted area only, so *you* are in control of which muscles you stretch or

strengthen. And because you'll be targeting specific muscles, the moves are small and gentle – perfect for helping you to get out of pain and back to full function.

You're probably eager to get going. But before you begin, you need to get a good understanding of the raw materials we'll be working with. Behold, the amazing mechanics of your spine.

THE DIFFERENT PARTS OF THE SPINE

Composed of 33 bones (vertebrae) all working in concert, the structure of the spine is really an amazing feat of biomechanical architecture. It is split into five parts: your neck, your midback, your lower back, your sacrum and your coccyx. Let's take a look at these five areas in more detail and explore some of the typical problems that clients of ours have encountered. We will also look at some of the other amazingly well-designed parts of the spine, specifically the vertebrae, discs and nerves.

▼ Understanding muscle groups
Sit-ups can actually accentuate existing weaknesses in the abdomen rather than strengthening the muscles. Active-Isolation exercises ensure that the right muscles get the right training.

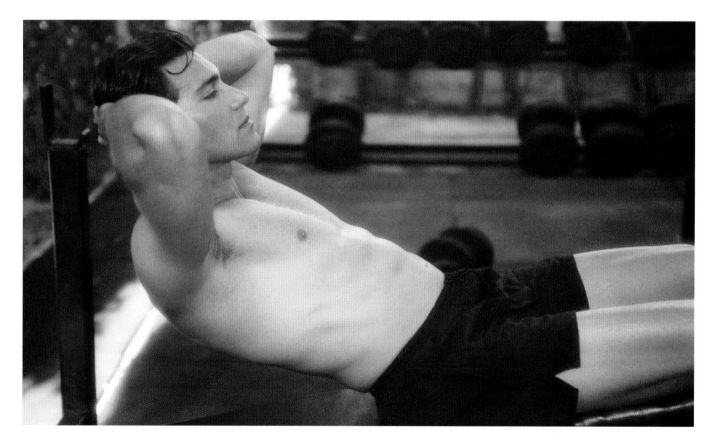

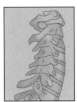

1. Your Neck

Yes, your neck *is* your back; it's the part that holds your head on.

This is the cervical spine, made up of seven vertebrae. The medical shorthand for this is C1 to C7, meaning cervical vertebra number 1 to cervical vertebra number 7.

The upper bones C1 and C2 are unique among all the other vertebrae, because they are in charge of head and neck rotation. C1, a ring of bone that supports the skull, is called the atlas, named after the mythical Greek god who supported the weight of the world on his shoulders. C2 is called the axis, because its function is literally that. It has a little blunt knob on the top that projects up into a hole in the atlas, allowing the neck to pivot. They are supported by special ligaments.

The cervical spine is highly mobile and busy all the time. The pressure of the weight of your head and the constant turning and bending of your head and neck can sometimes lead to wear and tear. This is why neck pain and problems are common.

Typical concerns: One of the problems that manifests in the cervical spine is locked neck. The symptoms are that the neck is contracted to either side and it seems to be locked into position.

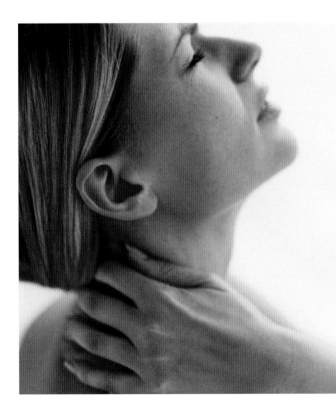

◄ Pain in the neck
Problems with the cervical spine – the neck – can cause extreme discomfort; symptoms may include throbbing headaches, a frozen shoulder or locked neck.

Another clue to the locked-neck condition is that one shoulder is cocked or carried a bit too high, as though the body is unbalanced. The smallest movement is not only painful but also impossible. It doesn't take long for that tension in the neck to cause a throbbing tension headache. Typically, the cervical spinal muscles are constricted and stressed, causing the spasm that reveals itself through pain and immobility.

Another malady of the cervical spine is frozen shoulder. Even though the shoulder is located beside the cervical spine and would seem to be unrelated, restriction of the cervical spine can most certainly cause muscles on each side to lock down, too.

The frozen shoulder is a loss of range of motion in the shoulder joint. Clients describe it as a knot of congestion, pain in the upper back, or a feeling that their shoulder blades are being drawn together. Frequently, the shoulder is not only locked up but also rolled forward in constriction.

When the cervical spine is contracted, the pectoralis major muscles in the upper chest fatigue and draw the shoulder forwards, causing the upper back to struggle to maintain upright posture and function. Then trapezius and rhomboid muscles in the upper back short out, and all muscles in the upper chest and upper back tighten to protect themselves. The tighter the front, the tighter the back. The tighter the back, the tighter the front. The result is pain, fatigue and a shoulder that seems to be frozen.

Getting the muscles to release is a matter of restoring circulation and range of motion, and keeping them flexible and strong enough to make sure that the structural integrity of the shoulder will be protected.

Thankfully, both of these painful situations can be completely avoided with the flexibility and strengthening exercises found in chapter 4.

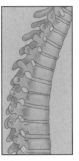

2. Your Midback

The longest designation of the spine is distinguished as the part of your spine that supports all your ribs, except the lower two (the 'floating ribs' that are fused to ribs above them rather than to vertebrae). It runs from below your cervical spine to your waist behind your chest. The upper part, between your shoulder blades, is typically the place where you carry all your tension.

The midback is known as the thoracic spine, made up of 12 vertebrae. The medical shorthand for this is T1 to T12 (thoracic vertebra number 1 to thoracic vertebra number 12). The thoracic spine has a very limited range of motion because the ribs provide support and the formation of each vertebra is designed to lock into place.

Typical concerns: The thoracic spine is particularly vulnerable to a knot of tension carried between the shoulder blades. This knot can cause a specific point of pain – a spasm of the deeper muscles in the back that feels tender to the touch.

The knot can occur from tension over a period of time, during which adhesions or scar tissue may set into the muscles and cause problems. Or it can occur in an instant, such as when a sprinter explodes off the starting block. When the body perceives that a muscle is injured instantly or over time, it builds a natural splint by creating a spasm to immobilise the area and protect it from further harm. If you want a spasm between your shoulder blades to

The Spine

The spine is a fascinating, miraculous system, but on the days it seems most painful, it can be hard to imagine that it's anything but a source of agony. But let's review the many ways that the spine helps you get through your day.

Support and Movement

- It keeps you upright so that you don't collapse on the ground in a heap (no small thing!).
- It is the base of attachment for connective tissue like tendons (which attach muscle to bone), ligaments (which attach bone to bone) and muscles. In fact, a *lot* of muscles attach to the spine.
- It directly supports your head, shoulders and chest and connects your upper body to your lower body.
- Its flexibility allows you to bend forwards and backwards and to both sides. It will rotate your upper half from side to side while your lower half stays still, and the other way around.
- It can and will combine any of the movements above.
- It has compensation systems that keep your weight distributed properly so that you can balance.

Protection and Renewal

- It houses and protects the spinal cord and nerve roots that communicate with your brain and then transmit messages to every part of your body – from the top of your head to the tips of your toes, and to many major internal organs in between – and back again.
- The individual vertebrae produce red blood cells in the marrow and store minerals. (And there you were thinking that your spine was just a source of excruciating pain!)

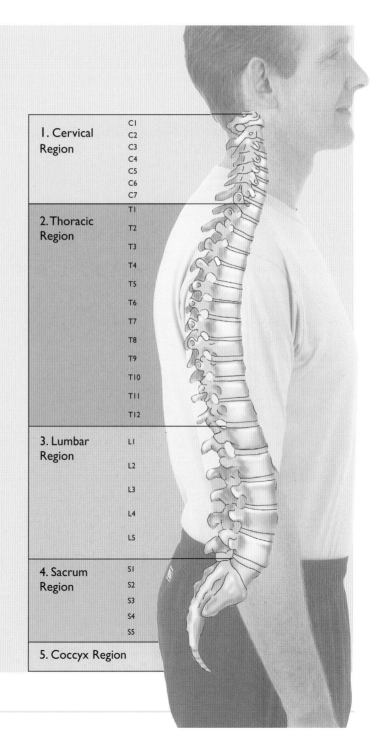

1. Cervical Region	C1
	C2
	C3
	C4
	C5
	C6
	C7
2. Thoracic Region	T1
	T2
	T3
	T4
	T5
	T6
	T7
	T8
	T9
	T10
	T11
	T12
3. Lumbar Region	L1
	L2
	L3
	L4
	L5
4. Sacrum Region	S1
	S2
	S3
	S4
	S5
5. Coccyx Region	

release, you have to convince the body that there is no injury. You have to relax the muscles and restore circulation and range of motion. We'll tell you how on page 207 in chapter 12.

Another complaint we get in our clinic is for non-specific backache in the thoracic region. General though this pain may be, it can throb. Intermittent or chronic, the pain can intensify with every breath because the ribs are connected at the thoracic spine and their expansions and contractions can irritate a back in trouble. It's just an ache that saps the energy and fun right out of life. The major stabilising muscles in the thoracic spine can weaken over time in the battle to 'brake' us, or hold us up against gravity. Preventing non-specific backache is a simple matter of getting strong and flexible. You have to get moving.

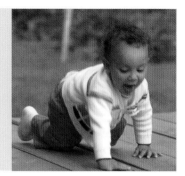

When we are born, we have shortened psoas and quadriceps; these held us in the foetal position in the womb. Crawling is our first attempt to elongate these two muscles so that we learn to stand erect.

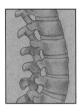

3. Your Lower Back

This notorious problem area, which runs from right below your lowest rib all the way to the top of your pelvis, is called the lumbar spine and is where strains most often cause pain. The lumbar spine is made up of five vertebrae. The medical shorthand for this is L1 to L5, meaning lumbar vertebra number 1 to lumbar vertebra number 5.

The lumbar vertebrae bear much of your weight and take most of the stress of movement. They are the largest and flattest of all the vertebrae, but, unfortunately, that doesn't always protect them from injury, fatigue and imbalance.

Typical concerns: When we see a client with one hip hiked up, we know that the lumbar spine is involved. As long as the pelvis is level and everything is working well, the body can move easily to the side. But when the body has a tight psoas – the primary hip flexor that helps us stand erect, which originates from L1 to L5, passes through the pelvis and attaches to the femur (thighbone) – it pulls the pelvis forwards and down, so the other erector muscles must struggle to compensate. When they tighten and fatigue, they can hike one hip up. The result is pain and fatigue caused by muscles trying to take up the slack and make up for immobility.

The most common complaint we hear is lower-back pain. It comes in all shapes and sizes: dull or sharp, chronic or intermittent. A confluence of muscles and connective tissue forms a band across your back just over your hipbone. When the lower back is injured or the muscles tighten, it causes pain, weakness and dysfunction. We attack this problem from the back *and* the front. Not only do we

restore range of motion and strength to stabilise the lumbar spine, but we also work on the abdominal muscles that support the back. If you suffer from lower-back pain and your doctor has ruled out injury, disease or dysfunction that must be medically treated, then getting fit can eliminate lower-back pain.

4. Your Sacrum

The sacrum is where the spine joins the pelvis down to the tailbone. These wide bones form a sort of solid inverted triangle. Made up of five fused vertebrae, the sacral spine's medical shorthand is S1 to S5.

Typical concerns: Because the sacrum is fused, it's rarely the source of problems, but occasionally we see people with piriformis syndrome. This is an acute inflammation of the sciatic nerve, a nerve that is actually woven through the bands of the inner fibres of the gluteal muscles – the muscles that run from the sacral spine through the buttocks. When the buttocks are bruised or weakened from sitting, the hip rotators beneath them can swell or spasm to compress that sciatic nerve. The result is a pain that shoots down the sacrum, through the buttocks and into the back of the leg. Releasing the nerve is a matter of relaxing the stranglehold of the muscles with Active-Isolated Stretching.

5. Your Coccyx

Pronounced 'COX-six', this is your tailbone. If the sacrum is an inverted triangle, the coccyx forms the point at the bottom.

The coccyx is made up of four vertebrae. No medical shorthand exists for the individual bones because the coccyx encases no spinal cord and is generally thought of as one unit. If you break your tailbone, it doesn't matter which of the bones broke. You only know you landed on it, it hurts like the dickens, and there's no way to put it in a cast.

Typical concerns: Because the coccyx is a relatively simple structure, the only injuries we ever see are bruising and fracturing. The coccyx completes the spine and certainly contributes to the shape of the body, but it is insignificant in terms of muscles and connective tissue that could be injured and cause dysfunction in related structures. When the coccyx is bruised or fractured, we merely advise our clients to protect it with padding on seats and to exercise extra care during activities that might further injure the bones. Ice and painkillers are the only other things that might help to relieve suffering.

Your Vertebrae

Each vertebra is shaped in a different way so that when they're stacked together, they interlock like 3-D puzzle pieces to protect the delicate spinal cord that runs up through their open centres. The interlocking positions must be perfect so that the spine can move but the cord is kept safe and secure without disruptions. The whole spine is held together by ligaments that allow the spine to bend and twist in a perfect balance of strength and mobility.

Although each vertebra is different, they all have a few things in common. Each is a rounded body with a hole in the centre called a foramen, through which the spinal cord runs. Most have bony processes coming off them – one at the rear and one on each side – that look a little like wings and act like brakes that stop the spine from moving too far backwards or to one side. Going too far would impinge or damage the spinal cord, so nature has designed this physical limit for each vertebra.

Your Discs

In between each vertebra is a joint called a facet. Within each facet is an intervertebral disc – a cushion that allows movement without rubbing the bones against each other.

The discs between the vertebrae have a fibrous outer lining and a gelatinous inner core. These discs basically function as spinal shock absorbers and account for about 20 per cent of the height of the spine.

Sometimes a disc can be injured or ruptured. Because the disc itself has few nerves and no blood supply of its own, it has no way to repair itself. When the disc is injured, a cascade of horrors can be set into motion, making life very miserable. Vertebrae rub together. Nerves can be pinched or inflamed by leaking inflammatory proteins, sending pain shooting all over the place and disrupting normal function in muscles and organs. Even though the disc itself can't feel pain, inflammation and pain can be rampant nearly everywhere else.

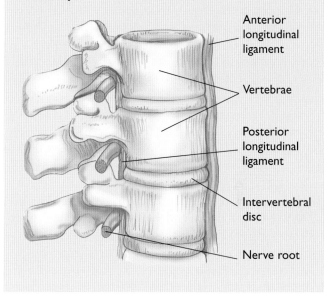

Side View of the Vertebra

The spine is split into five main sections made up of 33 vertebrae. Each of these are cushioned by discs and have nerves and nerve roots that branch off from the spinal cord and spread out through the body.

Anterior longitudinal ligament

Vertebrae

Posterior longitudinal ligament

Intervertebral disc

Nerve root

Discs get hammered every day. Subject to this wear and tear, they're the first to succumb to a lifetime of work and the first to show signs of ageing. At birth, the discs are 80 per cent water, but as life goes on, they dehydrate and deteriorate, gradually becoming less supple. For this reason, people get shorter as they age, and less supple. The good news is that as we age, there are fewer inflammatory proteins in the discs, so disc pain becomes pretty rare after the age of 60.

Your Nerves and Nerve Roots

Running through the centre of the spinal column is the spinal cord, starting at your brain and ending at the bottom of your lumbar spine in a bundle of nerves that looks a little like a horse's tail. For this reason, it's called the cauda equina (Latin for 'horse's tail').

These nerves are responsible for your leg muscle function, your ability to feel sensation all the way down to your toes, and your bladder, intestinal and genital function. That's why an injury in your lumbar region will radiate pain through your buttocks to your legs. In cases of severe injury, doctors will even look at disruption in the bladder, intestines and bowels as clues to locate the injury and determine its severity.

At each disc from the cauda equina up, a pair of nerve roots branch off from the spinal cord through a little opening in the vertebrae. These nerves transmit information from the brain through the spinal cord and out to the body and back again.

MUSCLE STRENGTH = STABILITY

The spine is a dynamic system designed to move. If it were meant to be completely stable, it would be a solid column of one thick bone with a hole bored through it for your spinal cord. But that's not the way it works. Stability means that the spine lets you move the way you're supposed to and stops you from moving the way you shouldn't.

When you straighten your spine and stand fully erect, your back muscles are not the only ones involved. You are also contracting opposing muscles at the same time: the abdominals and the erector spinae, which run up and down the spine. These oppositional forces balance each other and give you extra support. If you stand up and tighten up, front and back, you will notice how your back is rigid and erect.

Muscles are pivotal in holding everything together and are attached to every segmental level. The stronger the muscle, the better the support. Even muscles some distance from the spine itself can affect stability. For example, abdominal muscles are pivotal in holding the spine in place, although they're nowhere near it. But since they are attached to the sternum, the rib cage and the pelvis, contracting the abdominals results in flexion, or lateral bending, of the spine.

BACK PAIN IS AVOIDABLE

Too many people suffer from back pain needlessly. Although some back problems result from accident, disease or congenital deformity and will require medical intervention and surgery, most back problems are entirely preventable.

What we're telling you is that back pain might not be your fate. And surgery might not be your future.

It's up to you. You're in control. Make that leap. Stop thinking of yourself as a patient with a back problem – and start thinking of yourself as one of our athletes in training. You have the opportunity to correct a problem and get out of pain and, in doing so, become stronger, more flexible and more fit than you thought possible.

▶ Liberate yourself
The Whartons' programme will reduce back pain and give you increased flexibility and strength in 18 weeks.

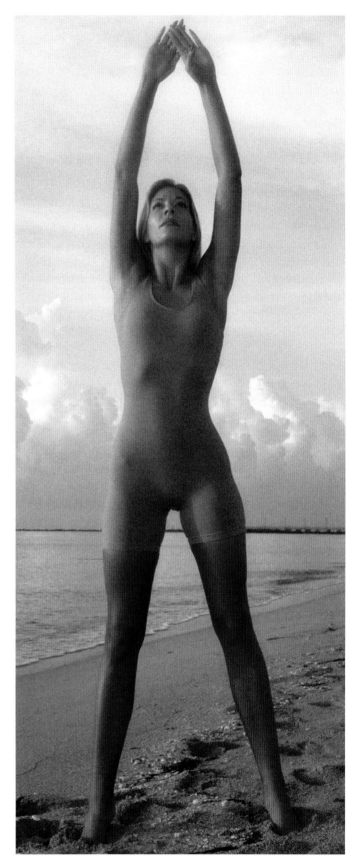

Trust us – we've seen it happen with our clients, hundreds of times. Join us and become more flexible, vital and pain-free than you've ever dreamed possible.

BEFORE YOU BEGIN

Before you begin our programme, make sure that your doctor says it's all right; take this book to him or her to get the green light – you might be surprised at the encouragement you'll receive. Long ago, back pain meant bed rest, but recent studies have shown that isn't the right answer for most back problems. In fact, it can make things worse. Moving is the order of the day.

We have designed a personal workout programme that will give you results in your first session. You'll feel better immediately, and feel progressively stronger, more flexible and have less pain over the next 18 weeks and beyond.

The programme has three components of a comprehensive workout: Active-Isolated Stretching; Active-Isolated Strengthening; and Cardio Training.

We'll begin with Active-Isolated Stretching, which is very quick and gentle. Rather than straining an injured back, it relaxes it and restores its range of motion. It gets things moving again.

When you're ready, we'll introduce Active-Isolated Strengthening, so you can slowly and gently become stronger and stronger.

And then when your body is really functioning, we'll introduce you to Cardio Training – primarily walking – to get your heart pumping and increase your endurance.

You'll go at your own pace at all times. We will coach you through each exercise individually and then teach you to put them all together into three six-week cycles that will take you from 'beginner' to 'advanced' level. Once you have mastered these exercises, you'll be able to refer back to the at-a-glance overview at the start of each routine, where all the exercises are combined onto a single page for quick reference.

You tailor the workout to your personal goals. It costs nearly nothing. There is really no special equipment required other than a stretch rope or strap and a set of ankle weights. There is no special clothing except a pair of comfortable shoes to walk in (and surely you already own a pair!). It's easy, fast and fun.

So, are you ready, athlete? Please prepare yourself to be amazed by how quickly, easily and comfortably you can completely rejuvenate your back, your body and your health.

The Benefits of the Whartons' Programme

The human body works hard to overcome every abuse and neglect; it is constantly trying to bring itself back to perfect function and form. Fortunately, the body is forgiving of mistakes and responds dramatically to training... and it's never too late to start exercising or to fine-tune an already effective training programme. Keeping your spine and back in good working order involves focused, efficient training; it's about enjoying the benefits of being an athlete rather than the miseries of a patient. If you follow our programme, you will become:

- **Lean,** so your spine doesn't have to support and balance excess weight.
- **Flexible,** so your spine can move within its full range of motion and keep blood flowing and muscles firing properly.
- **Strong throughout your entire body,** so your spine can handle the loads you put on it in bending forwards, backwards and sideways, in rotation, and in combination of all of these.
- **Balanced throughout your body,** so your back isn't called upon to compensate for weakened or shortened muscles.
- **Healthy,** so disease and deficiencies will not weaken your bones or impede you from activity.

- **Cardiovascularly strong,** so endurance is not a problem, and you can oxygenate your blood and maximise your body's ability to remove metabolic waste.
- **Smart,** so you'll avoid putting yourself and your back into situations where it can become stressed, overly fatigued or injured.

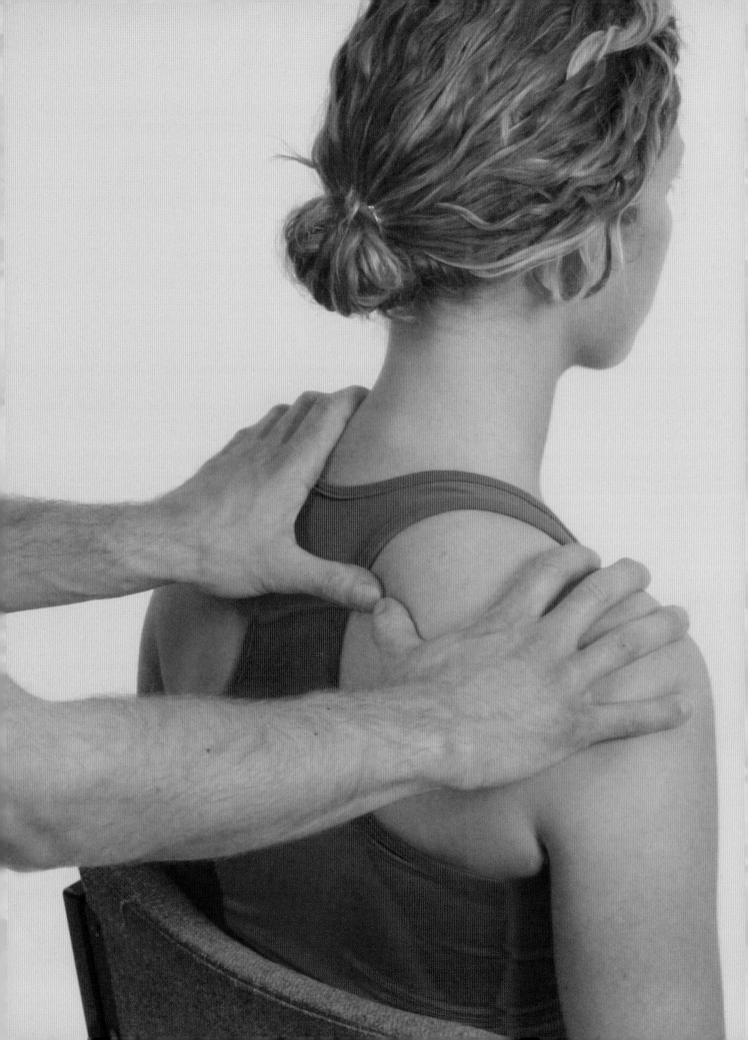

CHAPTER 2

POSTURE AND PRESSURES DOWN YOUR SPINE

We always tell our clients that, while the rest of the *body's parts may be on call, the back is always on duty. Unlike most other mammals, the human body was designed to stand upright, with the hands and arms free and the face oriented towards the front. In fact, almost all of our movement – from our sight to the reach of our arms to the way our knees and hips bend to propel us forwards – is directed to the front of our bodies.*

With all this forward movement, we need a stabilising force to keep us from falling on our faces. The back's job is to hold us upright and throw the brakes on to keep us from falling forwards. You might assume that such a stabilising system of bone and muscle would be tight and rigid – but it is quite fluid. Starting at the pelvis, the spine is continually adjusting, moving, stabilising and balancing against gravity so that we can move in an astonishing assortment of ways. Mastering the best ways to protect your posture from unnecessary pressure will help you make the most of this vibrant system for the long haul.

SITTING, STANDING, WALKING

Since the dawn of time, mothers have chanted a universal mantra, 'Stand up straight!' They couldn't be more *wrong*. In fact, straight is not the point. Being flexible and strong is the point. The spine is dynamic and always in motion, facilitating the countless positions and movements that our bodies are capable of making.

Gordon Gow is a Canadian kinesiologist who builds the weight equipment we use with our clients all over the world. One evening, when we were discussing spinal dynamics, he introduced us to a simple yet graphic representation of the spine, which showed how it works in relation to posture. Gordon balanced a broomstick by placing the end of the handle in his palm with the bristle end in the air. As it swayed from side to side and threatened to topple, he moved his palm swiftly from side to side to keep the broom in balance. He explained that this is the way a spine works in concert with the pelvis. The palm represents the pelvis – free-floating and serving as a sort of gyroscope for maintaining equilibrium – and the broomstick represents the spine.

In the early 1900s, physiologists set the standard for good posture by describing an alignment that was optimal for anatomical function. And, frankly, they did a pretty good job. Human bodies really have not changed that much in the last 100 years – but, my, the way in which we use them has. We have gone from a society of standing, walking, corn-harvesting, butter-churning, washboard-scrubbing people to a group of office-dwelling, car-driving, keyboard-tapping, television-watching sitters. And we pay a heavy toll for all this inactivity in terms of dysfunction and pain. It doesn't have to be that way. We are certainly capable of managing our bodies as nature designed them. But first, we have to know what nature had in mind. Try the alignment test below and see how good your posture is.

Few people have perfect posture. The good news is that minor postural anomalies are not necessarily associated with pain and dysfunction. The older we get, however, the more likely they are to become problematic to some degree.

SHAKE OFF THAT SLOUCH

Slouching is standing or sitting with a rounded upper back, a chest that caves in and shoulders that are rolled forwards. Nearly everything we do requires that we face forwards, reach forwards, bend forwards and move forwards. When combined with gravity, these activities make slouching seem like the natural result of a life lived in front of you. Remember, muscles work in opposition to each other. One flexes while the other extends. One contracts while the other relaxes. So when the muscles in your back (rhomboids and trapezius) are weak, the muscles in the front overwork and develop more strongly. They pull you forwards because your back isn't strong enough to hold you back.

When you're slouched, you force neck muscles to overwork to hold your face up. And you compress internal organs, including your lungs. You are not able to draw a full breath if your chest is compressed. If your slouch is pronounced, you can develop a hunchback – not good at all.

We make you this promise: if you'll do the flexibility and strengthening exercises we've outlined for you in chapter 4, you'll balance the strength and flexibility

How Do You Line Up?

An important first step in your PREhab programme is diagnosing your current posture. You can do this in one of two ways: clothed or, if you prefer, naked. All you will need is a clear wall to lean against or a full-length mirror. (Please note: this examination may not work for people outside a healthy weight range.)

CLOTHED

■ **Take your shoes off** and back up to a wall until your heels touch the skirting board. Working your way up your body, first put your bottom against the wall, then your shoulder blades and then the back of your head. Tighten your abdominals to stabilise yourself. Breathe deeply and relax for a moment as you notice how your body feels.

■ **Take two steps out** and stand with your feet slightly apart. If your body recognises this posture as its own and can maintain it, then you're probably doing a good job of staying in alignment. But if you hold this posture for a few seconds and then automatically adjust it – say by jutting your head forwards and dropping your chest – then you probably have a weakness and imbalance somewhere. Luckily, the Active-Isolated programmes will help you address both problems.

NAKED

■ **Find a full-length mirror** in front of which you can stand naked. Hang a weighted string down the centre of the mirror so that it's perpendicular to the floor but not touching it. Take off your clothes. Now, pull your hair back, if needed, and stand sideways to the mirror.

■ **Check to see** if your earlobe is in alignment with your shoulder. This may be difficult to do because you'll be turning your head to see yourself. Try using a second mirror in your hand, or merely use your hand to span between your ear and your shoulder to determine if they line up. Everything else will be easy to see: if you're in alignment, your shoulders will be lined up directly over the points where your thighbones connect to your pelvis. Those points on your pelvis will be lined up over the midpoints between the fronts and backs of your knees. And your knees will be lined up over your anklebones.

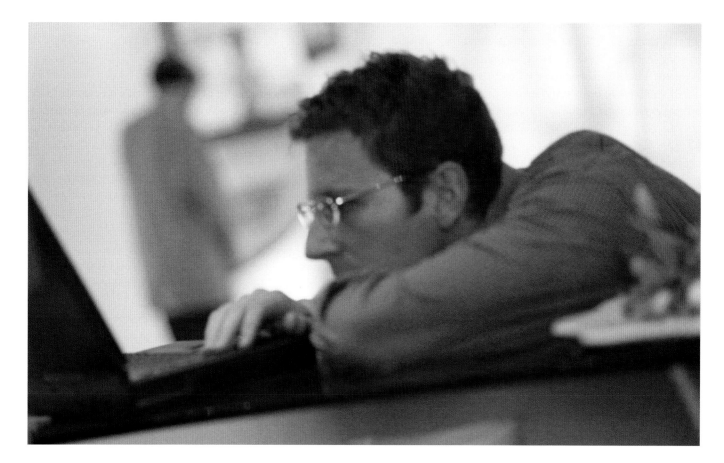

of the important muscles that hold you upright against the strength of those that pull you forward. Also, once you've done the 'How Do You Line Up?' test (see opposite) and you know what your trouble spots are, we would ask you to make a conscious effort to align your spine as you stand until you get used to the fun and ease of moving properly.

SITTING PRETTY

When most of us sit, we tend to sort of settle into a puddle. If the chair has a back, all the better. We lean back and in and curl up into relaxation. We roll our shoulders forwards, stressing the upper back and caving in our chest muscles. This posture might feel fine for a little while, but if you're in for the long haul, you're in trouble.

Let's start with a refresher course in gravity, the force of pull from 'out there' straight to the centre of the earth. When you're standing, the forces of gravity run through the top of your head and are absorbed and dissipated through your hips, knees, ankles and feet. But when you're sitting in perfect posture, those same forces run through the top of your head and are stopped at your buttocks, absorbed directly by your lower back and sacrum. That can be pretty

▲ Sit up and take note
Slouching is a common problem that leads to overworked neck muscles and compression of the lungs. In today's desk-bound society, computer users need to be particularly vigilant about their seated posture.

tough on the body, but it gets worse. When you curl up or swing your leg over the arm of the chair, then the body part that absorbs that same force of gravity will change, placing an odd strain on your back as it fights to keep you in balance.

Notice how you are sitting right now. Imagine gravity as a force in a line from 'out there' straight to the centre of the earth. If your spine isn't in alignment with your buttocks, where are the forces exerting themselves and which muscles in your back must compensate to hold you up in balance? Isn't it an amazing coincidence that these same muscles are the ones that always seem to be fatigued and strained?

When we're sitting, we are confining our bodies to small spaces. For the best result, sit with your bottom planted evenly on the seat. Put your feet flat on the floor, with your knees bent at 90-degree angles. We're designed to sit this way, but we weren't designed to sit as long as most of us do now. To maintain a seated posture, it's necessary to get that gravitational pressure relieved from time to time so that your back can rest. We encourage squirming and shifting in your seat. But better than this, you should take short, frequent breaks – say one every hour.

All you have to do is stand up and move a little. Take a few deep breaths and imagine that you have a helium balloon lifting your head off your shoulders. Tighten your abdominals and elongate your spine from the base of the sacrum all the way up. We call this 'resetting'. Move and reset. And plan to do it again in an hour.

STANDING TALL

For many people with back pain, everything feels better and more relaxed when standing with body weight distributed and the spine in alignment. But no one starts out standing – standing is a matter of lifting your body upright from another position, and this can be problematic. Just as we would coach an athlete to move from one position to another efficiently and powerfully, we're going to tell you how to manage these transitions safely so that you can spare your back and avoid injury.

Rolling out of bed: Lie on your back and tighten your abdominals. Roll to one side and push yourself up using your elbow, while at the same time pushing down with your opposite hand. Pivoting at the hip, drop your feet over the edge of the bed; your feet act as counterweights. Scoot your hips to the edge. Look around and get oriented. Keeping your feet spaced under your hips, put one foot in front of

Take a Load Off Your Back

All postures and body positions place different loads on the lumbar spine, which has to support the pressure of the forces. If you're looking to get the load off your back, consider these positions. They're listed from the least amount of pressure to the most.

- Lying flat on your back or lying on your side.
- Standing and relaxed.
- Sitting in a chair.
- Standing and bending forwards from the hips.
- Sitting in a chair and bending forwards from the hips.
- Standing and bending forwards from the hips while bearing weight.
- Sitting in a chair and bending forwards from the hips while bearing weight (astonishingly, up to 300 times the pressure of lying flat on your back!).

the other. Put your hands on the bed. Contract the abdominals. Push up with your hands until your back knee is locked. Now you're standing.

Getting up off the floor: If you're on the floor, roll over to the crawl position. Then rise up to your knees. Rock your buttocks back towards your heels. Bring up one knee until

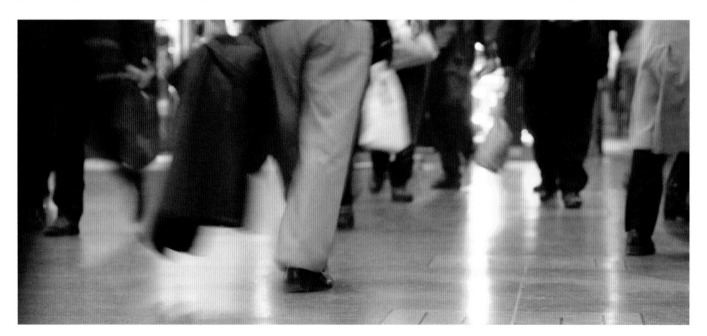

your foot is flat on the floor. Put the toes of your back foot on the floor. Put your hand on the same side, on your knee. Put the other hand on the floor. Rock back a little more and find your balance until you can rise. Use your hands for support and lift with your buttocks, otherwise known as the gluteal muscles, or glutes for short. Now you're standing.

Rising from your chair: Keeping your feet spaced under your hips, put one foot in front of the other. Put your hands on the seat beside your hips or on the arms of the chair. Flex your trunk forwards slightly. Contract the abdominals. Push up with your hands and glutes until your back knee is locked. Now you're standing.

Getting out of your car: Open the door, pivot on your buttocks until you're facing sideways, and swing your feet out of the car. Reach over your head with one hand and hold the door frame to pull yourself forwards. Reach down with your other hand and place it firmly on the seat to push off. Now you're standing.

WALKING UPRIGHT

Like all of us, you *think* you know how to walk. You've been walking since you were a toddler. Like many things you learned when you were in nappies, however, you probably missed some of the finer points.

A running coach we know argued rather credibly that walking is nothing more than catching yourself from falling in a series of self-rescues that move you forwards. She theorised that a walker leans forwards in the direction she wants to go, and, at the point of imbalance, she has two choices: either fall on her face or thrust one leg forwards and catch herself. Once she's on that out-thrust leg, she passes her torso over the top of it and then faces the choices again: flat on her face or throw her other leg out there.

She made the point by grabbing Jim by the front of his T-shirt and pulling him forwards. 'Make a choice!' she challenged. Jim toppled forwards and then caught himself by doing exactly what she thought he would do: he thrust his leg out. Our coach friend grinned in triumph and continued to pull him forwards by the T-shirt. Jim saved himself by taking another imposed step. Before he knew it, he was halfway across the floor. This was walking as our friend had

◀ **Walk the walk**
Many of us walk in such a way that we cause problems higher up, in the back. If a person's gait is initiated from the hip and not the buttock, muscular imbalances can occur.

Walking the Right Way

Before you teach yourself the correct way to walk, take a few steps as you normally would so that you'll remember how it felt. Now, the next step you take will open a whole new world of power and balance, because we're going to teach you to walk properly. Here's how walking should work.

- **Stand with your left foot forwards.** Contract your abdominals, and clench your right glute to lift your pelvis slightly forwards and up.
- **Your left arm,** the opposite to the walking leg, swings to mirror the move to balance you and help you move forwards.
- **The hip flexors –** the muscles that lift your thigh slightly to elevate and swing your leg – finish what the glute starts.
- **Your calf will help** by working with your hamstrings to extend your knee and propel you forwards.
- **You have just passed** your torso and centre of gravity over your supporting leg.
- **Your right foot should now** hit the ground at midfoot, not at your heel.
- **Your arch will flatten** slightly under the weight, but it is designed to spring back into shape to cushion the impact and give your step a little momentum as your ankle muscles stabilise your foot.
- **The forces of impact** from that step translate right up into your knee.
- **Your knee doesn't spring,** but it absorbs shock through muscles in the inner and outer thigh all the way to the hip.
- **Your right step is complete.** At this moment, engage your left glute to lift your pelvis slightly forwards and up, and start the next step with your left leg.

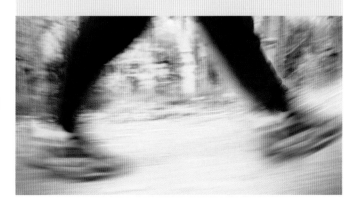

observed it – and as most people do it. But it's not right. The act of walking is not so much a question of constantly losing and regaining equilibrium, of pulling yourself forwards through space by catching yourself over each leg. It is actually more a function of being pushed. And this action comes primarily from your buttocks.

The point that really needs emphasising here is that this walking gait is distinctly different from the one that we have traditionally thought to be biomechanically efficient. The power in this gait is in your bottom – and this applies to both walking and running. By pushing from behind with your glute, rather than drawing forwards by raising your thigh from your hip flexors and extending your knee to get your foot out before you fall on your face, you're aiding your natural postural alignment and keeping the strain off your back.

SQUATTING FOR REST

As we've already established, one of the reasons that our backs are stressed is that we humans sit too much and for too long. The forces that translate down our spines and through our buttocks when they're planted in chairs are enormous. Although we think we are resting when we sit down, the act of sitting can actually tire our backs even more. Sitting down compresses vertebrae and fatigues the muscles. It can also have the detrimental effect of straining the connective tissues.

▼ Back to nature
In some cultures, squatting, as opposed to sitting, is still a preferred means of relaxation. This posture follows the body's own design for rest but has been all but forgotten in the West.

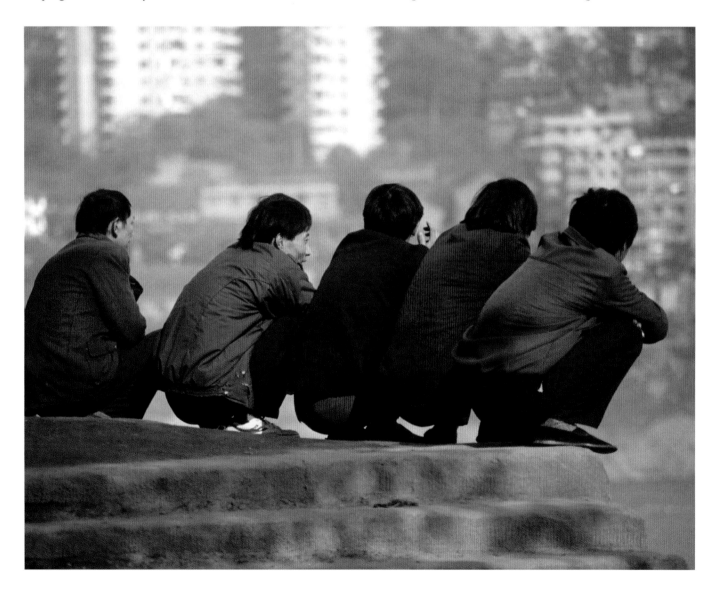

As human beings, we were designed to rest and relax from standing – and this was obviously a long time before chairs were invented. Although you wouldn't know it from habits witnessed in this country, our bodies were actually designed to squat for that much-needed rest and relaxation. In fact, when we're abroad and working in countries like Japan and Kenya, we observe a lot of people at rest by squatting… and we're very happy to join them. The act of squatting serves to relax your posture and elongate your spine like little else. For this reason, squatting is also a wonderful way to test how functionally flexible your back is. Only the flexible and fit can squat comfortably.

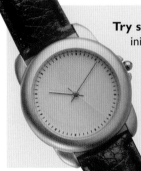

Try squatting for a minute or two initially, to see how adept you are at straightening up. As your legs get stronger, you'll be able to stay down longer, but don't push it at first. If you start the squat and it's not going well – you feel weak or something hurts – stop immediately and get back up.

It's probably been a long time since you've tried to squat, so it will take a little practice, particularly if you're inflexible or carrying a little extra weight. Squat only if you have healthy knees, because squatting requires them to support your weight on the way down and puts them into complete flexion while you're down, which can lead to strain. Also, what goes down must come up, so you need to be strong enough to make that happen. There's nothing more depressing than getting into an impressive squat and then having to roll over onto the floor before you can stand yourself up.

We call the full squat the 'complete collapse' phase. In other places around the world, people happily maintain the squat for long periods of time, but in our Western culture, we are accustomed to sitting in chairs and have abandoned one of the really great postures. In our clinic, we use it to test function in the back and to quickly stretch out. It's fun if you're in shape.

Squatting may not be for everyone, particularly if you're out of practice, but if you are able, we encourage you to join many cultures around the world and rediscover resting your back just the way nature intended it. If you manage to master the squat, you'll have yourself a wonderful way to rest. Your spine will elongate, and it will also relax your back muscles.

Squatting for Back Relaxation

Step 1

Stand with your feet shoulder-width apart; bend your knees and flex your trunk forwards.

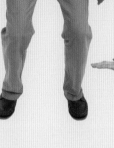

Step 2

Put your hands out in front of you and lean forwards; keep bending your knees until your hands touch the ground. Continue to bend your knees as you lower your buttocks towards the floor.

Step 3

You're all the way down when the backs of your thighs and the backs of your calves touch. Once you've mastered this position, your heels should be flat on the floor; hold your arms forwards to counterbalance.

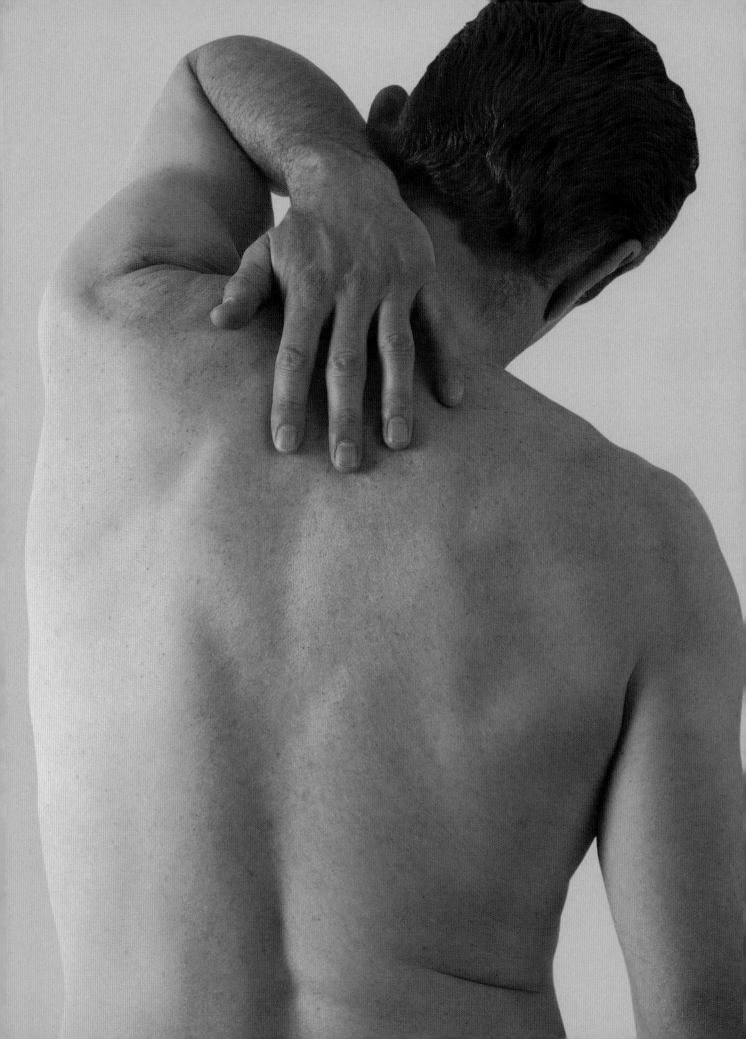

CHAPTER 3

TRACING PAIN'S MYSTICAL LINKS

The late astronomer Carl Sagan said, 'We are all *made of star stuff.' We think he's right. Each one of us is a universe, a perfectly calibrated, interwoven system. These bodies of ours are always thinking, even on the cellular level. Yet, when we feel pain, we usually point to the specific location of the pain and say, 'Here it is. This is the injury.' But that exact spot may not necessarily indicate where the injury really originated.*

An injury or an imbalance in one place can trigger pain or discomfort somewhere else entirely. Why is this? Because in this integrated organism, all parts work together, and every part is related to every other part. When we focus on one aspect, such as a 'contained' pain, we're forgetting that each of us is a whole system, perfect and miraculous, and that if one part of the system is disrupted, compressed or stressed, it affects everything else in the body.

Your body is only ever as strong and healthy as the weakest link in your system. It's constantly fighting against weakness to help you achieve perfection (or as close as you can get to it). Muscles recruit other muscles to compensate and counterbalance – whether you're moving or not. This constant shifting and balancing can create a whole litany of other complaints, and these, in turn, can often camouflage the origins of back pain. Because these origins can be so elusive at times, back pain can seem a touch more mysterious than other injuries and aches, but there's usually a very simple answer. Solving the mystery just takes a little detective work.

LABELLING THE PAIN

Whether you've had it for a long time or it suddenly strikes you, back pain can be specifically pinpointed or be so general and widespread that you can't spot the exact site. Sometimes you can move a certain way, and it disappears altogether. When you move another way, the pain shoots all over the place. A back problem can even cause pain somewhere else in the body.

One type of back pain, radicular pain, is a deep, steady pain that radiates from the spine and can run all the way to your foot. Sometimes it's accompanied by weakness, loss of function, tingling or numbness. Radicular pain usually results from inflammation of a spinal nerve root.

Referred pain is a dull ache that tends to travel around and is maddeningly inconsistent. Sometimes it hurts badly; sometimes it's not that bad. Referred pain starts in your lower back and radiates into the groin, buttocks and thighs.

The reason pain travels to and from your spine is that your spinal column is the conduit through which all messages are sent from the brain to the body and from the body to the brain. The area is rich in nerves and is linked everywhere, which makes it an excellent communications centre. Unfortunately, some of these messages are really bad news.

PAIN COULD BE A BLOCK IN YOUR ENERGY

We don't want to get all mystical on you, but even the most sceptical among us will admit that there's more to the universe than we can see. We think so, and, if we hadn't before, our experiences with our clients would have certainly changed our mindset. And we very much doubt that we're alone.

Several years ago, the Dalai Lama's personal doctor was invited to a prestigious hospital in New York City to diagnose a patient. This Tibetan physician was offered the use of the finest imaging and diagnostic equipment in the world. In fact, every lab test was at his fingertips. However, he chose otherwise; he politely declined and quietly approached the bedside. He examined the patient with *his* tools: his hands.

The doctor scanned and checked pulses – triggers of energy that run through meridians, which are channels of energy, or 'chi' (life force), just below the skin's surface. This procedure is standard in Chinese medicine and is used here in the West by practitioners of acupuncture. An experienced doctor or practitioner can detect blockages in energy and relate them directly to the source of injury or imbalance.

The Tibetan doctor worked for a few minutes and then gave his medical opinion, which turned out to be identical to the diagnosis determined earlier by New York doctors

Acupuncture is a holistic treatment that has been practised in the Far East for over 2,000 years and is today employed in the West as a complementary therapy – usually after medical diagnosis. It can be used to manage illness and maintain health.

Case Study: **Jill Nicklaus**

A Broadway dancer in a musical with back pain doesn't sound probable – but even the fittest and most supple of performers can suffer from a muscular imbalance.

When we met, Jill was a principal dancer in the musical *Cats*. She sometimes did two arduous, high-energy performances a day. She came to us with terrible back pain. Like most professional dancers, Jill is hypermobile – meaning that she's as flexible as a rubber band. And she's strong in all the muscles she uses to dance. But that's not all of them. Her quads, glutes and abductors (outer thighs) were extremely tight and compromised. All the lateral muscles in her hip and trunk were contracted and tight. Her lower abs and inner and outer thighs were extremely strong, but her lower back was weak. Over

time Jill had developed a series of damaging compensations. The other problem was the stage on which she performed – it slanted towards the audience. Dancing day after day on an uneven surface had thrown one side of her body out of balance.

In Jill's case, flexibility was less the issue than strength. Getting her out of pain was a matter of working fast to keep her on stage and giving her very light, small strengthening exercises to bring her back muscles up to par with her legs. We worked on glutes, lower abs and abductors. We did modified leg raises, using a pillow to take the strain off her back. We worked on

her neck for flexibility but emphasised strength for her upper back – trapezius and rhomboid muscles. We stabilised her from all angles.

We trained Jill's personal therapist to work with her three times a week with Active-Isolated Strengthening and Stretching. Her back let go. She was pain-free, strong and balanced within just four weeks. Jill realised that pain had ultimately been her friend. The pains she experienced had given her ample warning that she needed to balance muscles to become a better dancer. A cat might have nine lives, but a Broadway dancer has only one. Jill made sure she could enjoy hers.

with equipment and lab work. If the patient had been under the Tibetan doctor's care, the doctor would have unblocked the energy with acupuncture, by inserting small needles to stimulate the point of block called the gateway. Or he simply might have applied stimulating pressure with his hand. Either way, these methods have been practised for thousands of years, and they seem to work. And with all the medical mysteries that still remain, who are we to say it doesn't?

PAIN CAN ALSO BE EMOTIONAL

We know that pain is largely a matter of perception, so as long as most of it has to do with judgement, it stands to reason that pain isn't just affected by thoughts and feelings but can also be *caused* by thoughts and feelings. The human mind is capable of producing extreme pain. For example, think of the times you may have flinched when getting an injection, and the needle was still behind the back of the smirking nurse?

We don't understand how, but we know this to be true: the body remembers pain, fear and sorrow, and stores them. On an obvious level, you can observe this yourself. Walk into a restaurant and watch people for a few minutes. Without effort, you'll be able to pick out those people who are sad or afraid or are in some sort of pain. When we do deep-muscle massage or happen to agitate certain trigger points in a client, we sometimes accidentally unlock a muscle memory, where the body is storing emotion. It is not uncommon for the client to break the peaceful silence and comfort of a massage with an outburst of uncontrollable weeping.

Many is the time that we've had to stop and comfort. And although we are not qualified counsellors, we are the solitary witnesses to the body's release of a long-forgotten hurt, so we take the time to draw our clients into conversation. What just happened? What did you remember? What has caused you this much pain? Inevitably, the story is one of an incident so horrific that the mind suppressed it – or hid it somewhere in the body. When we release it, it doesn't go away, but it's better.

Such a trigger point in your back could be causing you to tense up and experience pain. Or maybe it's not one of these hidden memories, but, rather, carrying the figurative weight of the world on your shoulders has turned into literal slouching, slumping and hurting.

Getting to the bottom of emotional pain or disruptions in your energy are, no doubt, very worthy endeavours. But short of getting you on our table or into the hands of a

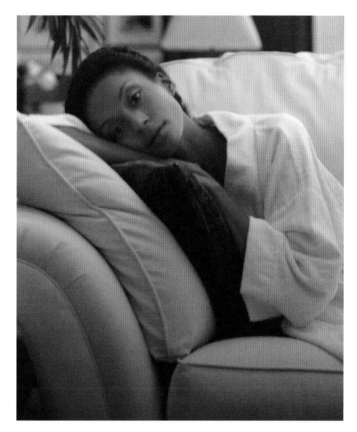

▲ Emotional healing
When investigating the root of muscular pain it is important to take into account possible psychological or emotional traumas the body may have stored up.

Tibetan physician, we really can't help you there. What we can do is help you connect the dots behind your own pain, narrow down where it's coming from, and help you chart a course for a new universe of pain-free living.

READING THE BODY'S MAP

If you're suffering from generalised back pain, you have to find the source of the pain before you can correct it. Surprisingly, the source of generalised back pain is seldom in the back. But how does one find the source?

The body is a unique flowchart, a sort of intricate web of connected systems. As we have explained, all muscles work in pairs, and the pairs work in teams to get you to move. When one muscle shorts out, it creates a point of tension and fatigue somewhere beyond itself. First, its companion muscle will strain. And when the pair is not doing its job, other muscles struggle to compensate. Eventually, a second short-out and a second compensation occur, setting off a chain reaction.

When we see unexplained pain or an overuse injury in the body, we start tracing it backwards to look for clues to the source of the problem. We ask, 'Why did this happen? What weak link in the chain caused this to short-out?' Very little is ever as it appears to be.

Really nailing down the origin of a back injury is important for a number of reasons. Soothing an injury is not enough if the source of the problem – the weak link – is not treated and corrected, because that weak link will continue to cause trouble and pain. Massages and chiropractic adjustments can provide your back with some relief, but the relief might not last long. Treating the problem without correcting the cause is a surefire guarantee that you'll be back in pain sooner or later.

When we are tracing an injury to its source, we put a mental dot on the source of pain and imagine lines radiating out from this point, from north to south and from east to west. Then we fill in the additional areas: northwest, southwest, northeast and southeast. The result is an imaginary yet detailed star-shaped compass with its centre right on the injury.

From a back injury, most of the weak links are to the south, more often than not below the pelvis. If the pain is on the right, the weak links are probably on your left. If the pain is on the left, the weak links are probably on your right. In the case of the upper back, neck and shoulders, their weak links are sometimes revealed when you look for clues to both the east and west.

Flat Feet and Your Back

It is difficult to imagine but flat feet – or fallen arches – are often responsible for problems or pain experienced in the back. This seemingly trivial complaint, far away from the back, actually magnifies as it travels through the muscles and ligaments of the leg and, before you know it, your back is manifesting the problem.

- **Ideally, when your foot rolls forwards** through your step, the compressed arch springs back into position to give you a little push off for your next step. But when the arch is flattened, the ankle rolls to the inside.
- **Without the support of the ankle,** the whole leg rotates towards the midline of the body. When the ankle and lower leg are rolled inwards, the knee is thrown out of alignment. The stabiliser and cushion for the knee is the medial meniscus, a pad on the inside of the upper kneecap. Over time, strain from the imbalance imposed by the ankle compromises the medial meniscus.
- **Without full function of the medial meniscus,** your knee loses its ability to stabilise and cushion, and the joint becomes stressed. Eventually, the pressure will blow out the anterior cruciate ligament, the attachment that holds the bones in your thigh to the bones in your shin through your knee.
- **As the knee is the juncture between** your lower and upper leg, it's the joint responsible for moving the body forwards. When the anterior cruciate ligament is compromised and becomes lax, pain, irritation and weakness make a proper gait impossible.
- **As we move up the chain** from the weak link, we see that if the knee can't create a proper gait, the hip muscles

take over in a series of compensations. The quadriceps and hamstrings contract to protect the knee. But they're not designed to move the leg forwards and do the knee's job. So they, too, become fatigued and weakened.

- **Continuing up the chain,** when the quadriceps and hamstrings are compromised, the hip flexors take over to try and help lift the leg up from the thigh so that you can move forwards.
- **Outer and inner thigh muscles** struggle to stabilise the pelvis, which will have to rotate now to move that leg forwards.
- **Underneath the glutes** in the buttocks, six deep rotators, which are involved with internal and external rotation of the hip, finally fatigue and lose function.
- **If we go one step further** up the chain, we find the lower back kicking in to stabilise the pelvis. And, suddenly – you guessed it – you have back pain.

Starting at the point of your back pain, test your muscles and joints one at a time by isolating them and activating them with the simple exercises in this book (see chapter 4). Test how flexible and strong each area is individually. When you find a muscle that seems weaker than those surrounding it, or you have very little range of motion in one position, you might have the culprit.

Still, keep going. Keep testing down the line, moving on to the next set of muscles and the next joint. Often you'll find yourself going from the point of pain in your back, right through your buttocks, down your thigh, past your knee, through your ankle, and right to the bottom of your foot. It's important to keep going until you pass over the last weak muscle and inflexible joint in the line.

Once you've figured out exactly where your weak link is, make a point during your exercise sessions to focus on strengthening and unlocking from that point *up* to the injury in your back.

STANDING ON YOUR OWN WEAK LINKS: YOUR FEET

One of our favourite songs begins, 'The foot bone's connected to the anklebone; the anklebone's connected to the shinbone; the shinbone's connected to the kneebone…' (you get the picture). We sing this to our baffled clients who can't believe that a fallen arch can cause a back spasm.

When one of our clients comes in with back pain, we begin by whipping his or her shoes off. Why such interest in the foot when the back is in pain? Believe it or not, one of the biggest culprits in back pain is the flat foot. When the arch has 'fallen' and rocked the ankle inwards, the flat foot basically has ensured that the body will be unable to absorb shock.

Sometimes, the culprit isn't all the way down in the feet. You could have a weak muscle somewhere up the line – like quadriceps – that's causing the back pain. But the best way to start checking for weakness and imbalance is to track it through the chain, from the back downwards.

HAS A WEAK LINK THROWN YOU OUT OF BALANCE?

Therapists and trainers often used to blame simple leg-length discrepancy for pain in the back. An athlete was evaluated by lying flat on a table with an observer at the foot of the table. The observer took both of the athlete's feet in his hands, pressed the ankles together, eyeballed the soles of the feet, and finally declared, 'You're out of whack. Your

left anklebone is a full inch below your right one. Your left leg definitely is longer.' Then the athlete would go out and get a 1-in (2.5cm) lift for the right shoe so that both legs could be even.

This apparent leg-length discrepancy probably was caused not by a leg bone that was longer, but by an imbalance in the muscles and tendons of the pelvis. And the source of this imbalance might surprise you. A tight hamstring at the back of one thigh can jack up the opposite side of the pelvis. A tight iliotibial band in the knee on one side could jack up the other side of the pelvis.

When the lower extremities are in balance and the pelvis is free-floating and flexible, the leg-length discrepancy may disappear. All you have to do is follow the injury from your back to the source and correct the problems all the way down the line with stretching and strengthening.

If your back hurts and you suspect that the pain might be the result of a weak link somewhere down the line, remember that your pelvis is the foundation of the body. It connects and balances your lower extremities against your upper body and your back. If your back is in pain above the foundation, it's possible that the culprit is below, throwing your pelvis out of kilter and straining your back. The only way to find out is to check for imbalance (see page 36).

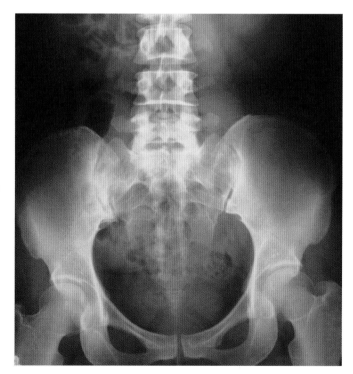

▲ **Well grounded?**
Muscular problems in the legs or feet can imbalance the pelvis, the foundation of the body, leading to back pain.

Checking for Pelvic Imbalance

First, ask a friend to help you. It's important that you feel comfortable with this person because relaxation is a big part of this process. It should take around a minute.

Step 1

Lie on your back on a flat surface with your legs together and have your partner press down with the palms of the hands on your hipbones, one hand on the left and one hand on the right.

Step 2

Your partner should rock you back and forth, pressing left, right, left, right, until you are fully relaxed.

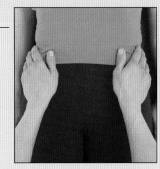

Step 3

Now have your partner look down to see if your anklebones are even. If they're not, do a full Active-Isolated Stretching routine (see page 48) and repeat these three steps. In the majority of cases, leg-length differences are caused by tight muscles in lower extremities.

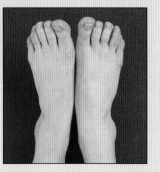

If you've checked your body against pelvic imbalance and your anklebones are even, or closer after the Active-Isolated training, you don't have a leg-length discrepancy. The imbalance will be somewhere between your back and your feet, caused by muscles and connective tissues that have been compromised, weakened and tightened in their efforts to compensate. You now have a great opportunity to do some work to get that back out of pain.

PUTTING THE MAP TO WORK

Let's look at the experience of one of our clients, Gene Pressman, a New York businessman. He decided that he wanted to run the New York City Marathon and came to us to help him put together a training programme.

We put him on a precise schedule. We worked with him in our clinic and in the gym. We sometimes accompanied him on long runs, and a warm friendship developed. Gene worked hard, and it paid off. He competed in the marathon and did very well. We didn't see him for a while.

One day he phoned to say that he'd put his back out and was in real pain. At our clinic, Gene disclosed that he had suffered a knee injury in a skiing accident that had resulted in surgery but that his doctor had not really stressed rehab much, so Gene went about his business, thinking everything was all right.

Bingo. His knee had been weakened and sore from surgery, so he favoured the other leg. He limped. It didn't take much time for this imbalance to translate right up to his back.

Limping had weakened the muscles below the injured knee and had gone all the way down to his foot. The arch had given way from stress and could no longer absorb shock. So with each step, the shock was translating all the way up through his ankle to his knee.

The fallen arch had fatigued and strained Gene's ankle, and this had further aggravated his knee, which had weakened his adductors – the inner-thigh muscles. His abductors, the muscles on the outsides of his thighs, were so weak that he was unable to stabilise his pelvis.

Instead of using his glutes when he walked, Gene was using his hip flexors. From the pain in his back, we could easily trace backwards to the glutes, hip flexors, abductors, adductors, knee, lower leg, ankle and arch. The knee started it. The limp aggravated it. The arch finished it. And the back felt it.

Gene's recovery started with three simple exercises to strengthen his ankles and arch. We're going to give them to you in detail here, because we'll mention them a couple of times later in case studies, and we want you to know what they are.

1. To strengthen his ankles, we put an ankle weight in the toe of a long tube sock and tied the sock around his ankle, threading the weighted end of the sock between his big toe and the toe next to it (like a flip-flop) and letting it dangle. He sat upright on the edge of one of our tables with the weight just above the floor. We put a rolled towel under his knee to take the strain off his kneecap. He extended his ankle and pointed his toes towards the floor. From this starting position, he brought his foot straight up, leading with his toes. The little weight provided resistance. He angled his foot to the inside and lifted in a sweep, leading with his toes. He lowered the weight to the starting position and then angled his foot to the outside and lifted in a sweep, leading with his toes. He did 10 on each side.

2. To strengthen his ankle evertors and invertors (the muscles that turn the ankle), we simply laid him on his side and wrapped a single ankle weight around both of his feet under the arches and over the tops. He relaxed his feet and let them hang off the table. Then, without moving his legs, he lifted both feet from the ankles up towards the ceiling. He did 10 repetitions on each side.

3. To strengthen his arches, we put a towel on the floor, vertically in front of Gene, and had him sit in a chair at the edge of it. He worked with one foot at a time without moving his heel, contracting all his toes to bunch the towel up and draw the far edge towards him in a series of 'grips'. When he was finished, we straightened the towel out and placed it horizontally in front of him. He put his foot on it. He started with his little toe and, without moving his heel, contracted all his toes to bunch the towel up and sweep it towards the midline of his body in a series of 10 contractions. This strengthened his supinators, the muscles in the ankle that turn the forefoot inwards. Finally, we straightened the towel and had him lead with his big toe and, without moving his heel, sweep the towel to the outside of his body. This strengthened his pronators, the muscles in the ankle that turn the forefoot outwards.

For Gene, getting well was a matter of getting back to basics. In addition to these three small exercises, we reintroduced Gene to all the stretching and strengthening exercises you'll find in this book – the same ones he had used to train for a successful marathon.

Although he felt better after the first session, it took six weeks to get him fully well. Now he's free from back pain and back into a regular training programme, but the moral of his story is that he is a solid athlete who got derailed by a deceptively small injury. By tracing back the mystical links, we were able to get him out on the trails again. The same detective methods can work for you.

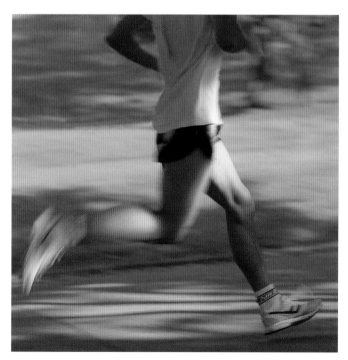

▲ Getting back on your feet
Treating the source of back pain, often elsewhere in the body, helps most people return to exercise and greater flexibility.

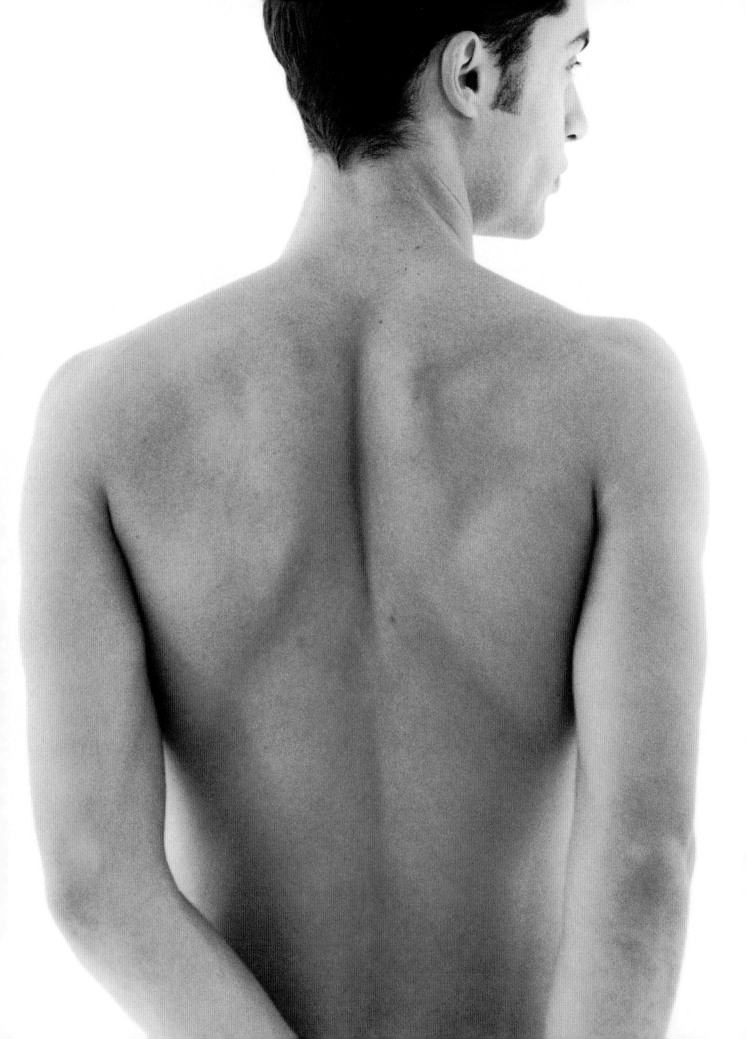

2

TRY PREHAB, NOT REHAB

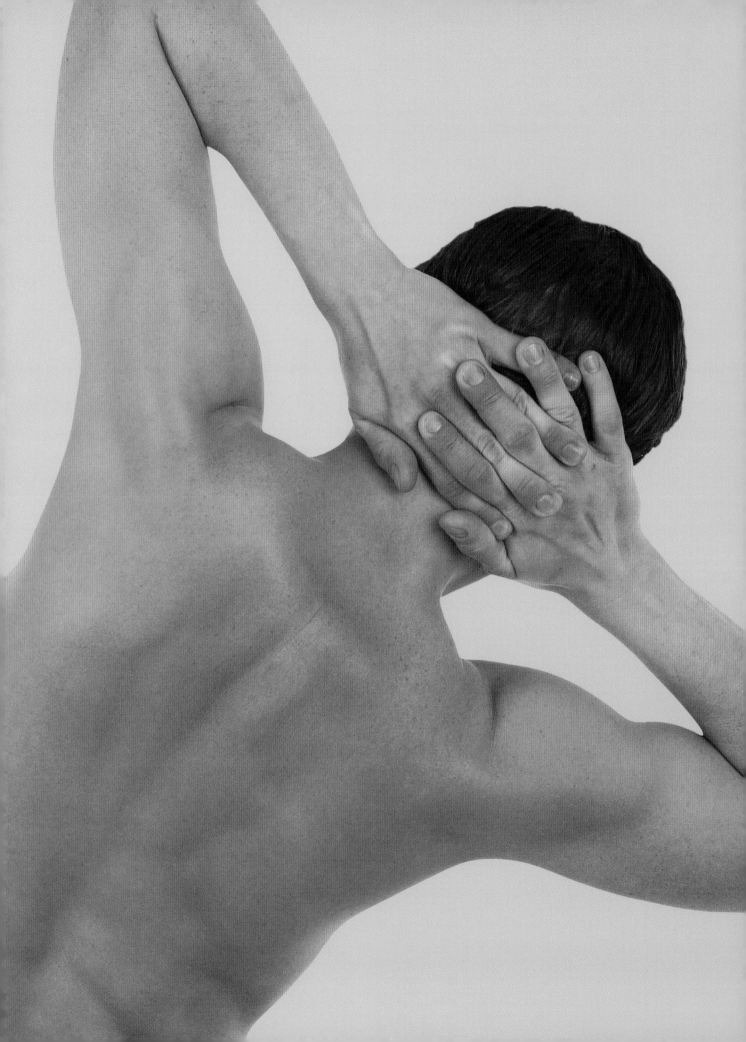

CHAPTER 4

THE ACTIVE-ISOLATED PLAN FOR FLEXIBLE, STRONG, PAIN-FREE BACKS

We've spent a great deal of our careers repairing *athletes' injuries. Unless they are caused by accidents, they're usually the products of mistakes in training or performance. The need for intense rehabilitation is, in our view, tragic: most injuries can be prevented through better training and preparation. Instead of rehab, we would much rather do PREhab – that is, help athletes prepare properly so that injuries never happen.*

These same principles can help you in everyday life. It's tough out there. You are making extraordinary demands on your body all day and every day. And you're going to live for a long time, which means that your body has to adapt to your changing lifestyles and activities – and hold up through it all. You have to be prepared, just as a professional athlete has to be.

If you don't at the moment suffer from chronic back problems and you never want to, you have added incentive to avoid trouble. By following our programme, you'll get all the benefit of exercise – as well as the satisfying security of knowing that you've headed problems off at the pass. With PREhab, your fit, lean and healthy body will have you living life more fully and powerfully than you ever thought possible.

If you are one of the many unfortunate people who do suffer from chronic back problems, and your doctor has ruled out any disease, injury and genetic anomalies, rehab may be in order. It may be time for you to take some action, literally. Get moving. Gone are the days when you'd be relegated to your bed for days or weeks on end. In fact, research tells us that bed rest for a bad back is bad advice – you'll probably get better faster if you move.

Maximum function in your back is, more often than not, a matter of being lean, flexible, strong, balanced and healthy. With our programme, you have the simple tools you need to achieve revolutionary results in less than 30 minutes a day.

Trust us – this investment in yourself can pay huge dividends. Within just a few days of beginning our programme, our clients report that they are feeling more energetic, have a greater range of motion, and are even experiencing blissful relief from chronic pain. And now it's your turn – so let's get started!

THE PRINCIPLES OF ACTIVE-ISOLATED TRAINING

The foundation of our programmes is flexibility – specifically, Active-Isolated Stretching – and this is where we'll begin. It's impossible to overestimate the importance of being flexible. When your joints are able to move through their full ranges of motion, your body moves the way it was designed: completely, easily, painlessly and efficiently. You may have forgotten the joy of living in such a body, but you're about to rediscover that freedom.

The principles of 'Active-Isolated' are remarkably simple. As we've explained, muscles work in pairs of opposites. When one muscle lengthens, the *opposite* muscle shortens to make movement happen. If you want that one to lengthen or stretch, you have to relax it, but that muscle can't relax if it's working. That's where the opposite muscles come in. When you fire, engage and activate those muscles, they shorten. Then, the muscles you intend to stretch are *relaxed* because they are isolated. As a result, they get stretched very efficiently and precisely.

Let's look at an example. Picture a runner preparing to do laps at the track. He throws his heel up on the bench, straightens his knee, bends over, takes hold of his ankle and pulls himself 'nose to toes'. He can't quite get there because he's not warmed up yet, so he bounces, trying to go lower with every bounce.

You've seen it. You've probably even done it. Our runner was doing the hamstring stretch. Or was he? With his leg up and his knee straight, his quadriceps (the muscle group in the front of his thigh) is totally relaxed. Those muscles are ready to be stretched. The hamstrings (the muscle group in the back of his thigh, opposing the relaxed quads) are activated and firing. In fact, they're tightening up to protect themselves from being overly stretched and ripped. And they're contracting to help our well-intentioned runner hold his body in balance as he teeters from his heel on the bench. From his upper back all the way down to his ankle, every muscle behind him is firing, tightening, activating, protecting, recoiling, working. Not stretching. And most muscles in front of him are relaxed and ready for a stretch that will never happen.

So let's flip our thinking upside down and get this right. If you want to stretch the hamstrings, you have to relax them by firing the opposite muscles – the quads. This is Active-Isolated Stretching.

We have expanded the principles of Active-Isolated Stretching to Active-Isolated Strengthening exercises. The principles are identical, but the focus of your intention is opposite. In Active-Isolated Strengthening, when one muscle lengthens and stretches in relaxation, the opposite muscle shortens to make that movement possible. That shortened muscle is working and being *activated*. (If you add a weight, then it's lifting.) At the same time, the opposite, relaxing muscle is *isolated* and stretched.

▼ Loosen up the right way
Many athletes mistakenly prepare for exercise by warming up 'nose to toes' – with the leg straight and head forwards. This has the opposite effect of a beneficial stretch and tightens the muscles.

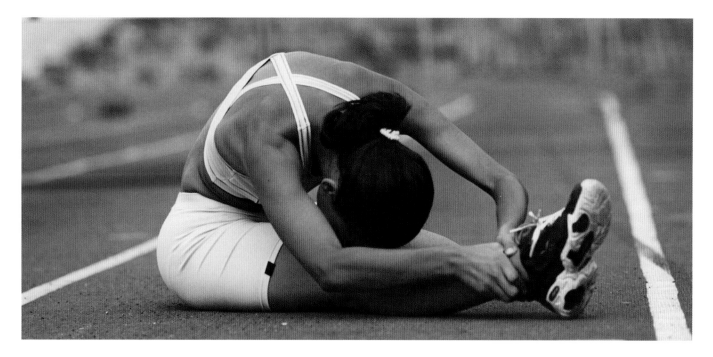

When to Throw the Brakes on a Workout

Athletes describe working out as 'effort'. No doubt about it, effort can be uncomfortable. You'll learn to live with that, and even like it. But there are signals that tell you your workout must cease immediately. If you experience any of the following, take action without delay.

■ **Discomfort in any degree of severity in the upper body: chest, arms, neck and jaw**
The symptoms of a heart attack are described as an ache, burn, tightness, pressure, a sensation of fullness or an overwhelming sense of unexplained dread. The sensations can be very subtle – don't dismiss them. Dial 999 for an ambulance, take an aspirin, and lie down immediately.

■ **Faintness, dizziness, light-headedness or nausea**
Feeling faint or light-headed is a signal that your brain isn't getting enough blood and oxygen. You have two immediate problems: you have to prevent blacking out and falling on your face, and you have to figure out what's happening. You don't have a lot of time – stop whatever you're doing and 'go to ground'. Lie down and get your feet higher than your head. Often, lying down will relieve the symptoms. If you don't recover while lying down, dial 999. Even if the symptoms go away, tell your doctor.

■ **Shortness of breath, effort, wheezing or inability to recover to easy breathing within five minutes**
When you start an exercise programme, or you work out harder than usual, breathing a little hard is quite normal. If you're panting and gasping so hard that you can't speak or control your breath, stop and settle down. If, after five minutes of rest, you still can't catch your breath, call an ambulance, take an aspirin, and lie down.

■ **Pain in your back, bones or joints during or after exercise**
Nothing should hurt in these workouts. Muscle aches and slight discomfort as you push yourself from level to level are normal, but pain in your back, bones and joints is *not*. Pain is nature's way of telling you something is wrong. We always pay attention to pain and react quickly. If it hurts, stop. Take a few days off, lower the intensity of the exercise, and try it again. If it still hurts, see your doctor.

A COMPLETE BACK PROGRAMME

We have designed a programme that will give you real results immediately. In contrast to other programmes that can take weeks to see results, the benefits of these exercises start to kick in after your first session. From the first day, you'll understand why the deceptively simple principles of Active-Isolated Stretching and Strengthening have revolutionised the world of sports performance.

The programme contains three components of a comprehensive workout.

■ Active-Isolated Stretching
■ Active-Isolated Strengthening
■ Cardio Training

We will coach you through each exercise individually and then we'll teach you to put them all together into three cycles, or phases, that will take you from 'beginner' through 'intermediate' to 'advanced'. The three cycles allow us to adjust workout patterns so that you can progress steadily and safely. You'll see results that will amaze you, especially when we start combining workout components for maximum benefit in minimum time.

The first component of the programme is Active-Isolated Stretching. In our programme, you'll start as a beginner, no matter how fit you are. You'll determine your own starting point, depending on how tight your joints are when you start. Within one session, you'll feel your joints begin to unlock, allowing you a measure of freedom of movement within your body that you may not have felt in a long time. As your programme progresses, you will improve significantly on the first workout, but at your own pace. You'll feel more relaxed as your joints move through their full ranges of motion in the way they were intended to. Your circulation will improve. You'll sleep better. You'll feel better.

Once we have you moving, we'll add some weight lifting with Active-Isolated Strengthening, to give your muscles strength and tone. You'll start with weights that feel right for you and you will advance when you're ready. You'll build the muscles that will support and protect your back from future pain and injury. Within a few sessions, you'll feel power and real energy kick in.

When you're strong and moving easily, we'll add a walking programme to burn calories, boost your cardiovascular system and give you back your stamina. At this point in the programme, we consider you an 'advanced' athlete, meaning that you've mastered the same tools that have helped dozens of Olympians keep their backs healthy and strong.

THE TOOLS YOU'LL NEED

Two reasons why Active-Isolated workouts are so popular? They're simple, and they're fast. They fit right into a tight space and an even tighter schedule. You don't need a special gym; all the exercises can be done almost anywhere. Here's what you'll need.

- A bed or enough open floor space to lie down and extend your arms out to your sides
- A sturdy chair
- An 8ft (2.4m) strap or stretch rope, narrow enough in diameter to wrap around your hand
- A set of attachable weights (see page 66 for information on choosing weights) for use on wrists and ankles

With the most effective workout system in the world in your hands, you'll find you even have the time to get it done. You'll need only 30 minutes a day for the first two of the three, six-week cycles. In the last six-week cycle, when we add walking to your programme, you'll enjoy an extra 20 to 30 minutes of 'me' time, two or three days a week. By the time you get to that last six weeks, you'll be so excited about your revitalised body that you'll be bounding down the street.

We're here to coach you – we'll teach you each exercise, one at a time. Once you've mastered the exercises, you'll be able to use the at-a-glance pages – the first of which you'll find on page 48 – for quick reference.

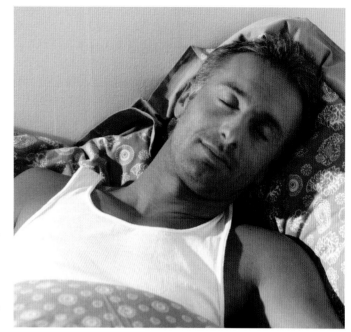

▲ You'll sleep much better
Research has proved that correct exercise helps you sleep soundly. In turn, a good night's sleep will make you feel relaxed, energetic and motivated to build up your strength even further.

YOUR WHARTON JUMP START

You're about to embark on a programme that's identical to the one we use to train elite athletes. It's the one we use ourselves. We're going to show you how to unlock your joints, strengthen your muscles and increase your stamina using principles that take advantage of the way your body was designed. This is fitness the way nature intended it. Simple. Fun. Fast. And revolutionary. But before we begin, here are a few thoughts about getting your programme off to the best start possible.

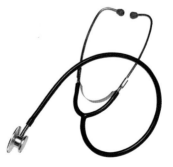

First, get your doctor's approval. There are times when fitness programmes should be approached with caution, and having a back injury tops that list. Take this book to your doctor and, together, outline the best plan for your situation.

Just begin. Getting started on a fitness programme is pretty simple. Forget having to start on a Monday. Forget the list of things that you have to complete first. Forget waiting for your best friend to get ready so that you can do it together. Forget having to lose 10lb (4.5kg) first. Starting an exercise programme begins with a decision to do it. Now.

Make an appointment. Until you are comfortable with integrating workouts into your daily life, we urge you to block out the time each day on a diary or calendar, as though you were scheduling an appointment that you must keep. Before you know it, you'll be looking forward to the time that is yours.

Swap activities. We ask some of our new clients to keep time logs for a few days, so they can examine exactly how they're spending time. Only after the schedule is on paper in 15-minute increments can they see blocks of time that could be easily traded for a workout. Sometimes, the trade-off involves a bit of sacrifice but, more often than not, it's a matter of tightening up some inefficiencies to free an hour to train. Watch a little less television. Read on the exercise bike instead of in your armchair. Get up 30 minutes earlier.

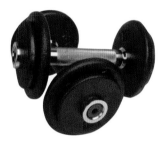

Get your clothes and equipment together. All your good intentions will fall by the wayside if you realise that you can't lift a weight because you forgot to get one. Get everything together before you start.

Start slowly and progress gradually. One of the greatest myths in training is that it has to hurt in order for it to be doing your body any good. That little catchphrase, 'Go for the burn!' has ruined a generation of good trainers and hapless clients.

Athletes describe a good workout not as 'pain', but as 'effort'. You know you're working when you're pushing a little. Anything beyond this is risking injury. When your workout no longer challenges you, and is so easy that you're not putting any effort into it, then it's time to slightly increase weight, time or duration. We'll show you how.

Exercise between meals. If you're planning a no-holds-barred workout, wait a couple of hours after eating. After you've eaten, your body puts its energy and blood supply into digesting food in your stomach. If you divert that energy and blood supply into large muscles, then you inhibit your body's ability to digest. A common reaction is vomiting. We don't know about you, but we think nothing spoils a good workout like being sick.

Adjust your workout to suit the weather and time of day. Working out raises your metabolism and your body temperature, so dress to stay cool. But keep your common sense: if you're going for a brisk walk, don't wear shorts in a snowstorm. When in doubt, wear layers of clothing that you can peel off. Also, be mindful of your safety. Changing light conditions alter your depth perception, and a path that looks flat at 7:00 in the morning might look like tossed rubble at noon.

We're often asked, 'When is the best time of day to work out?' Our answer is, 'Any time you can'. Although some literature suggests that working out right before bedtime

The 21-Day Guarantee

If it's been a while since you've worked out, we know that starting can sometimes feel overwhelming. But we know that you will succeed with the Active-Isolated programme, even if you've bailed out of others in the past. Here's why:

- **You're going to feel better** from your first workout, and you'll feel even better every day. You'll be stronger and more flexible, and will have more stamina. You'll be able to move with energy and power. That relief and freedom from pain will probably be more than enough to keep you going.
- **Researchers also tell us** that it takes 21 days for a habit to take hold. If you stay on track for only 21 days, you'll have made working out a habit – an integral, joyful and important part of your life. You'll already have seen amazing results and will be well on your way to having the body that you deserve.

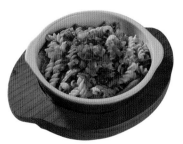

revs you up so that sleeping is difficult, we do it every night and sleep fine. In fact, we rely heavily on exercise to diffuse the stresses of the day and relax us right before bed.

One word of caution about early-morning workouts: please be careful about rocketing right into a hard cardio workout. Going from 0 to 60 is tough on the heart. Warm up first and start slowly.

Muscle Tear

Stretching will not tear your muscles – in fact you can stretch a muscle 1.6 times its length. The joints of your body have limited ranges of motion to keep you from flopping all over the place. Also, nature designed you to have a built-in range-limit detector – it's called *pain*.

■ **As you approach the limit of your** range of motion in a stretch, you experience the sensation of tightness, followed by discomfort, then pain. In fact, your joints have sensors that tell your body to draw back from being overly stretched, in order to prevent tearing. That's why the first sensation is tightness: the muscle is contracting back to protect itself. (While it's true that you can stretch a muscle until it tears, this is due to trauma and will not happen during a normal Active-Isolated Stretching workout.)

■ **So how flexible can you expect to be?** It depends on where you start. Some people were born flexible and have remained so all their lives. And some of us started out with flexibility, but lost it as we aged. No matter how flexible you are right now, you'll see tremendous gains as you work out.

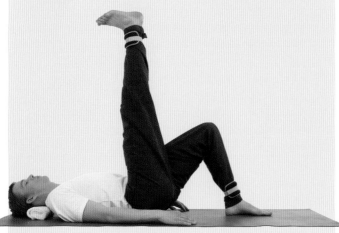

Divide your workout for convenience. Research assures us that two or three short workouts can be as beneficial as one longer one, provided that all the workouts are equal in intensity. If you don't have time to do it all in one workout, divide it into two or three parts and save some of it for later.

Keep a record of your workouts. You'll find a personal workout log on page 93. Make photocopies of it for your own use. Keeping a log helps you to stay on track and gives you a clear picture of your progress.

Do your exercises in order. The workouts are specifically organised to warm up and unlock muscles first and then to engage them when they're ready to fire. Don't skip around; follow the sequence of exercises presented in the Stretching and Strengthening programmes in the order specified.

Don't rush a move or a release. In both stretching and strengthening, bring a movement to its finish. Extend all the way out, hold, and flex all the way back as far as you can go. If you cut a movement short, you'll deprive all the muscle fibres of participating, and they will then become weaker.

Rather than rock 'n' roll, think of this as a waltz. We help our clients to break their gym-music habit (pounding, driving rhythms are good for excitement but bad for pacing), and teach them to adjust to a slower, more effective pace.

Know your own limits. How will you know that you're working hard enough to make it count? We've organised the individual exercises to contain guidelines. Stretches (or flexes) require a little tug of the rope or strap at the end of each move. Strengthening exercises (or lifts) are a matter of judgement on your part. The lifts should take effort, but not pain and extreme exertion.

If you run out of steam, cut back. If you get midway through a workout and decide that you can't do more, quit. Do as much as you can and be proud of it. Don't worry. You'll soon have built up to the point where you can handle the whole workout without difficulty.

There are days when even the thought of working out seems overwhelming. The question to answer is, 'Am I really too tired to work out, or do I just think I am?' If you're too tired, forget the workout. If you're not sure, start the workout and see how you feel after 5 or 10 minutes. Remember that working out can energise you when your energy is low. Once you get moving, you might feel better and discover that the workout is no problem. If you don't feel more energised, cut the workout short.

If it hurts, stop immediately. As you progress, you'll learn to distinguish between the discomfort of exertion and real pain. Until you know the difference, treat all pain the same. It's a message from your body that you're doing (or are about to do) damage and you need to back off. If backing off alleviates the pain immediately, you might test the exercise again, with fewer repetitions or less weight (if you're lifting). If the pain is acute or persists, see your doctor.

Remember to breathe. Time exercise naturally: exhale as you stretch and inhale as you return to the neutral position.

MAKING SPACE

Where's the best place to do your Active-Isolated Stretching routine? We like to stretch on the floor or on a bed, but anywhere is all right. (When you are beginning, we advise you to pick a place close to a large mirror, where you can properly check your form.) You'll be sitting and lying down, so you want to make sure you'll be as comfortable as possible. Extend that feeling into your dress – wear loose-fitting, comfortable clothing. And don't forget to keep a bottle of water within easy reach. Now you're ready to begin!

Please note: we've included the complete series of exercises here. Please see pages 48 and 58 for easy, at-a-glance references to the exact exercises that you'll do each day of the programme.

▼ Getting off to a good start
It's important that you feel comfortable while you exercise. This means wearing loose clothing, having enough space to lie down and ensuring that you have some water close to hand.

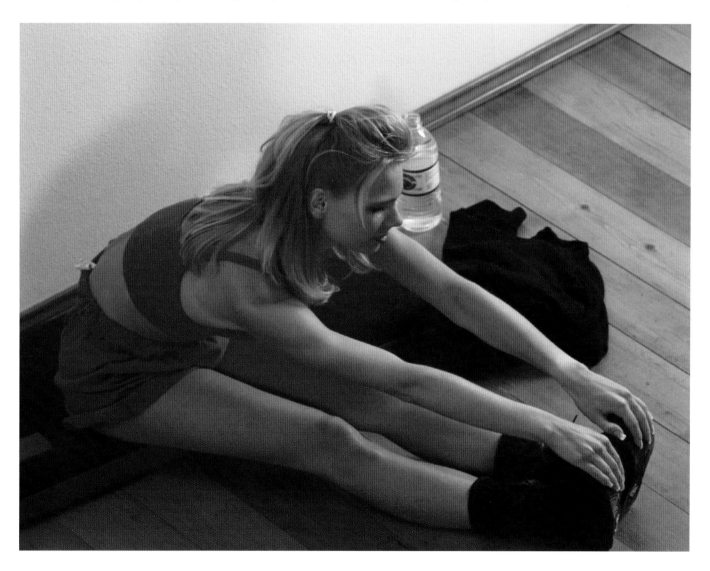

STRETCH 1:
ACTIVE-ISOLATED STRETCHING
(HIP AND TRUNK)

This workout is the foundation of the Active-Isolated Stretching method and is featured in each week of the plan. Follow each exercise in the order specified here. Detailed step-by-step illustrations appear over the following pages. For information on the names and locations of the muscle sets involved in these exercises, please see pages 274–275.

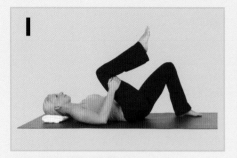

Single-leg Pelvic Tilts

Hold Each stretch: 2 seconds
Reps: 10 right, 10 left

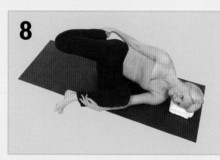

Double-leg Pelvic Tilts

Hold Each Stretch: 2 seconds
Reps: 10

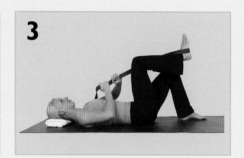

Bent-leg Hamstrings

Hold Each Stretch: 2 seconds
Reps: 10 right, 10 left

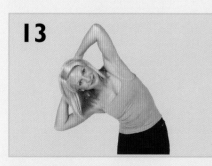

Psoas

Hold Each Stretch: 2 seconds
Reps: 10 right, 10 left

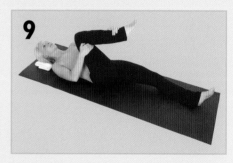

Quadriceps

Hold Each Stretch: 2 seconds
Reps: 10 right, 10 left

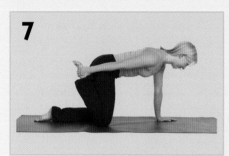

Gluteals

Hold Each Stretch: 2 seconds
Reps: 10 right, 10 left

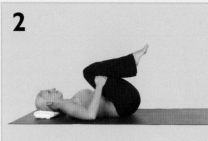

Trunk Lateral Flexors

Hold Each Stretch: 2 seconds
Reps: 10 right, 10 left

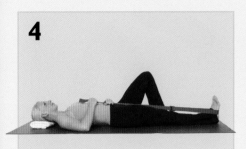

Straight-leg Hamstrings

Hold Each Stretch: 2 seconds
Reps: 10 right, 10 left

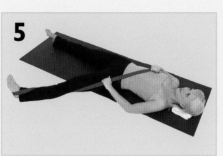

Hip Adductors

Hold Each Stretch: 2 seconds
Reps: 10 right, 10 left

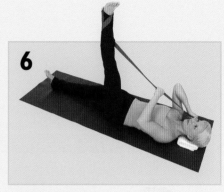

Hip Abductors

Hold Each Stretch: 2 seconds
Reps: 10 right, 10 left

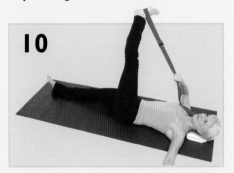

Piriformis

Hold Each Stretch: 2 seconds
Reps: 10 right, 10 left

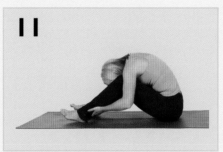

Trunk Extensors

Hold Each Stretch: 2 seconds
Reps: 10

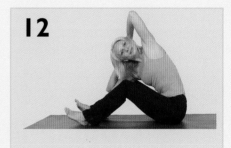

Thoracic-lumbar Rotators

Hold Each Stretch: 2 seconds
Reps: 10 right, 10 left

1

Single-leg Pelvic Tilts

Active Muscles You Contract: Abdominals and muscles from the fronts of your hips down the fronts of your thighs

Isolated Muscles You Stretch: Lower back and buttocks

Hold Each Stretch: 2 seconds **Reps:** 10 right, 10 left

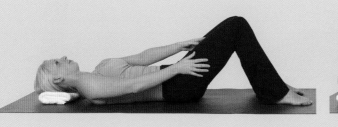

1 Lie on your back on a flat surface. Tuck a rolled towel or small pillow under your neck and head. Bend your knees to keep the pressure off your back. Reach down to weave your fingers together behind the knee of your exercising leg. If you can't reach all the way to your knee, hold the back of your thigh as close to your knee as you can.

2 Using your abdominals and hip flexors (muscles along the fronts of your hips), lift your exercising leg towards your chest as far as you can. At the end of your stretch, gently assist with your hands, but don't force it. Add slight pressure, extending the range of the stretch a little more. Hold it for two seconds and then relax in preparation for the next stretch.

2

Double-leg Pelvic Tilts

Active Muscles You Contract: Abdominals and muscles from the fronts of your hips down the fronts of your thighs

Isolated Muscles You Stretch: Lower back and buttocks

Hold Each Stretch: 2 seconds **Reps:** 10

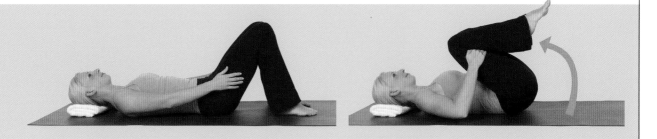

1 Lie on your back on a flat surface. Tuck a rolled towel or small pillow under your neck and head. To relax your back, bend both knees, with your feet flat on the surface. Reach down and place one hand behind each knee. If you can't reach all the way to your knees, hold the backs of your thighs as close to your knees as you can.

2 Using your abdominals, and your quadriceps (muscles down the fronts of your thighs), lift your legs towards your chest as far as you can. At the end of your stretch, gently assist with your hands, but don't force it. Add the slightest pressure, extending the range of the stretch just a little more. Hold for two seconds and then relax in preparation for the next stretch.

3

Bent-leg Hamstrings

Active Muscles You Contract: Muscles in the fronts of your thighs

Isolated Muscles You Stretch: Large muscles in the backs of your thighs, just behind your knees

Equipment: Strap or rope　**Hold Each Stretch:** 2 seconds　**Reps:** 10 right, 10 left

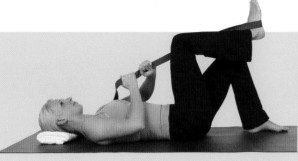

1 Lie on your back on a flat surface. Bend both knees and keep your feet flat. Hold the ends of your strap together to form a loop. Slip it under the arch of one foot. Hold the strap taut. Keeping your knee bent and relaxed, lift your exercising leg until your thigh is perpendicular to the surface.

2 Keeping the loop taut, straighten your leg by contracting your quadriceps until your knee is locked. Gently assist with your strap, but don't force it. With practice, the sole of the foot will point at the ceiling. Hold for two seconds. Relax.

4

Straight-leg Hamstrings

Active Muscles You Contract: Muscles from the fronts of your hips down the fronts of your thighs

Isolated Muscles You Stretch: Large muscles in the backs of your thighs

Equipment: Strap or rope　**Hold Each Stretch:** 2 seconds　**Reps:** 10 right, 10 left

1 Lie on your back on a flat surface. Tuck a rolled towel or small pillow under your neck and head. Your exercising leg should be straight out. The other leg should be bent at the knee, with your foot down flat. Hold the ends of your strap together to form a loop. Slip it under the arch of the foot of your exercising leg. Take out the slack and hold it tight. Lock your knee.

2 From your hip, using your quadriceps, aim the sole of your foot towards the ceiling and lift your leg straight up as far as you can. Grasp the ends of the strap with both hands and 'climb' up it as your leg lifts. Gently assist with your strap, but don't force it. With practice, the sole of the foot will point at the ceiling. Hold for two seconds. Relax.

5

Hip Adductors

Active Muscles You Contract: Muscles on the outsides of your thighs, in the middle of your buttocks, and across your front thighs

Isolated Muscles You Stretch: Muscles on the insides of your thighs

Equipment: Strap or rope **Hold Each Stretch:** 2 seconds **Reps:** 10 right, 10 left

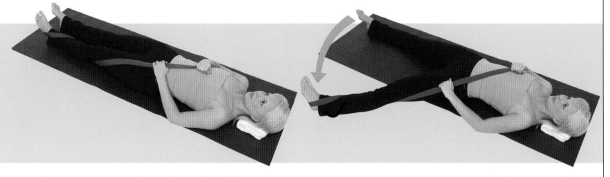

1 Lie on your back on a flat surface with both legs straight out. Make a loop with your strap and slip it under the arch of one foot. Wrap the strap round the inside of the ankle so the ends are on the outside. Lock your knee. Lift your heel very slightly off the floor and pull the strap tight. Rotate your non-exercising leg inwards slightly, to stabilise your body.

2 From your hip, using your abductors (on the outside of your thigh), extend your leg out to the side, leading with your heel. Keep slight tension on the strap. Sliding the same-side hand down the strap, hold the top with the other hand. At the end of your stretch, gently assist with your strap, but don't force it. Hold for two seconds. Relax.

6

Hip Abductors

Active Muscles You Contract: Muscles on the insides of your thighs

Isolated Muscles You Stretch: Muscles on the outsides of your thighs and hips

Equipment: Strap or rope **Hold Each Stretch:** 2 seconds **Reps:** 10 right, 10 left

1 Lie down on your back on a flat surface with both legs extended. Make a loop with your strap and slip it under the arch of one foot. Wrap it round the outside of the ankle so the ends are on the inside. Lock your knee. Rotate your non-exercising leg inwards slightly and your exercising leg outwards slightly. Take the slack out of your strap and hold it tight.

2 From your groin, using your adductors (on the inside of your thigh), sweep your leg across the midline of your body, leading with your heel, just above your non-exercising leg. Keep your knee locked. Keep slight tension on the strap. At the end of the stretch, gently assist with your strap to extend the stretch a little more. Hold for two seconds. Relax.

7

Psoas

Active Muscles You Contract: Muscles in your buttocks and the backs of your thighs

Isolated Muscles You Stretch: Muscles in your groin and the fronts of your upper thighs

Hold Each Stretch: 2 seconds **Reps:** 10 right, 10 left

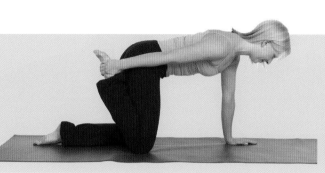

1 Get on your hands and knees. With the knee bent, extend your exercising leg until your foot is off the floor. Bring that foot up behind you until you can reach back with your hand and grasp your ankle. Get a firm grasp, but don't strain your back. If you can't reach your ankle, settle for your shin. In time, the ankle will be within reach.

2 Using your hamstrings and gluteal muscles, lift your exercising leg up until your thigh is parallel to the ground or horizontal with your body. Be careful not to arch your back. Go as far as you can. At the end of your stretch, gently assist with your hand, but don't force it. Extend the range of the stretch just a little more. Hold for two seconds. Relax.

8

Quadriceps

Active Muscles You Contract: Muscles in your buttocks and the backs of your thighs

Isolated Muscles You Stretch: Muscles in the fronts of your thighs

Hold Each Stretch: 2 seconds **Reps:** 10 right, 10 left

1 Lie on your side in a foetal position with your knees curled up. Rest your head on a small pillow. Lock your lower arm under the knee of your bottom leg and tighten your abdominals.

2 With your upper hand grasp your top ankle. If you can't reach, use your strap. Keep the top knee bent and your leg parallel to the surface.

3 Contract your hamstrings and glutes, extending the top leg back as far as you can. Gently assist but don't force it. Hold for two seconds and do reps. Roll over to repeat on the other side.

9

Gluteals

Active Muscles You Contract: Abdominals and muscles from the fronts of your hips down the fronts of your thighs

Isolated Muscles You Stretch: Muscles in your lower back that rotate your torso, muscles that rotate your hips, and buttocks

Hold Each Stretch: 2 seconds **Reps:** 10 right, 10 left

1 Lie on your back with both legs extended. Point the toes of your non-exercising leg inwards to stabilise your hips. Bend the other leg.

2 Using your abdominal muscles and hip flexors, lift your bent knee towards the opposite shoulder. Keep your pelvis flat. When you can, put your hand on the outside of your knee and gently guide the stretch.

TIP: For a deeper stretch, grasp your shin with the opposite hand. As the knee nears the shoulder, press your heel towards the floor and gently assist the stretch with your hand. Keep your pelvis on the floor. Hold for two seconds. Relax.

10

Piriformis

Active Muscles You Contract: Lower abdominals, muscles in the hips that rotate the legs, muscles on inside and front of the thigh

Isolated Muscles You Stretch: The muscle that lies underneath the big muscle in your buttock

Equipment: Strap or rope **Hold Each Stretch:** 2 seconds **Reps:** 10 right, 10 left

1 Lie down on a flat surface with both legs extended. Hold the ends of your strap together to form a loop. Slip it under the arch of one foot. Hold the strap taut. Lock the knee of your exercising leg so that it is straight and turn the foot of your non-exercising leg inwards slightly.

2 From your hip and using your quadriceps and hip flexors, pull the strap to lift your leg straight up until it is perpendicular to your body. Point the bottom of your foot towards the ceiling.

11

Trunk Extensors

Active Muscles You Contract: Abdominals

Isolated Muscles You Stretch: Muscles that run from your pelvis to the base of your skull along the spine, lower-back muscles

Hold Each Stretch: 2 seconds **Reps:** 10

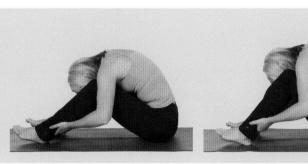

1 Sit on a flat surface with your back straight, your knees slightly bent, your feet hip-width apart, your toes pointed slightly up and your feet resting on your heels, as shown.

2 Tuck your chin down, contract the abdominal muscles, bend at your hips and pull your torso down as far as you can. Grasp the sides of the lower legs to assist at the end of each stretch.

TIP: (For a deeper lower-back stretch, or if your hamstrings are tight, bring your heels closer to your body.) Add slight pressure to extend the stretch a little more. Hold for two seconds. Relax.

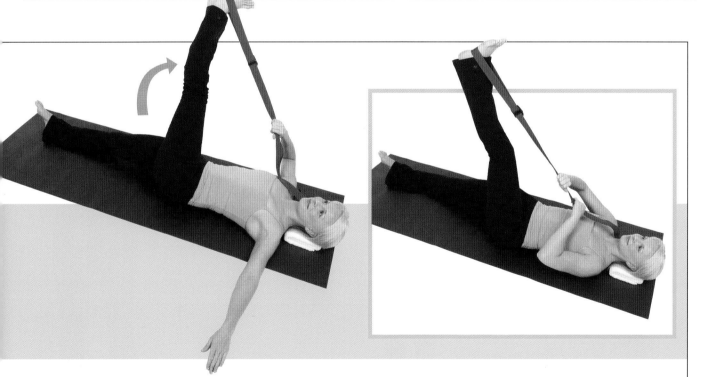

3 Hold the loop tight. Extend your other hand straight out to keep you from rolling. Contract your inner-thigh muscles. Bring your leg across your body and down towards the floor until your hip begins to roll up. Assist the stretch gently with the strap. Hold for two seconds. Relax.

TIP: If you're in any discomfort when you lock your knee straight, try relaxing the knee very slightly. You can use the strap to lift your leg by drawing up its ends with both your hands, in a hand-over-hand manoeuvre.

12

Thoracic-lumbar Rotators

Active Muscles You Contract: Abdominals; muscles on the sides of your chest; thoracic-lumbar rotators (muscles on the sides of your back)

Isolated Muscles You Stretch: Muscles up the spine; stabilising, rotating and balancing muscles in the back and sides; lower-back muscles

Hold Each Stretch: 2 seconds **Reps:** 10 right, 10 left

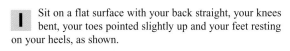

1 Sit on a flat surface with your back straight, your knees bent, your toes pointed slightly up and your feet resting on your heels, as shown.

2 Lock your hands by lacing your fingers together behind your head with your elbows out. Tuck your chin down.

13

Trunk Lateral Flexors

Active Muscles You Contract: Abdominals; muscles on the sides of your chest; thoracic-lumbar rotators

Isolated Muscles You Stretch: Muscles along the spine, muscles in the sides of your trunk

Hold Each Stretch: 2 seconds **Reps:** 10 right, 10 left

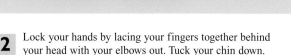

1 Stand straight, with your legs shoulder-width apart and both arms relaxed down by your sides.

2 Raise one arm, placing your hand behind your head with your elbow pointed away from your body.

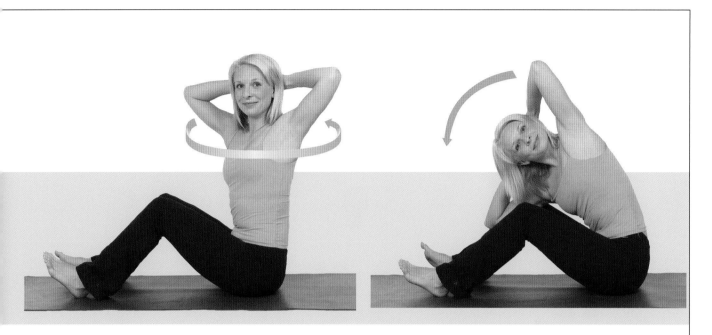

3 Contracting your entire abdomen, including the muscles in your side and the opposite thoracic-lumbar rotator muscles, rotate your upper body in one direction until you have rotated as far as you can go. Do this four or five times until you feel loosened up.

4 When you're ready, rotate once more, hold, and flex your body forwards, leading towards the surface with your elbow. Hold for two seconds. Return to an upright position. Relax. Work one side at a time, completing all repetitions before beginning the opposite side.

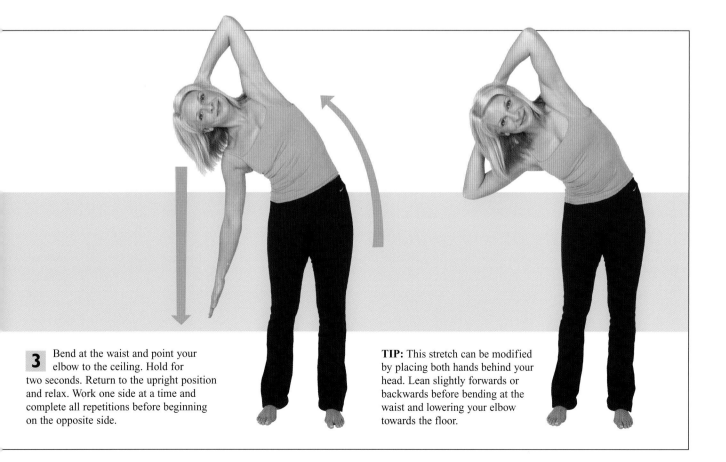

3 Bend at the waist and point your elbow to the ceiling. Hold for two seconds. Return to the upright position and relax. Work one side at a time and complete all repetitions before beginning on the opposite side.

TIP: This stretch can be modified by placing both hands behind your head. Lean slightly forwards or backwards before bending at the waist and lowering your elbow towards the floor.

STRETCH 2: ACTIVE-ISOLATED STRETCHING

(SHOULDERS AND NECK)

The plans on pages 90 to 92 will tell you when to do this workout, which is essential for keeping your upper body supple. Follow the exercises in the order specified here. Detailed step-by-step illustrations appear over the following pages. For information on the names and locations of the muscle sets involved in these exercises, please see pages 274–275.

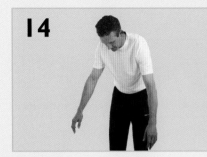

14

Shoulder Circumduction

Hold Each Stretch: Technically there is no stretch here
Reps: 10 clockwise, 10 anticlockwise

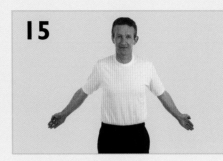

15

Pectoralis Majors

Hold Each Stretch: 2 seconds
Reps: 10

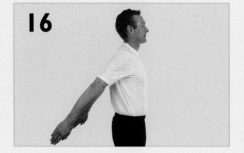

16

Anterior Deltoids

Hold Each Stretch: 2 seconds
Reps: 10

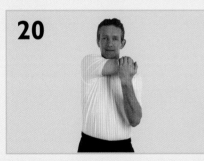

20

Rotator Cuff 2 (Trapezius)

Hold Each Stretch: 2 seconds
Reps: 10 right, 10 left

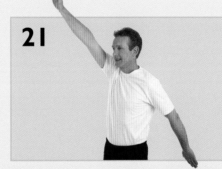

21

Forward Elevators of the Shoulder

Hold Each Stretch: 2 seconds
Reps: 10 right, 10 left (in opposition)

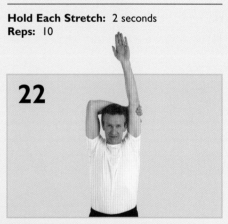

22

Side Elevations of the Shoulder

Hold Each Stretch: 2 seconds
Reps: 10 right, 10 left

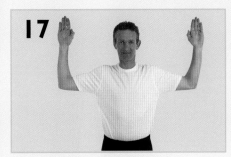

Shoulder Internal Rotators

Hold Each Stretch: 2 seconds
Reps: 10

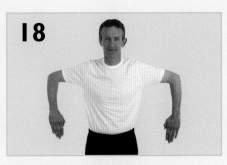

Shoulder External Rotators

Hold Each Stretch: 2 seconds
Reps: 10

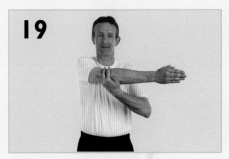

Rotator Cuff 1 (Rhomboids)

Hold Each Stretch: 2 seconds
Reps: 10 right, 10 left

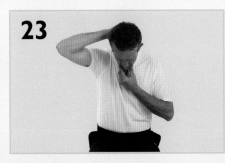

Neck Extensors

Hold Each Stretch: 2 seconds
Reps: 10

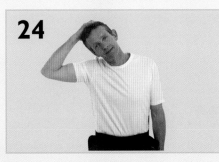

Neck Lateral Flexors

Hold Each Stretch: 2 seconds
Reps: 10 right, 10 left

14

Shoulder Circumduction

Active Muscles You Contract: Shoulders

Isolated Muscles You Stretch: No muscles are specifically isolated. This is a warm-up exercise

Hold Each Stretch: Technically, there is no stretch **Reps:** 10 clockwise, 10 anticlockwise

1 Stand and bend forwards at the waist. Allow your arms to dangle loosely from your shoulders. Relax as completely as you can. Bend your knees slightly to keep tension out of your back.

2 Move your arms in small circles – the right arm rotating clockwise, the left arm circling in an anticlockwise motion…

15

Pectoralis Majors

Active Muscles You Contract: Backs of your shoulders and the area between your shoulder blades

Isolated Muscles You Stretch: Muscles in your chest and shoulders

Hold Each Stretch: 2 seconds **Reps:** 10

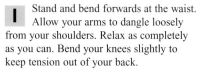

1 Stand on a flat surface with your feet slightly apart. Relax your knees, straighten the arms, lock your elbows. Swing your arms forwards so that your fingertips touch. Inhale.

2 Use the muscles in the backs of your shoulders and between your shoulder blades to swing your arms straight back until they can go no further. Exhale.

TIP: This stretch is done in progressive stages, with each swing a little higher than the one before it.

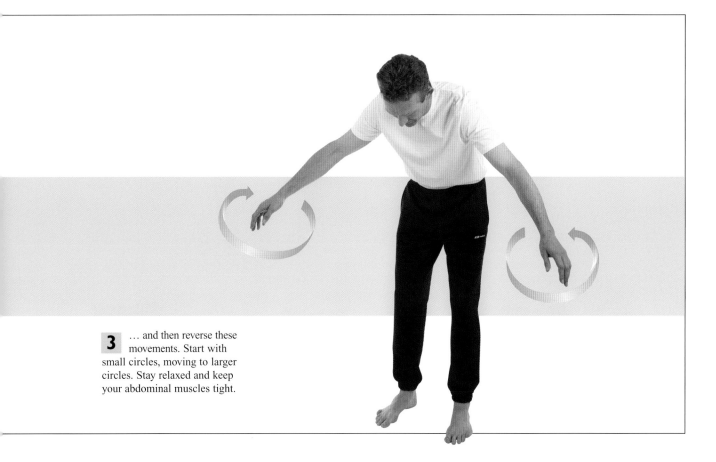

3 … and then reverse these movements. Start with small circles, moving to larger circles. Stay relaxed and keep your abdominal muscles tight.

16

Anterior Deltoids

Active Muscles You Contract: Backs of your shoulders and the triceps

Isolated Muscles You Stretch: Upper arms and fronts of your shoulders

Hold Each Stretch: 2 seconds **Reps:** 10

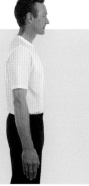

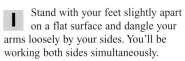

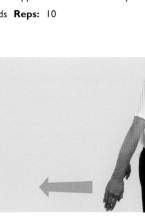

1 Stand with your feet slightly apart on a flat surface and dangle your arms loosely by your sides. You'll be working both sides simultaneously.

2 Swing your arms back, palms facing, keeping your elbows locked. Warm up with 10 gentle repetitions.

3 For a deeper stretch, bring fingertips together behind your back, with elbows locked. Raise your arms. Hold for two seconds, relax, repeat.

17

Shoulder Internal Rotators

Active Muscles You Contract: External rotator muscles in the backs of your shoulders

Isolated Muscles You Stretch: Internal rotator muscles in your shoulders

Hold Each Stretch: 2 seconds **Reps:** 10

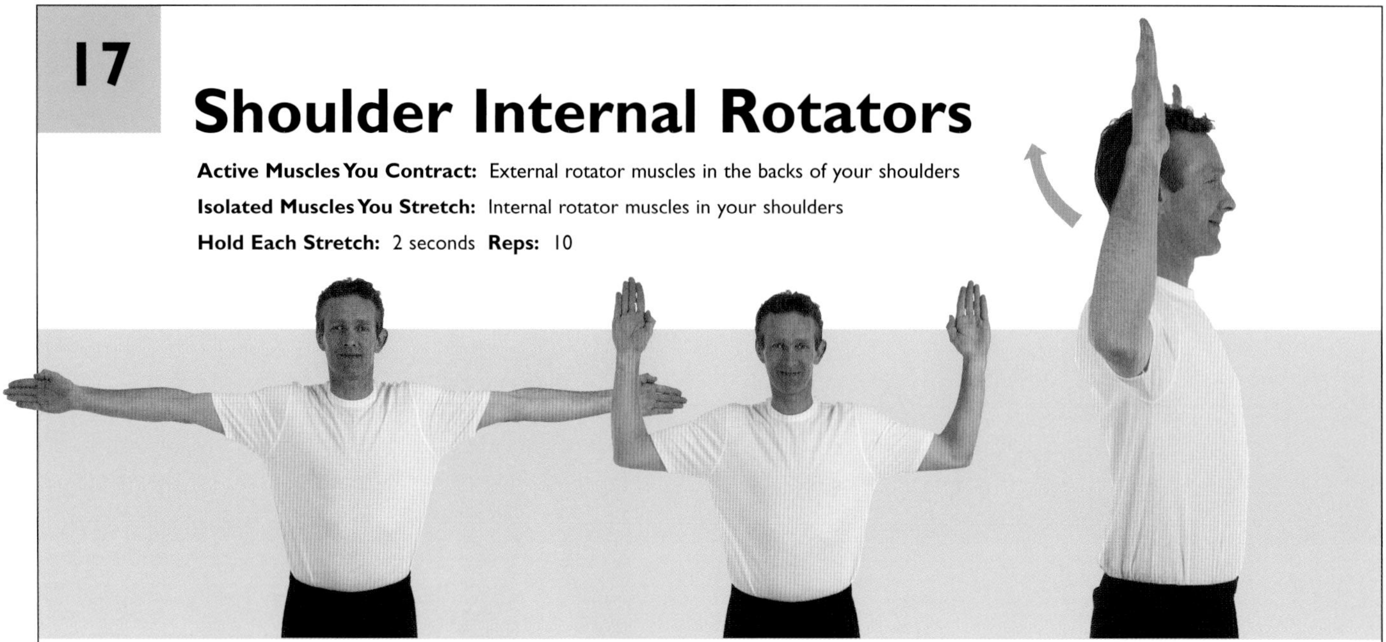

1 Stand on a flat surface with your feet slightly apart. Raise your arms out to the sides so that your elbows are level with your shoulders.

2 Point your forearms, hands and fingertips towards the ceiling, palms facing forward. Your elbows should be at 90-degree angles, still level with your shoulders.

3 Lock the angle of your elbows. Keeping the shoulders steady, pivot so that your forearms and hands move up and back, passing behind your head. Hold for two seconds, relax, then repeat.

18

Shoulder External Rotators

Active Muscles You Contract: Internal rotator muscles in your shoulders

Isolated Muscles You Stretch: External rotator muscles in the backs of your shoulders

Hold Each Stretch: 2 seconds **Reps:** 10

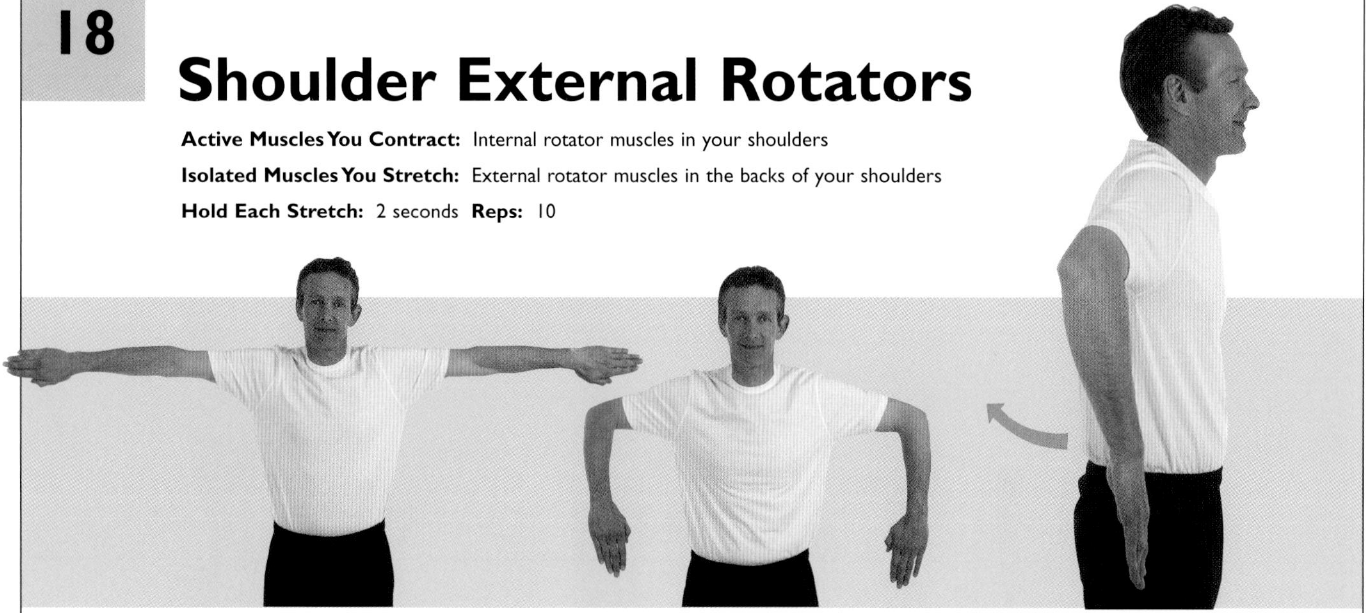

1 Stand on a flat surface with your feet slightly apart. Raise your arms out to the sides so that your elbows are level with your shoulders.

2 Point your forearms, hands and fingertips towards the floor, palms facing backwards. Your elbows should be at 90-degree angles, still level with your shoulders.

3 Lock the angle of your elbows. Keeping the shoulders steady, pivot so that your forearms and hands are behind the midpoint of your body. Hold for two seconds, relax, then repeat.

19

Rotator Cuff 1 (Rhomboids)

Active Muscles You Contract: Muscles in the fronts of your shoulders and your chest

Isolated Muscles You Stretch: Rotator cuffs (muscles in the shoulders)

Hold Each Stretch: 2 seconds **Reps:** 10 right, 10 left

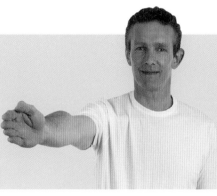

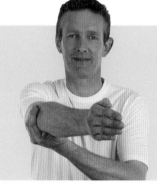

1 Stand on a flat surface with your feet slightly apart and your arms relaxed at your sides. Lift one arm straight up until it is level with your shoulder. Lock your elbow.

2 Start to pass your arm across your chest towards the opposite shoulder and place your opposite hand at the elbow.

3 Pass your arm as far as it can go, making sure you keep your shoulder down. Hold for two seconds, then relax and repeat.

20

Rotator Cuff 2 (Trapezius)

Active Muscles You Contract: Muscles in the fronts of your shoulders

Isolated Muscles You Stretch: Rotator cuffs and muscles below the shoulder blades

Hold Each Stretch: 2 seconds **Reps:** 10 right, 10 left

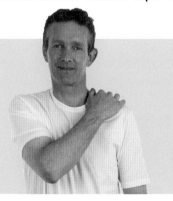

1 Stand on a flat surface with your feet slightly apart and your arms relaxed at your sides. Lift one arm with your elbow bent. Pass it straight across the chest towards your opposite shoulder.

2 Keep your torso stationary and relaxed; gradually stretch until your hand reaches down your back or as far as it can go.

3 Assist the stretch gently at the end with your opposite hand at your elbow. Hold for two seconds and then relax in preparation for the next stretch.

STRETCH 2: SHOULDERS AND NECK

21

Forward Elevators of the Shoulder

Active Muscles You Contract: Muscles in your shoulders

Isolated Muscles You Stretch: Muscles in your shoulders

Hold Each Stretch: 2 seconds **Reps:** 10 right, 10 left (in opposition)

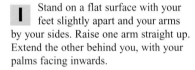

1 Stand on a flat surface with your feet slightly apart and your arms by your sides. Raise one arm straight up. Extend the other behind you, with your palms facing inwards.

2 Using one arm then the other, repeat several times. Now do the same exercise again but with the palm of your raised hand facing outwards.

3 Repeat with the palm of your raised hand facing forwards. Stretch your shoulders in opposition until you can go no further. Hold for two seconds, relax and repeat.

22

Side Elevators of the Shoulder

Active Muscles You Contract: Muscles in your shoulders

Isolated Muscles You Stretch: Muscles in your shoulders

Hold Each Stretch: 2 seconds **Reps:** 10 right, 10 left

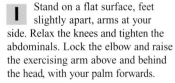
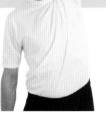

1 Stand on a flat surface, feet slightly apart, arms at your side. Relax the knees and tighten the abdominals. Lock the elbow and raise the exercising arm above and behind the head, with your palm forwards.

2 Hold your exercising arm between your elbow and shoulder, and assist the stretch until you feel it beneath your shoulder blade. Learn to bring your exercising arm straight over and back without having to nod your head. Hold for two seconds, relax, repeat.

23

Neck Extensors

Active Muscles You Contract: Muscles in the front of your neck

Isolated Muscles You Stretch: Muscles in the back of your neck

Hold Each Stretch: 2 seconds **Reps:** 10

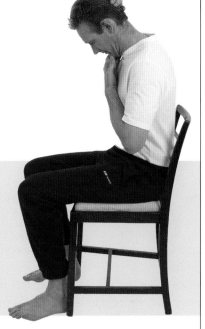

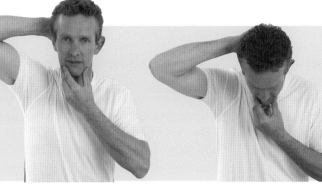

1 Sit in a chair with your back straight and your feet flat on the floor. Face forwards. Place one hand on the back of your head and one hand on your chin to assist the stretch.

2 Tuck your chin down, roll the head forwards until your chin meets your chest. Keep your shoulders relaxed and your torso straight – the stretch is in the neck only.

3 Assist the end of the movement by pressing your head forwards and down with your hand at the back of the head. Be careful not to strain your neck. Hold for two seconds, relax, repeat.

24

Neck Lateral Flexors

Active Muscles You Contract: Muscles in the opposite sides of your neck

Isolated Muscles You Stretch: Muscles in the sides of your neck

Hold Each Stretch: 2 seconds **Reps:** 10 right, 10 left

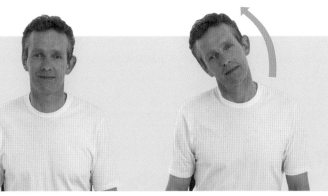

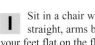

1 Sit in a chair with your back straight, arms by your side and your feet flat on the floor. Face forwards.

2 Cock your head to one side by bringing your ear straight down towards the top of your shoulder. Keep your shoulders down and relaxed and your torso still.

3 Place your fingertips lightly on the side of your head over your ear, and pull your head down towards your shoulder. Be careful not to strain your neck. Hold for two seconds, relax, repeat.

THE ACTIVE-ISOLATED STRENGTHENING ROUTINE FOR BACKS

You already understand the principles of Active-Isolated Stretching. Now it's time to apply those principles to strengthening your muscles. Using small amounts of weight and the resistance of your own body to work out, you isolate specific muscles or groups of muscles and 'fire' them one at a time in a specific sequence. By bolstering weakened muscles, you'll relieve the strain on other, compensating muscles; help remedy current aches; and prevent back pain in the future.

As we discussed earlier, muscles work in pairs. When you fire one muscle, the opposite muscle will relax. When one is fatigued or struggling, your body automatically deploys other muscles to kick in and assist. The irony of this is that you might be able to get the job done – lift something – but still have a weak muscle, because all the *real* work was done by other recruited muscles. When you work out using conventional methods, there's no accommodation for this phenomenon. That's what's different about Active-Isolated Strengthening: you actually strengthen a specific muscle, instead of just lifting a weight. By isolating the targeted muscles, your body cannot recruit help, so the intended muscle is truly strengthened, precisely and efficiently.

As with the stretching routines, you should always work out in comfortable clothing that allows you to move freely and keeps you cool. We suggest shorts and a T-shirt. Wear non-skid shoes or go barefoot.

Keep your trusty bottle of water by your side, and find two small towels or pillows to use during your workouts.

You'll also need two attachable weights. In order to select a starting weight, first lift a 1lb (455g) weight. If it's too light, move to one weighing 2lb (910g). Continue moving up until you find a weight that's fairly easy to lift but still gets your attention. Try it on both your wrist and ankle, because you're going to use the same weight on both.

Don't be a hero. Don't overestimate your ability just because the number is smaller than you think worthy. Don't buy a weight that you can 'grow into' or 'work up to'. You need to be able to work with the weight *straightaway*. Remember that the weight will be attached to one of your limbs, which will provide even more weight to lift when the time comes. You'll work with this weight until your strength increases. When this weight no longer feels heavy, go back to the store and move up to the next denomination, looking for the same sensation you had with the first weight. (Some shops may even allow you to do an exchange.)

For the first week, do one set of each exercise. If the exercise calls for the use of weights, start with 1lb (455g) weights. In the beginning, your single set will teach your body to repattern your neurological pathways. When that set becomes easy, add another set. When *that* set is easy, add more weight (if applicable), in 1lb (455g) increments. As always, if you need to do so, rest between sets.

◀ Fire those muscles
Some Active-Isolated Strengthening techniques involve using small amounts of weight to isolate and strengthen specific muscles.

STRENGTH 1:
ACTIVE-ISOLATED STRENGTHENING
(MUSCLES BELOW THE BELT LINE)

You'll start this workout during the fourth week and continue through all three phases of your plan, as prescribed on pages 90 to 92. Follow the exercises in the order specified here. Detailed step-by-step illustrations appear over the following pages. For information on the names and locations of the muscle sets involved in these exercises, please see pages 274–275.

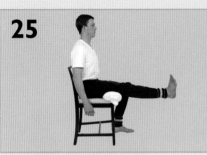

25

Quadriceps – Knee Extensors

Reps: 10 right, 10 left

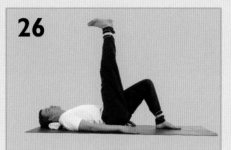

26

Quadriceps – Hip Flexors

Reps: 12 right, 12 left
(Remember: three positions!)

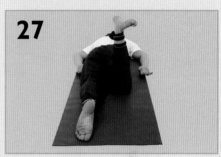

27

Hamstrings

Reps: 12 right, 12 left
(Remember: three positions!)

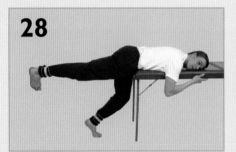

28

Hip Extensors and Hamstrings

Reps: 10 right, 10 left

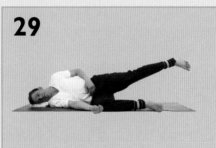

29

Hip Abductors

Reps: 10 right, 10 left

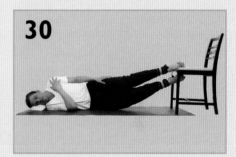

30

Hip Adductors

Reps: 10 right, 10 left

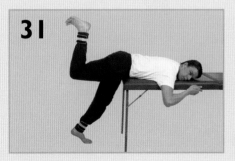

31

Gluteals

Reps: 10 right, 10 left

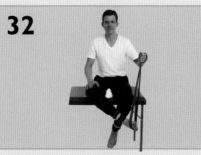

32

Hip External Rotators

Reps: 10 right, 10 left

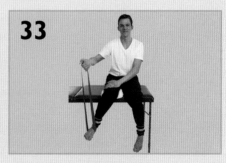

33

Hip Internal Rotators

Reps: 10 right, 10 left

25

Quadriceps – Knee Extensors

Active Muscles You Strengthen: The four muscles in the 'quad' group that run from underneath your kneecap to your hipbone

The Basic Lift: Extend your knee   **Pace of Lifting:** Up slowly, pause, down slowly

Equipment: Rolled towel or small pillow, ankle weights   **Reps:** 10 right, 10 left

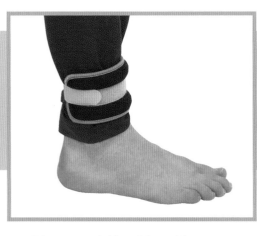

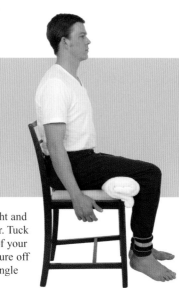

I Take your attachable weights and fasten one to each of your ankles.

2 Sit with your back straight and your feet flat on the floor. Tuck a rolled towel under the knee of your exercising leg to take the pressure off your back. Your foot should dangle above the floor slightly.

26

Quadriceps – Hip Flexors

Active Muscles You Strengthen: Muscles in the top of your thighs from underneath your kneecap to the front of your hip

The Basic Lift: Flex your hip   **Pace of Lifting:** Up slowly, pause, down slowly

Equipment: Rolled towel or small pillow, ankle weights   **Reps:** 12 right, 12 left

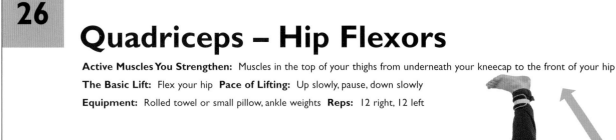

I Put weights on both ankles. Lie on your back on a flat surface. Tuck a rolled towel behind your neck. Bend your non-exercising leg at the knee and place your foot flat on the surface. Straighten your exercising leg by extending your knee. Lock your knee. Keep your foot relaxed.

2 **Front:** Lifting from the hip, use your quadriceps to power the move, bringing your leg up towards your head as far as you can. Aim the bottom of your foot towards the ceiling. Pause and return slowly to the starting position in preparation for the next rep. There is no need to rest between repetitions. Keep it going for 12, then move on to the inside exercise.

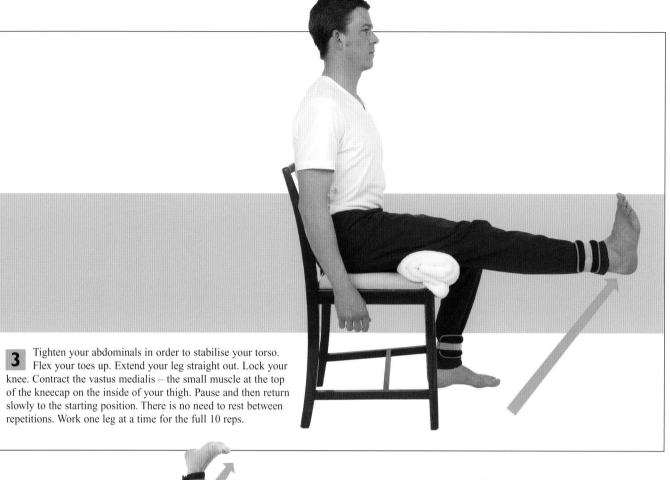

3 Tighten your abdominals in order to stabilise your torso. Flex your toes up. Extend your leg straight out. Lock your knee. Contract the vastus medialis – the small muscle at the top of the kneecap on the inside of your thigh. Pause and then return slowly to the starting position. There is no need to rest between repetitions. Work one leg at a time for the full 10 reps.

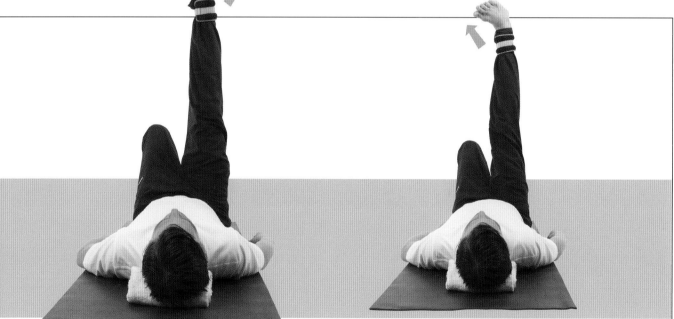

3 **Inside:** Without adjusting your basic position, rotate your exercising leg from your hip by pointing your toes to the outside. Keep your knee locked. From your hip, and contracting your front and inner thigh muscles, lift your leg straight up towards your head as far as you can. Aim your foot towards the ceiling. Pause and return slowly to the starting position. There is no need to rest between repetitions.

4 **Outside:** Repeat step three but this time rotate your exercising leg from your hip by pointing your toes to the inside. From your hip and contracting your front and outer thigh muscles, lift your leg straight up towards your head as far as you can. Once you have done the reps, change legs and move through the three variations again – doing 12 reps for each.

27

Hamstrings

Active Muscles You Strengthen: Muscles in the rear of your thighs from behind your knee to your buttocks

The Basic Lift: Flex your knee **Pace of lifting:** Up slowly, pause, down slowly

Equipment: Ankle weights **Reps:** 12 right, 12 left

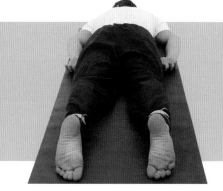
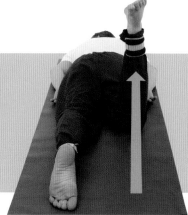

1 Do each of the following three exercises 12 times per leg. Put weights around both your ankles. Lie on your stomach on a flat surface. Keep your hips flat on the surface and your feet straight.

2 **Straight up and back:** Flex your knee by contracting your hamstrings and bringing your foot towards your buttocks. This isolates the muscles in the middle of the rear thigh. Pause and return slowly to the starting position in preparation for the next rep. There is no need to rest in between repetitions.

28

Hip Extensors and Hamstrings

Active Muscles You Strengthen: Muscles in the rear of your thighs that attach to the head of your gluteals at the fold of your buttocks

The Basic Lift: Extend your hip **Pace of Lifting:** Up slowly, pause, down slowly

Equipment: Ankle weights **Reps:** 10 right, 10 left

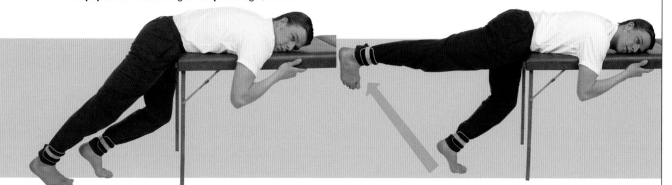

1 Put ankle weights around both ankles. Lean forwards over a workout table or bed with hips at the edge, your abdomen flat on the surface, and feet as near to flat on the floor as you can manage. Bend the non-exercising leg to a 90-degree angle; it should not be supporting your weight. Straighten the exercising leg, extend it out behind you, and rotate it inwards from the hip.

2 With your foot turned inwards and your knee straight, lift your exercising leg towards the ceiling, leading with your heel, until the muscles in your buttocks engage, but not beyond parallel with your back and hips. Pause, then lower your leg slowly to the starting position. There is no need to rest between reps. Work one leg at a time for the full 10 reps.

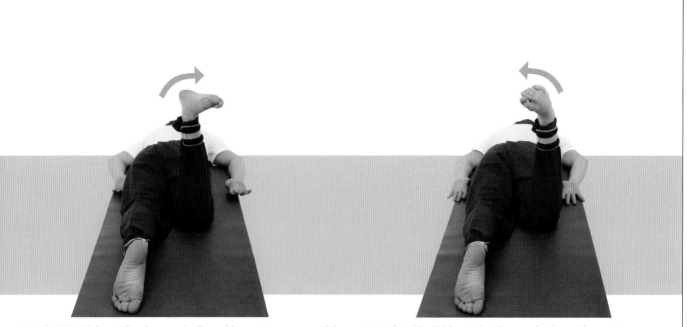

3 **Inside:** Without adjusting your body position, rotate your exercising foot out. Keep your hips flat and your foot turned out. This isolates the muscles on the inside of the rear thigh. Bring your foot towards your buttocks by contracting your hamstring muscles. Pause and return slowly to the starting position. There is no need to rest between repetitions.

4 **Outside:** Without adjusting your body position, rotate your exercising foot in. Bring your foot towards your buttocks by contracting your hamstring muscles. Keep your hips flat and your foot turned in, to isolate the muscles on the outside of the rear thigh. Pause and return slowly to the starting position.

29

Hip Abductors

Active Muscles You Strengthen: Muscles in the top of your thighs from the top of your knee to your groin

The Basic Lift: Lying on your side, lift your leg towards the ceiling   **Pace of Lifting:** Up slowly, pause, down slowly

Equipment: Rolled towel or small pillow, ankle weights   **Reps:** 10 right, 10 left

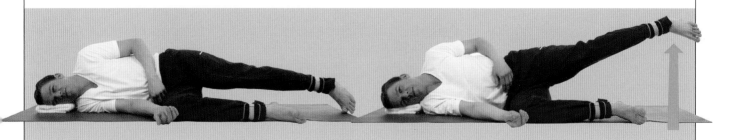

1 Lie on your side on a flat surface with both legs extended and your body straight. Put a rolled towel or small pillow under your neck and head. Fasten weights on both ankles, but work only one leg at a time. Bend the knee of your bottom leg 90 degrees towards your chest to take pressure off the back. Keep the knee of your top (exercising) leg straight.

2 Lift your foot straight up towards the ceiling, leading with your heel. This keeps your leg internally rotated. Lift as far as you can go, pause, and lower your leg slowly to the starting position. Be careful not to slam your toes to the floor. There is no need to rest between repetitions. Keep it going. Work one leg at a time for the full 10 reps.

30

Hip Adductors

Active Muscles You Strengthen: Muscles in the insides of your thighs from your knee to the top of your groin area

The Basic Lift: Lying on your side, lift your inner thigh towards your midline **Pace of Lifting:** Up slowly, pause, down slowly

Equipment: Rolled towel or small pillow, ankle weights, chair or some other stable surface of moderate height next to which you can lie

Reps: 10 right, 10 left

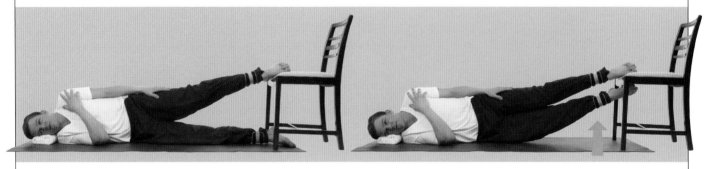

1 Fasten weights around the ankles. Put a rolled towel under your neck. Lie on your side on a flat surface with knees and legs straight out. Lift the top leg to rest the foot or ankle on a chair. Your leg should be at a 45-degree angle to the floor. Contract your abdominals and position arms comfortably.

2 Keeping your knee locked, contract the inner thigh muscles to bring the exercising leg up to meet your top leg. Keep your arms relaxed. Pause, then lower slowly. Work one leg for the full 10 reps.

31

Gluteals

Active Muscles You Strengthen: Buttocks

The Basic Lift: Extend your hip **Pace of Lifting:** Up slowly, pause, down slowly

Equipment: Ankle weights **Reps:** 10 right, 10 left

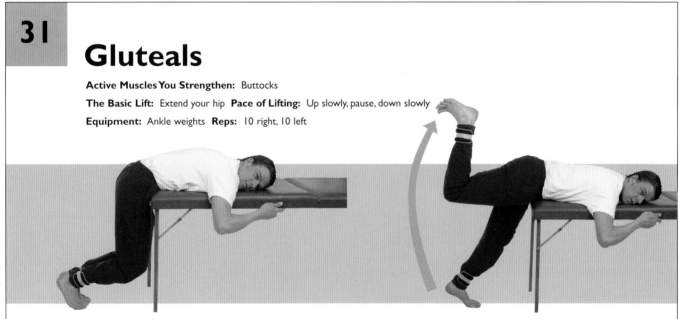

1 Put the weights around both ankles. Lean forwards over a workout table or bed, with hips poised at the edge, your abdomen flat, and feet as near flat on the floor as you can manage. Bend your non-exercising leg to a 90-degree angle and relax it. The leg should not support your weight or serve as a brace. Bend your exercising leg to 90 degrees. Hold the angle.

2 Lift your leg up, leading with the foot and your heel aimed towards the ceiling, until you feel your gluteals engage. You should be able to get your thigh parallel with your hips. Pause, then lower your leg slowly back to the starting position. There is no need to rest between reps. Work one leg at a time for the full 10 reps.

32

Hip External Rotators

Active Muscles You Strengthen: Deep muscles in your buttocks that externally rotate your hips

The Basic Lift: Rotate your hips internally and rotate your thighbone externally   **Pace of Lifting:** Up slowly, pause, down slowly

Equipment: Rolled towel, ankle weights, stretch rope or strap   **Reps:** 10 right, 10 left

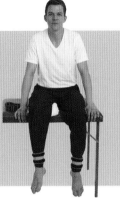 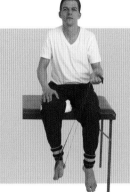 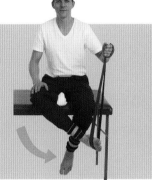

1 Fasten weights around both ankles. Place a rolled towel under the knee of the exercising leg. Sit on a bed or table with the backs of the knees at the edge and the lower legs dangling.

2 Loop the rope around the foot arch of your exercising leg. Hold the rope ends to the inside with the opposite hand. Use the other hand to stabilise the thigh of your exercising leg.

3 Rotate your lower exercising leg towards the middle of the body, leading with the foot, then pulling upwards on the rope. Pause, then lower the leg. Do the 10 reps, then swap legs.

33

Hip Internal Rotators

Active Muscles You Strengthen: Deep muscles in your buttocks that internally rotate your hips

The Basic Lift: Rotate your hips externally and rotate your thighbone internally   **Pace of Lifting:** Up slowly, pause, down slowly

Equipment: Rolled towel, ankle weights, stretch rope   **Reps:** 10 right, 10 left

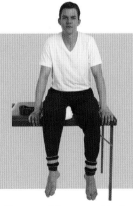 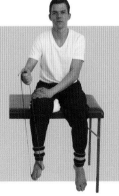 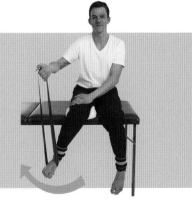

1 Fasten weights around both ankles. Place a rolled towel under the knee of the exercising leg. Sit on a bed or table with the backs of the knees at the edge and lower legs dangling.

2 Loop the rope around the foot arch of your exercising leg. Hold the rope ends to the outside using the hand on the same side. Use the other hand to stabilise the thigh of your exercising leg.

3 Rotate your lower exercising leg away from the middle of the body, leading with your foot then pulling upwards on the rope. Pause, then lower the leg. Do the 10 reps, then swap legs.

STRENGTH 2:
ACTIVE-ISOLATED STRENGTHENING
(MUSCLES BELOW THE PELVIC CORE)

You'll start this workout during the fourth week and continue through all three phases of your plan, as prescribed on pages 90 to 92. Follow the exercises in the order specified here. Detailed step-by-step illustrations appear over the following pages. For information on the names and locations of the muscle sets involved in these exercises, please see pages 274–275.

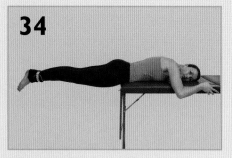

34

Sacrospinalis

Reps: 10, right and left simultaneously

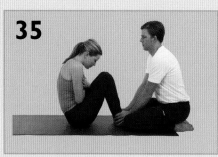

35

Upper Abdominals

Reps: 10

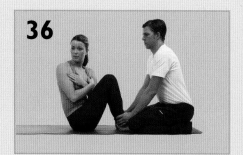

36

Oblique Abdominals

Reps: 10

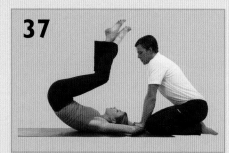

37

Lower Abdominals

Reps: 10

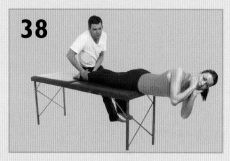

38

Trunk Extensors and Rotators

Reps: 10 of each position – straight, right, left

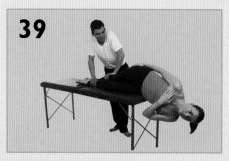

39

Trunk Lateral Flexors

Reps: 10 right, 10 left

34

Sacrospinalis

Active Muscles You Strengthen: Lower back

The Basic Lift: Extend both hips with straight legs   **Pace of Lifting:** Up slowly, pause, down slowly

Equipment: Ankle weights   **Reps:** 10, right and left simultaneously

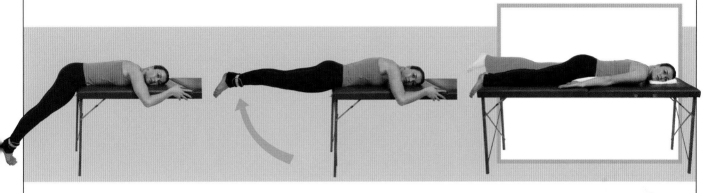

1 Attach one weight to each ankle. Bend over a bed or table with your pelvis at the edge and feet on the floor. Grip the table edge to stabilise your body. Lock your knees. Keep your feet together.

2 Leading with your heels, lift your legs towards the ceiling until you feel your gluteals engage. Pause, then slowly lower the leg. Do the 10 reps.

TIP: Beginner? Use a body-length surface, a towel under the hips and no weights. Raise the legs until the gluteals engage, pause, then lower. Work both legs together, doing 10 reps.

35

Upper Abdominals

Active Muscles You Strengthen: Muscles in your upper abdomen

The Basic Lift: Flex your trunk with bent knees   **Pace of Lifting:** Up slowly, pause, down slowly

Equipment: Furniture or a companion to hold your feet down. When you are advanced, you can hold an ankle weight in your hands against your chest to add more resistance   **Reps:** 10

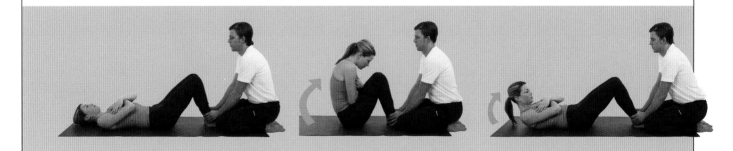

1 Lie flat. Bend the knees and tuck your feet under something to keep them down. Fold your hands across your chest and gently tuck your chin in. This will lift the back of your head up.

2 Continue this into a roll until the back is vertical and the chest is at the knees. Pause, then roll back, placing one vertebra at a time on the surface until the head is down. Do 10 reps.

TIP: Beginner? Tuck your chin in until the head lifts and the abdominals contract. Don't roll up. Keep your back flat on the surface. Pause, then roll back until your head is down. Do 10 reps.

36

Oblique Abdominals

Active Muscles You Strengthen: Muscles on the sides of your abdomen

The Basic Lift: Flex your trunk with bent knees and rotate your torso   **Pace of Lifting:** Up slowly, pause, down slowly

Equipment: Heavy furniture or a companion to hold your feet down. When you are advanced, you can hold an ankle weight in your hands against your chest to add more resistance   **Reps:** 10

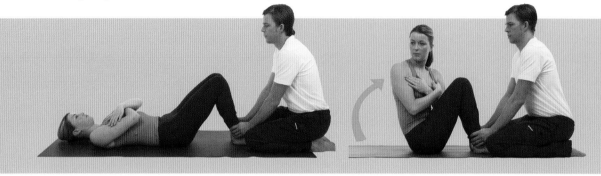

1 Lie flat on a surface. Bend your knees and tuck your feet under something that will help you keep them firmly down. Fold your hands over your chest.

2 Tuck your chin towards your chest. Rotate your torso to one side. Roll up slowly until you're upright. Use a folded towel or a mat under your bottom if you're uncomfortable.

37

Lower Abdominals

Active Muscles You Strengthen: Muscles in your lower abdomen

The Basic Lift: Curl up, leading with your pelvis   **Pace of Lifting:** Up slowly, pause, down slowly

Equipment: Heavy furniture or a companion to support your weight. When you are advanced, you can strap an ankle weight to both ankles to add more resistance   **Reps:** 10

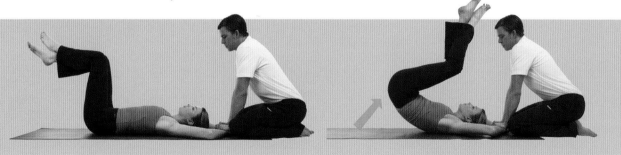

1 Lie flat on your back. Bend your knees and cross your feet at the ankles. Reach back over your head and slip your hands under something heavy that will lock you down and resist your weight as you lift. Bring your knees up until your upper legs are perpendicular to the surface with which your lower legs are parallel.

2 Pause for a second to make sure you're balanced and stable, and then thrust your lower body straight up towards the ceiling. Your buttocks will follow your knees and feet, and you'll feel the lower abdominals engage.

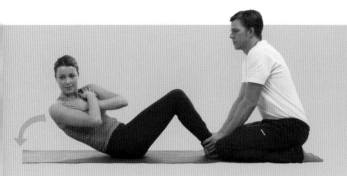 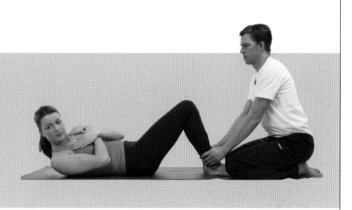

3 Pause and then, still in rotation, roll back down, placing one vertebra at a time on the surface until your is back on the floor. Pause, then rotate to the opposite side and begin an upward roll.

TIP: Beginner? Rotate your torso and lift until your head leaves the surface and your oblique abdominals engage. Don't roll up. Keep your back flat on the surface. Pause and then, keeping your torso in rotation, roll slowly back down until the side of your back is flat and your head is back down. Do the next rep on the opposite side.

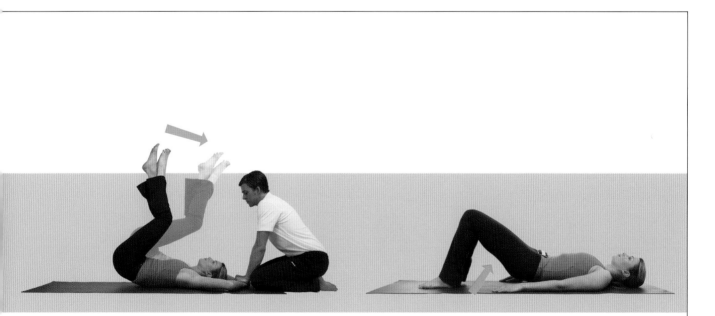

3 When you're up as far as you can go and you're up on your shoulders, roll back down ever so slightly. Pause and then return slowly to the starting position. Remember to keep your knees bent and avoid arching your back. There is no need to rest between repetitions. Use a folded towel or a mat under your bottom if you're uncomfortable.

TIP: Beginner? Lie flat on a surface, placing an ankle weight on your abdomen right below your tummy button if you want to increase resistance. Bend your knees and place your feet flat. Keep your back on the surface, contract your lower abdominals, tilt your pelvis slightly, and lift your buttocks 5–8cm (2 to 3 inches). Pause, then return to the starting position.

38

Trunk Extensors and Rotators

Active Muscles You Strengthen: All the muscles of your back

The Basic Lift: Roll your shoulder blades up towards the ceiling **Pace of Lifting:** Up slowly, pause, down slowly

Equipment: You need a helper with this one **Reps:** 10 of each position – straight, right, left

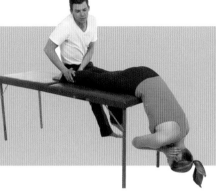 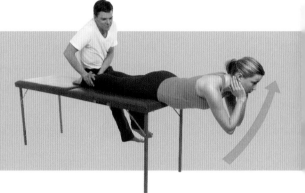

1 Lie flat on your front on a bed or a table with your legs and pelvis on the surface and your upper body over the edge. You need a helper to hold your lower legs or ankles. Place your hands on your cheeks and tuck your elbows in tight. Relax and tuck your head down.

2 Lift your upper body up from your waist until you're cantilevered straight out. Hold your position. Lift your head. Pause. Slowly lower yourself back to the starting position.

39

Trunk Lateral Flexors

Active Muscles You Strengthen: Sides of your back

The Basic Lift: Lifting your trunk up from the side **Pace of Lifting:** Up slowly, pause, down slowly

Equipment: You need a helper with this one **Reps:** 10 right, 10 left

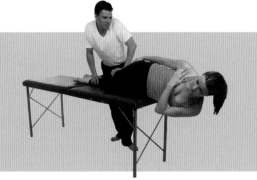

1 Lie on your side on a bed or a table. With a partner holding your lower calves and ankles, move over the edge until you are cantilevered straight off the surface from your waist. Keep your top arm and hand straight and on your side. Tuck your lower arm out of the way by holding it across your chest.

2 Bend and lower your torso, leading with your head, towards the floor. Remember to keep your body relaxed and in alignment. Go down as far as possible. You'll feel a stretch along your side.

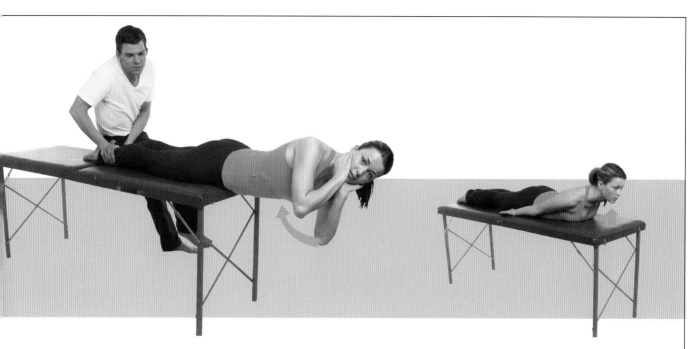

3 Rotate your upper torso to one side as far as you can and lift your upper body while still in rotation. Pause. Return to starting position slowly. Rotate to opposite side and repeat.

TIP: If your back is weak, or you don't have a partner to help you, lie flat on your stomach with your arms at your sides. Relax everything below your waist. Lift the head and chest off the surface and roll the shoulders back. Your back will be arched. Hold, then slowly lower yourself back to the starting position.

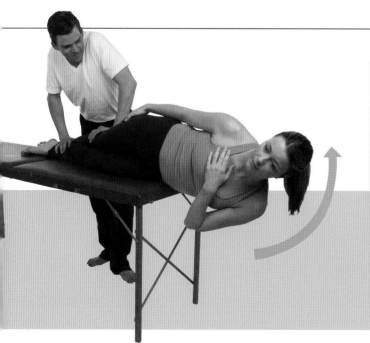

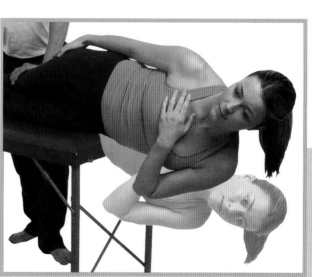

3 Slowly lift your upper torso back up until your body is back in a straight line. Lift your head up and slightly incline it towards your body at the end of the movement. Pause. Repeat by lowering your torso slowly.

TIP: Keep your body in alignment at all times and you'll really reap the benefits of this trunk-strengthening exercise.

STRENGTH 3:
ACTIVE-ISOLATED STRENGTHENING
(MUSCLES IN UPPER TRUNK AND SHOULDERS)

You'll start this workout during the fourth week and continue through all three phases of your plan, as prescribed on pages 90 to 92. Follow the exercises in the order specified here. Detailed step-by-step illustrations appear over the following pages. For information on the names and locations of the muscle sets involved in these exercises, please see pages 274–275.

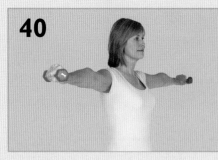

Deltoids

Reps: 10 of each of the three parts in the sequence

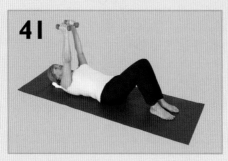

Pectoralis Majors

Reps: 10, right and left simultaneously

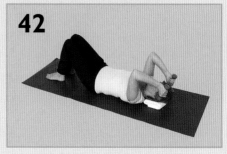

Triceps – Supine Position

Reps: 10, right and left simultaneoulsy

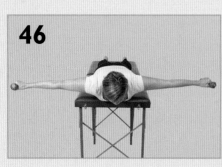

Trapezius

Reps: 10, right and left simultaneously

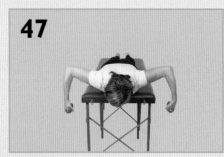

Rhomboids

Reps: 10, right and left simultaneously

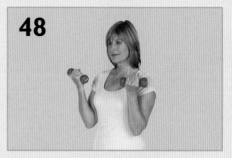

Biceps

Reps: 10, right and left simultaneously

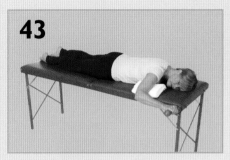

Shoulder External Rotators

Reps: 10 right, 10 left; or 10 both sides simultaneously

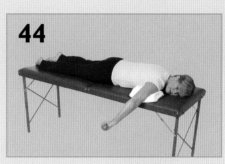

Shoulder Internal Rotators

Reps: 10 right, 10 left; or 10 both sides simultaneously

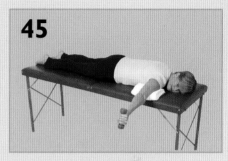

Triceps – Prone Position

Reps: 10 right, 10 left; or 10 both sides simultaneously

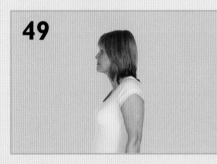

Shoulders (The Roll)

Reps: 10

40 Deltoids

Active Muscles You Strengthen: Front, back and the middle of your shoulders, your upper back and upper arms

The Basic Lift: Lifting your arms in sequence: up and forwards, up and sideways, and up and backwards **Pace of Lifting:** Up slowly, pause, down slowly **Equipment:** Handheld weights, a chair (optional) **Reps:** 10 of each of the three parts in the sequence

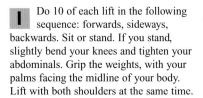

1 Do 10 of each lift in the following sequence: forwards, sideways, backwards. Sit or stand. If you stand, slightly bend your knees and tighten your abdominals. Grip the weights, with your palms facing the midline of your body. Lift with both shoulders at the same time.

2 **Shoulder front:** With your arms straight at your sides, slowly swing the weights straight up from your shoulders in arcs in front of you until they're level with your shoulders. Pause and then slowly return to the starting position. Hold your form and control the weights on the way back down.

41 Pectoralis Majors

Active Muscles You Strengthen: Front of your chest

The Basic Lift: Lifting your arms straight up from a supine position **Pace of Lifting:** Up slowly, pause, down slowly

Equipment: Rolled towel or small pillow, handheld weights or ankle weights held in your hands **Reps:** 10, right and left simultaneously

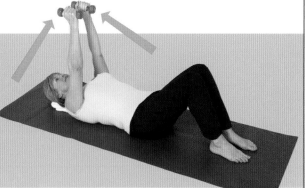

1 Lie flat on your back with your knees bent and relaxed and your feet flat. Tuck a rolled towel or small pillow under your neck and head. With weights in each hand, extend your arms straight out to your sides with your elbows locked and your palms up.

2 Lift from both sides at the same time and with equal weights. Bring your hands straight up towards the ceiling to meet above your face. Pause and then slowly return to the starting position. Hold your form and control the weights on the way back down.

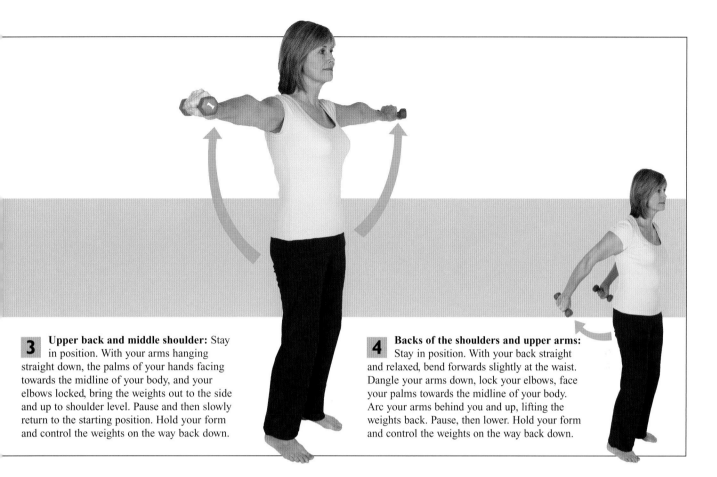

3 **Upper back and middle shoulder:** Stay in position. With your arms hanging straight down, the palms of your hands facing towards the midline of your body, and your elbows locked, bring the weights out to the side and up to shoulder level. Pause and then slowly return to the starting position. Hold your form and control the weights on the way back down.

4 **Backs of the shoulders and upper arms:** Stay in position. With your back straight and relaxed, bend forwards slightly at the waist. Dangle your arms down, lock your elbows, face your palms towards the midline of your body. Arc your arms behind you and up, lifting the weights back. Pause, then lower. Hold your form and control the weights on the way back down.

42

Triceps – Supine Position

Active Muscles You Strengthen: Muscles in the backs of your upper arms

The Basic Lift: From supine position, extending your arms from bent elbow **Pace of Lifting:** Up slowly, pause, down slowly

Equipment: Rolled towel or small pillow, handheld weights or ankle weights held in your hands **Reps:** 10, right and left simultaneously

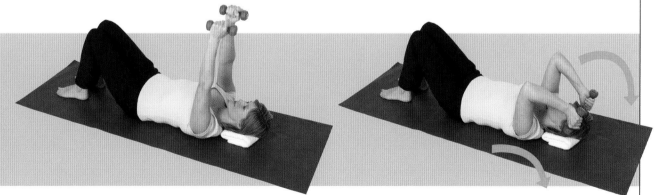

1 Lie flat on your back with knees bent, and your feet flat. Tuck a rolled towel or small pillow under your neck. Hold the weights up over your shoulders, perpendicular to the surface, with your palms facing to the midline of your body. Lock your elbows. Work both sides at the same time and with equal weights.

2 Bring the weights down by keeping your upper arms straight up and flexing your elbows until the weights are near your ears. Pause, then return to the starting position. Hold your form and control the weights on the way back up. Be careful when you are holding the weights above your face.

STRENGTH 3: MUSCLES IN UPPER TRUNK AND SHOULDERS

43

Shoulder External Rotators

Active Muscles You Strengthen: Deep shoulder or rotator cuff

The Basic Lift: Externally rotate your shoulders **Pace of Lifting:** Up slowly, pause, down slowly

Equipment: Handheld weights or ankle weights held in your hands, one or two rolled towels or small pillows **Reps:** 10 right, 10 left

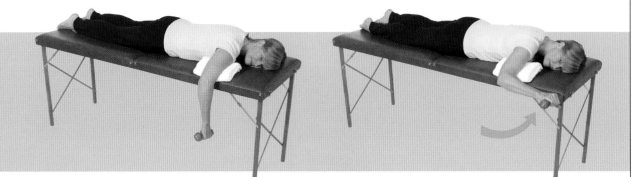

1 Lie on your front on a bed or a table. Place a rolled towel under your shoulder to take the strain off. Turn your head to one side and relax your neck. Extend your upper arm straight out from your shoulder over the edge and dangle your lower arm, hand holding a weight, towards the floor. Your elbow should be at 90 degrees with your knuckles facing forwards.

2 Rotating from the shoulder, arc the weight straight up until it's level with your head. (Be careful not to hit your face.) Pause and then slowly return to the starting position. Hold your form and control the weight on the way back down. You can work both shoulders simultaneously if the surface is narrow and your weights are equal.

44

Shoulder Internal Rotators

Active Muscles You Strengthen: Deep shoulder or rotator cuff, and sides of your chest

The Basic Lift: Internally rotate your shoulders **Pace of Lifting:** Up slowly, pause, down slowly

Equipment: Handheld weights or ankle weights held in your hands, one or two rolled towels or small pillows **Reps:** 10 right, 10 left

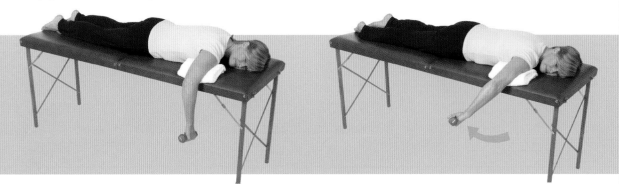

1 Lie on your front on a bed or a table. Place a rolled towel under your shoulder. Turn your head to one side and relax your neck. Extend your upper arm straight out from your shoulder over the edge and dangle your lower arm, hand holding a weight, towards the floor. Your elbow should be at 90 degrees with your knuckles facing forwards.

2 Lock your wrist and bring your hand straight back, leading with your palm. Do not use back muscles to help lift this load. Pause and then slowly return to the starting position. Hold your form and control the weight on the way back down. You can work both shoulders simultaneously if the surface is narrow and your weights are equal.

45

Triceps – Prone Position

Active Muscles You Strengthen: Muscles in the backs of your upper arms

The Basic Lift: From face down, extending your elbows **Pace of Lifting:** Up slowly, pause, down slowly

Equipment: Handheld weights or ankle weights held in your hands, one or two rolled towels or small pillows **Reps:** 10 right, 10 left

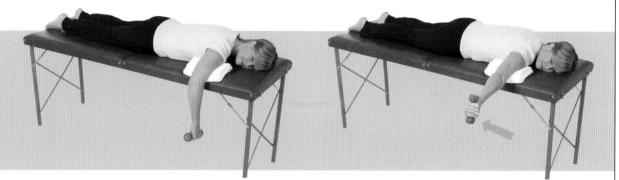

1 Lie on your front on a bed or a table. Place a rolled towel under your shoulder to take the strain off. Turn your head to one side and relax your neck. Extend your upper arm straight out from your shoulder over the edge and dangle your lower arm, hand holding a weight, towards the floor. Your elbow should be at 90 degrees with your knuckles facing forwards.

2 Lock your wrist, straighten out your elbow, and bring your hand straight out and up until your elbow is locked. Pause and then slowly return to the starting position. Hold your form and control the weight on the way back down. You can work both shoulders simultaneously if the surface is narrow and your weights are equal.

46

Trapezius

Active Muscles You Strengthen: Outer group of muscles that stabilise and control your upper back and your shoulder

The Basic Lift: From face down, lifting up and out from your shoulders **Pace of Lifting:** Up slowly, pause, down slowly

Equipment: Handheld weights or ankle weights held in your hands **Reps:** 10, right and left simultaneously

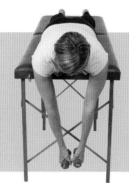

1 Lie on your front on a bed or a table, with your face and shoulders over the edge. Work both arms simultaneously with equal weights. Dangle your arms straight down from your shoulders. Keep your head and neck aligned straight with your body. Start with the weights directly below your nose. Keep your arms straight, your elbows locked and your knuckles facing out.

2 Leading with your knuckles and rotating from your shoulders, arc the weights out to your sides and up as far as you can go. Pause and then slowly return to the starting position. Hold your form and control the weights on the way back down.

47

Rhomboids

Active Muscles You Strengthen: Inner group of muscles that stabilise and control your upper back and your shoulder

The Basic Lift: From face down and with elbows bent, lifting up and out from your shoulders **Pace of Lifting:** Up slowly, pause, down slowly

Equipment: Handheld weights or ankle weights held in your hands **Reps:** 10, right and left simultaneously

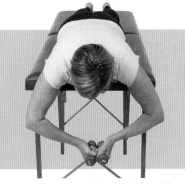 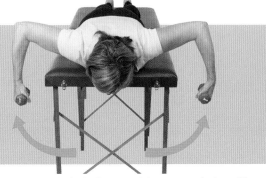

1 Lie on your front on a bed or a table, with your face and shoulders over the edge. Work both arms simultaneously with equal weights. Dangle your arms over the edge and nod your head forwards. Your knuckles should face each other, with palms face up and thumbs pointing forwards. Lock the elbows at 90-degree angles and bring the weights together until they touch.

2 Arc your locked elbows straight up towards the ceiling as far as you can go, separating the weights. Pause and then slowly return to the starting position. Hold your form and control the weights on the way back down.

48

Biceps

Active Muscles You Strengthen: Fronts of your upper arms

The Basic Lift: Flex your elbow **Pace of Lifting:** Up slowly, pause, down slowly

Equipment: Handheld weights, a chair (optional) **Reps:** 10, right and left simultaneously

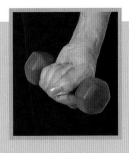 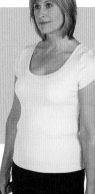 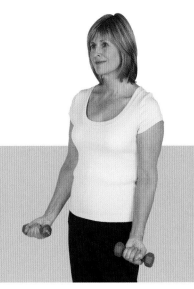

1 Stand on a flat surface with your feet apart and your knees relaxed, or sit on a chair. Start by holding the weights in your hands down at your sides with your elbows straight and your wrists locked. Your palms should face forward with your thumbs to the outside.

2 To stabilise the lift, lock yourself into position by keeping your elbows tight against your torso between your hipbones and waist.

49

Shoulders (The Roll)

Active Muscles You Strengthen: Inner group of muscles that stabilise and control your upper back and shoulder

The Basic Lift: Rotate your shoulder joint   **Pace of Lifting:** This is a continuous roll

Equipment: Handheld weights or ankle weights held in your hands   **Reps:** 10

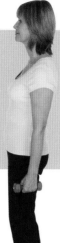

1 Stand with your back straight, feet slightly apart and knees slightly bent. Contract the abdominals. Take a weight in each hand, with palms facing in and thumbs facing forwards. Hold your arms down at your sides. Straighten your elbows.

2 Roll your shoulders forwards, then up and over, then roll backwards and lower them down. This should all happen in one continuous roll. Pause and repeat.

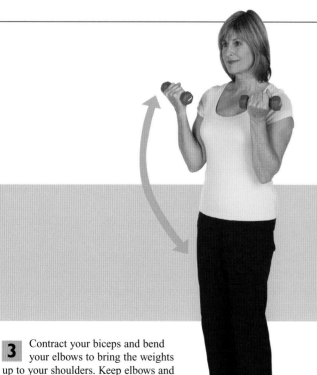

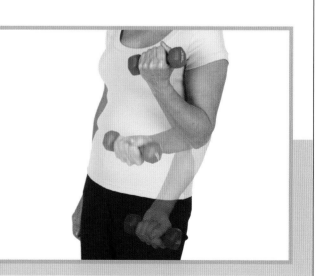

3 Contract your biceps and bend your elbows to bring the weights up to your shoulders. Keep elbows and upper arms against your body. Pause, then lower. Hold your form and control the weights on the way back down.

TIP: As you progress to lifting heavier weights, you can work both arms at once with equal weights, or one at a time.

YOUR CARDIO PROGRAMME

While there are almost endless possibilities for boosting your heart rate for a good cardio workout, we've selected the most basic: walking. Despite being so basic that it's elemental to human activity, walking is a guaranteed blood-pumping, heart-pounding, energy-lifting, muscle-building, fat-melting, joint-pampering, metabolism-raising, mood-elevating workout. Unparalleled, in fact.

Dress so that you'll be comfortable and can move easily. When the weather is cool, you might start out dressed warmly and peel the layers down. You can tie your jacket or sweatshirt around your waist when it's too warm to wear. Although you can walk barefoot – and many people do on the beach – most of us prefer shoes that are specifically

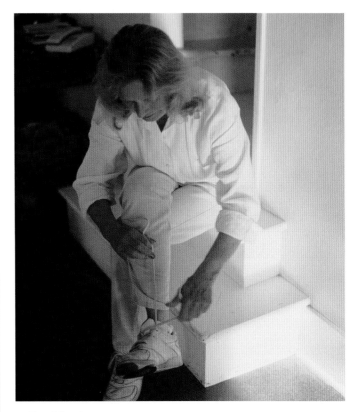

▲ Good footing
You can walk in any shoes that are comfortable, provided they offer your feet proper support.

Your Own Two Feet

When you shop for walking shoes, take along a pair of socks like the ones you intend to wear when you walk. Experts suggest that you try the shoes on at the same time of day that you intend to do your walking workout, because the size of your foot may vary as much as half a size during the course of your day.

- When you find some shoes you like, lace them all the way up, and walk around the sales floor.
- Put the shoes through their paces – slow, fast, left turn, right turn, pivot and about-face.
- Don't be swayed by what they look like; you care only about how they feel.
- Use your own judgement and buy the shoes you like, rather than simply taking the advice of a sales assistant.
- Buy snug-fitting socks that are free from raised seams and designed to wick sweat away from your foot. This will prevent blistering, skin irritations, and odour. A clean pair of socks with every workout is a must.

designed for walking. If you don't have walking shoes, you can walk in any shoe that is comfortable and provides support for your feet.

When enjoying your status as an 'advanced' Active-Isolated-method athlete, try to remember these suggestions.

Keep it simple. Walk as you normally do. Stride evenly and smoothly. Start off slowly, and gradually build to the pace at which you intend to walk. We suggest a good clip at a conversational pace, meaning that you can walk and still speak in full sentences without gasping between words. When you're experienced, you can push this pace slightly so that conversation is a little more difficult, but still not impossible. Keep your torso upright, with your shoulders relaxed and back, and your head up, so that you can get good deep breaths. Relax your hands and swing your arms rhythmically. As you speed up the pace, your arms will come up and 'pump' energy into your stride. This means you're working.

Be alert to your environment. Keep an eye on your walking surface so that you don't hit a rock or a pothole. Also, unless you're in a protected place (like an indoor track), remain alert to potential dangers such as cars that come too close, snarling guard dogs who don't like the look of you, and ill-intentioned strangers. If you walk on the pavement and are nervous about people driving up behind you, cross to the side of the approaching traffic. You'll see everyone before they see you.

Entertain yourself. If walking isn't stimulating enough for you and you enjoy listening to music or recorded books, try a non-skip CD player designed for working out. If you are listening to music, make sure it has a beat that's in sync with your pace. It's nearly impossible to clip along when you're listening to Zen chants or to keep a slow pace when you're listening to salsa. Just make sure that you're matched in rhythms.

Observe track etiquette. If you walk on a track, remember that walkers are considered to be at the bottom of the pile among athletes who use the track. Be courteous and safe, and walk in a counterclockwise direction in the far outside lane, leaving the inside lanes for the runners. If you hear someone coming up behind you yelling, 'Track!' you are being told that someone is trying to pass you, and you are being asked to get out of the way.

Drink water. Be sure to hydrate before, during and after your walk.

Leave your weights at home. Do not carry hand weights. They don't add any benefit to walking and, in fact, may even be harmful during the unpredictable ups and downs of a cardio workout.

Bring a pal. Take your dog. Invite friends and family. Turn these brief moments of invigorating exercise into a mobile social club. Walking is wonderful fun to share.

▶ **The more the merrier**
Walking need not be a solitary activity. Take the family pet or invite friends to come along – conversation will help you to find a good pace and breathing rhythm.

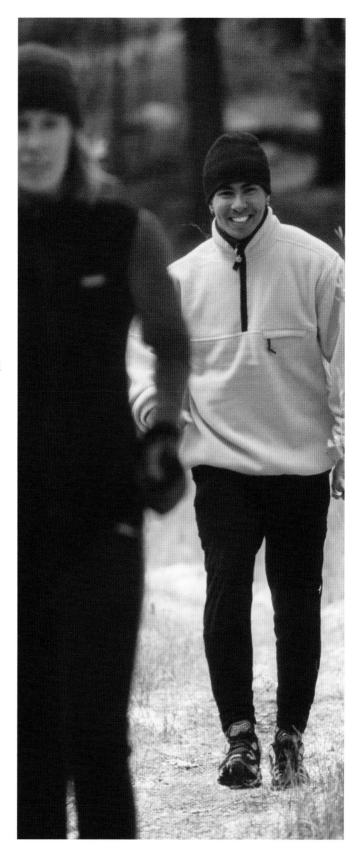

Your Complete Programme

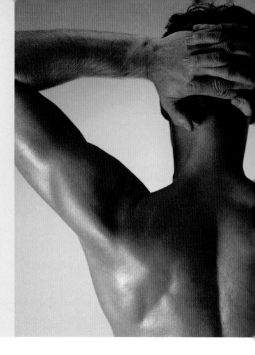

You now have your complete programme. We've assembled an at-a-glance chart so that you can see your workouts for each phase of our plan. Phase 1, the beginning six weeks, emphasises Active-Isolated Stretching (see pages 48 and 58 for details of each workout). Phase 2, the intermediate six weeks, increases the number of Active-Isolated Strengthening workouts (see pages 67, 74 and 87 for details of each workout). Phase 3, the advanced six weeks, completes the programme by adding cardio for total-body conditioning (see pages 88–89). There you have it – flexibility, strength and cardiovascular endurance – your complete fitness programme for a healthy back.

Phase 1: Beginning 6 Weeks

Week 1	SUNDAY	MONDAY	TUESDAY	WEDNESDAY	THURSDAY	FRIDAY	SATURDAY
	Rest	Stretch 1 & 2	Stretch 1 & 2	Stretch 1 & 2	Stretch 1 & 2	Stretch 1 & 2	Stretch 1 & 2

Week 2	SUNDAY	MONDAY	TUESDAY	WEDNESDAY	THURSDAY	FRIDAY	SATURDAY
	Rest	Stretch 1 & 2	Stretch 1 & 2	Stretch 1 & 2	Stretch 1 & 2	Stretch 1 & 2	Stretch 1 & 2

Week 3	SUNDAY	MONDAY	TUESDAY	WEDNESDAY	THURSDAY	FRIDAY	SATURDAY
	Rest	Stretch 1 & 2	Stretch 1 & 2	Stretch 1 & 2	Stretch 1 & 2	Stretch 1 & 2	Stretch 1 & 2

Week 4	SUNDAY	MONDAY	TUESDAY	WEDNESDAY	THURSDAY	FRIDAY	SATURDAY
	Rest	Stretch 1	Stretch 1	Stretch 1	Stretch 1	Stretch 1	Stretch 1
	Rest	Strength 1	Strength 2	Strength 3	Strength 1	Strength 2	Strength 3

Week 5	SUNDAY	MONDAY	TUESDAY	WEDNESDAY	THURSDAY	FRIDAY	SATURDAY
	Rest	Stretch 1	Stretch 1	Stretch 1	Stretch 1	Stretch 1	Stretch 1
	Rest	Strength 1	Strength 2	Strength 3	Strength 1	Strength 2	Strength 3

Week 6	SUNDAY	MONDAY	TUESDAY	WEDNESDAY	THURSDAY	FRIDAY	SATURDAY
	Rest	Stretch 1	Stretch 1	Stretch 1	Stretch 1	Stretch 1	Stretch 1
	Rest	Strength 1	Strength 2	Strength 3	Strength 1	Strength 2	Strength 3

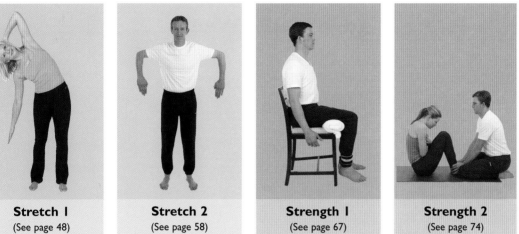

Stretch 1	**Stretch 2**	**Strength 1**	**Strength 2**	**Strength 3**
(See page 48)	(See page 58)	(See page 67)	(See page 74)	(See page 80)

Phase 2: Intermediate 6 Weeks

	SUNDAY	MONDAY	TUESDAY	WEDNESDAY	THURSDAY	FRIDAY	SATURDAY
Week 7	Rest	Stretch 1	Stretch 1	Stretch 1	Stretch 1	Stretch 1	Stretch 1
	Rest	Strength 1	Strength 2	Strength 3	Strength 1	Strength 2	Strength 3

	SUNDAY	MONDAY	TUESDAY	WEDNESDAY	THURSDAY	FRIDAY	SATURDAY
Week 8	Rest	Stretch 1	Stretch 1	Stretch 1	Stretch 1	Stretch 1	Stretch 1
	Rest	Strength 1	Strength 2	Strength 3	Strength 1	Strength 2	Strength 3

	SUNDAY	MONDAY	TUESDAY	WEDNESDAY	THURSDAY	FRIDAY	SATURDAY
Week 9	Rest	Stretch 1	Stretch 1	Stretch 1	Stretch 1	Stretch 1	Stretch 1
	Rest	Strength 1	Strength 2	Strength 3	Strength 1	Strength 2	Strength 3

	SUNDAY	MONDAY	TUESDAY	WEDNESDAY	THURSDAY	FRIDAY	SATURDAY
Week 10	Rest	Stretch 1	Stretch 1 & 2	Stretch 1	Stretch 1 & 2	Stretch 1	Stretch 1
	Rest	Strength 1	(no strengthening)	Strength 2	(no strengthening)	Strength 3	(no strengthening)

	SUNDAY	MONDAY	TUESDAY	WEDNESDAY	THURSDAY	FRIDAY	SATURDAY
Week 11	Rest	Stretch 1	Stretch 1	Stretch 1	Stretch 1	Stretch 1	Stretch 1
	Rest	Strength 1	Strength 2	Strength 3	Strength 1	Strength 2	Strength 3

	SUNDAY	MONDAY	TUESDAY	WEDNESDAY	THURSDAY	FRIDAY	SATURDAY
Week 12	Rest	Stretch 1	Stretch 1	Stretch 1	Stretch 1	Stretch 1	Stretch 1
	Rest	Strength 1	Strength 2	Strength 3	Strength 1	Strength 2	Strength 3

Phase 3: Advanced 6 Weeks

Week 13	SUNDAY	MONDAY	TUESDAY	WEDNESDAY	THURSDAY	FRIDAY	SATURDAY
	Rest	Stretch 1	Stretch 1 & 2	Stretch 1	Stretch 1 & 2	Stretch 1	Stretch 1 & 2
	Rest	Strength 1	Strength 2	Strength 3	Strength 1	Strength 2	Strength 3
	Rest	Cardio (20 minutes)		Cardio (20 minutes)		Cardio (20 minutes)	

Week 14	SUNDAY	MONDAY	TUESDAY	WEDNESDAY	THURSDAY	FRIDAY	SATURDAY
	Rest	Stretch 1	Stretch 1 & 2	Stretch 1	Stretch 1 & 2	Stretch 1	Stretch 1
	Rest	Strength 1	Strength 2	Strength 3	Strength 1	Strength 2	Strength 3
	Rest	Cardio (25 minutes)		Cardio (25 minutes)		Cardio (25 minutes)	

Week 15	SUNDAY	MONDAY	TUESDAY	WEDNESDAY	THURSDAY	FRIDAY	SATURDAY
	Rest	Stretch 1	Stretch 1 & 2	Stretch 1	Stretch 1 & 2	Stretch 1	Stretch 1
	Rest	Strength 1	Strength 2	Strength 3	Strength 1	Strength 2	Strength 3
	Rest	Cardio (30 minutes)		Cardio (30 minutes)		Cardio (30 minutes)	

Week 16	SUNDAY	MONDAY	TUESDAY	WEDNESDAY	THURSDAY	FRIDAY	SATURDAY
	Rest	Stretch 1	Stretch 1 & 2	Stretch 1	Stretch 1 & 2	Stretch 1	Stretch 1
	Rest	Strength 1		Strength 2		Strength 3	
	Rest		Cardio (30 minutes)		Cardio (30 minutes)		Cardio (20 minutes)

Week 17	SUNDAY	MONDAY	TUESDAY	WEDNESDAY	THURSDAY	FRIDAY	SATURDAY
	Rest	Stretch 1	Stretch 1 & 2	Stretch 1	Stretch 1 & 2	Stretch 1	Stretch 1 & 2
	Rest	Strength 1	Strength 2	Strength 3	Strength 1	Strength 2	Strength 3
	Rest	Cardio (30 minutes)		Cardio (30 minutes)		Cardio (30 minutes)	

Week 18	SUNDAY	MONDAY	TUESDAY	WEDNESDAY	THURSDAY	FRIDAY	SATURDAY
	Rest	Stretch 1	Stretch 1 & 2	Stretch 1	Stretch 1 & 2	Stretch 1	Stretch 1 & 2
	Rest	Strength 1	Strength 2	Strength 3	Strength 1	Strength 2	Strength 3
	Rest	Cardio (30 minutes)		Cardio (30 minutes)		Cardio (30 minutes)	

Training Log

(PHOTOCOPY FOR YOUR USE)

Date	
Week	

Notes	

	Sunday	Monday	Tuesday	Wednesday	Thursday	Friday	Saturday
Stretch 1							
Stretch 2							

	Sunday		Monday		Tuesday		Wednesday		Thursday		Friday		Saturday	
		weight used		weight used		weight used		weight used		weight used		weight used		weight used
Strength 1														
Strength 2														
Strength 3														

	Sunday	Monday	Tuesday	Wednesday	Thursday	Friday	Saturday
Cardio Training							
Time Walked							
Route and Remarks							

	Sunday	Monday	Tuesday	Wednesday	Thursday	Friday	Saturday
Water Drunk	Litres	Litres	Litres	Litres	Litres	Litres	Litres

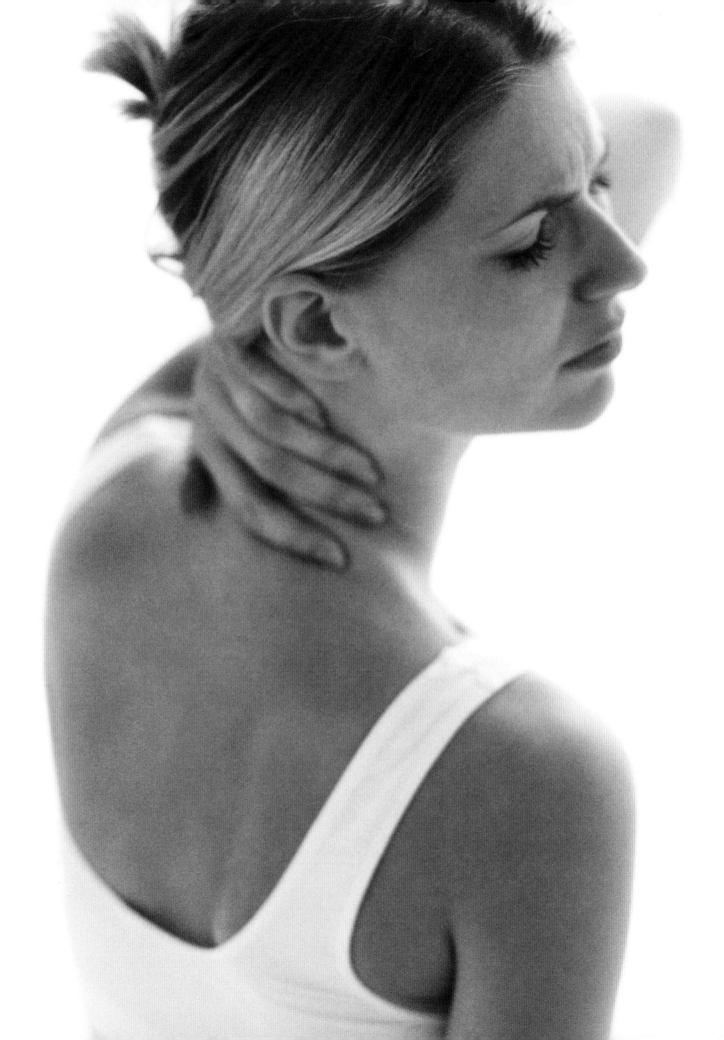

3

STOPPING THE PAIN

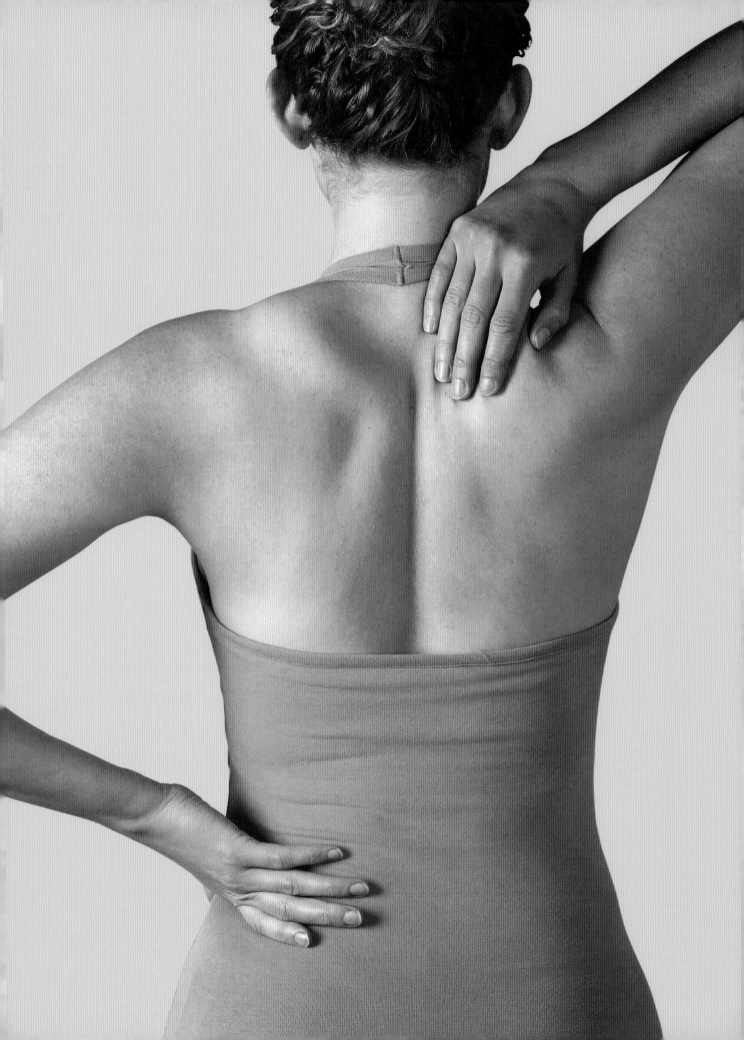

CHAPTER 5

NAMING – AND TAMING – YOUR MOST COMMON ACHES

Pain is Mother Nature's clear signal that your body *is being damaged. In fact, your brain is programmed to instantaneously react to wrench you away from pain stimulus. In rehabilitation, pain is used as a diagnostic tool for pinpointing injury, getting an initial measure of its severity, and following up with subsequent readings on the progress of healing to see how things are going. Pain can be a very good and necessary thing.*

About two-thirds of us will experience lower-back pain within our lifetimes. A recent survey conducted by market researchers NOP revealed that 30 per cent of people in the UK suffer regularly from back pain, and that conditions such as arthritis and osteoarthritis cost the economy 700 million working days a year.

Doctors know, as we do, that most back problems can be mitigated or prevented altogether if people are lean, fit, flexible and healthy. Acute pain is a warning, an attention-getting mechanism that the mind and body use to sound the alarm that something is terribly wrong. The person in pain responds by jerking away from the source of the pain and doing something about it, such as yelling for help or running the injury under cold water. The medical response to acute pain is to quickly relieve it. From both the patient's point of view and the doctor's point of view, acute pain is actually useful.

But when pain is chronic – continuing for more than three months – it outlives its usefulness. There's no need for nerves to sound an alarm to the brain to alert it to an injury that can't be healed or pain that can't be relieved by immediate response.

Chronic pain can set off a cascade of problems like depression, sleep disturbance and anxiety. If chronic pain disrupts a person's ability to function, feelings of hopelessness can set in. Even with professional help, it's not easy to live with pain, because it grabs all the attention.

Pain management centres do everything medically possible to relieve pain and depression, redirecting attention, reframing the problem and rehabilitating the patient so that as much function as possible is restored. Counselling and fitness training are key components in the programme. Let's look at some suggestions for what you can do when you've just begun to experience back pain.

Check your life for stress. Pain can be very real, but there could be reasons for it that are not physical. Stress and tension head straight for the back. We seldom see back spasms in happy, relaxed people. Check for things that are bothering you or causing you anxiety. If you can 'fix' some of these, you might discover that your pain will decrease or disappear altogether. Get a little more aerobic exercise, during which the body is likely to release endorphins – hormones that are nature's tranquillisers and painkillers. Your sense of well-being will be enhanced, and you'll work off any pent-up tension.

Consult your doctor to ensure that pain does not equal damage. No matter what the diagnosis or treatment, a person must not leave a doctor's office until absolutely clear about which activities are allowed or advisable. When activity will cause more harm, lay off. If the activity will cause pain but no additional damage, the doctor will allow the patient to 'push through' the pain.

Include stretching and light lifting in your workout. A fit, healthy, flexible, strong person doesn't suffer from frequent back pain. The programme in this book is guaranteed to put you in that category.

If you're depressed or anxious, get medical treatment. Depression and anxiety are both a cause and an effect of back problems. It's not unusual for a back patient to walk out of a doctor's office with prescriptions for depression and anxiety as well as pain.

One of the best ways to cure a bad back is to lose weight by adjusting your diet and revving up your metabolism with exercise. Every extra pound of fat fatigues and strains the back, which is why doctors often refer patients to a dietitian, who can develop a suitable diet plan.

Get enough rest. We work hard, we get exhausted, we rest for a day and come back stronger. With a back injury, however, it's nearly impossible to have a hard day followed by an easy day. Every day is hard, so nothing ever regenerates and recovers fully to come back stronger. You must give your back the opportunity for that necessary time to repair.

Pace yourself. Sometimes people just overdo it. They're having fun and get carried away. When this happens, they pay the price. Often it's a back spasm. There's nothing wrong in pushing your own physical limits, but be sensible about it.

Muscles get stronger by working hard to the point of breaking down, then recovering through rest. During the period of rest and inactivity, the muscle fibres reorganise, regenerate and get stronger. When the muscles are tested again, they can take a heavier load. When stressed harder, they break down again. In recovery, they come back even stronger.

TAMING BACK SPASMS ON YOUR OWN

Most of the time, back pain is merely muscle spasm in response to an injury or an inflammation. A spasm is the involuntary contraction of a muscle (like a clenched fist that you can't open) and is nature's way of immobilising muscles to serve as a sort of 'splint' around an injury. If a spasm occurs in your back, it's doing its job: to freeze your spine and protect you from further injury.

The reasons that spasms occur are as varied as the injuries. Some are caused by overuse (like swinging a golf club all day when you're out of condition), an imbalance or a single traumatic incident (like falling, or suddenly changing direction). You can also suffer a spasm if muscles are fatigued from poor posture or from holding a position too long (like typing all day). Spasms can be generated from injury or inflammation of the vertebrae, muscles, ligaments, tendons or the discs between the vertebrae.

Spasms can be severe when they're in neutral position and intense when they're strained by movement. Although they usually clamp down, spasms can fool you by letting go. You think you're better, but, when you move, they grab you again.

Don't suffer endlessly: the 'I Can Take It' syndrome is bizarre. What's the matter with us? We shouldn't view pain as a chance to prove how tough we are.

When your back is in pain or in spasm, the whole body tenses, causing imbalances that torture other muscles recruited to help you move. Blood flow is impeded. Metabolic waste isn't properly flushed. The area becomes irritated. Your adrenaline rises, your heart rate increases, your breathing becomes rapid, and you become exhausted.

In our clinic, we use the following 10 steps to help alleviate a patient's pain and get the back moving once again.

1. Take over-the-counter pain medication. Aspirin and non-steroidal anti-inflammatory drugs (NSAIDs) such as ibuprofen might be your first line of defence when your back is hurting. Taken properly, these can help to reduce pain and inflammation in the muscles that support your spine and the soft tissues that surround it, such as tendons and ligaments, by blocking the production of prostaglandins

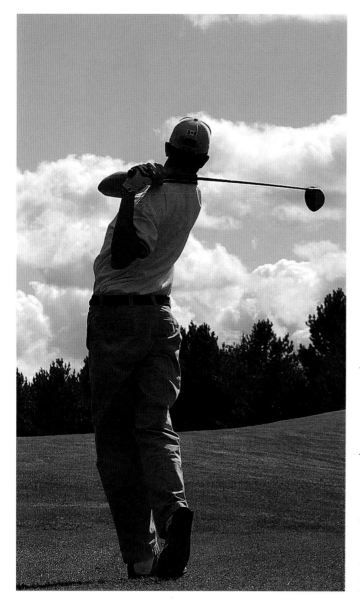

▲ Driving pain
Back spasms have a host of different causes but overuse is a common one — as seen in the occasional golfer who spends all weekend swinging a golf club.

(chemicals that cause inflammation and trigger transmission of the pain signal to the brain).

When you are in pain, you tense up to protect the injury from further harm. Protection takes enormous energy and causes imbalances and tension everywhere. Relieving the pain, even temporarily, can allow you to move or flex the injured muscle just a little, because you have less need to protect yourself. You'll increase your range of motion and pump blood to the injury to promote healing and restore function. You'll also be more relaxed, sleep better and allow your body to rejuvenate more quickly.

A few little words of caution: pain is your body's way of communicating clear messages to you about the status of an injury. Don't use painkillers to mask pain that you need to be evaluating and using for information. And if you have had to take painkillers for a long period of time in order to be comfortable, there's something wrong and you need to take a different approach to deal with the pain.

NSAIDs have possible side-effects of which you need to be aware: nausea, indigestion, diarrhoea and peptic ulcers. Aspirin could impede your blood's ability to clot and cause prolonged bleeding, colitis, gastrointestinal disorders, ringing in the ears and aggravation of asthma, hives and gout. Be careful.

2. Breathe and relax. Panic and tension can amplify pain to an astonishing extent. Stop making any voluntary sound that expresses pain. Relax your face completely and get rid of the grimace. Unclench your hands. Shake out your arms. Tell yourself that you can get this pain under control. Breathe deeply with your hand over your upper abdomen, just below your breastbone at your diaphragm. Exhale deeply so that your abdomen moves your hand in to the count of four. Push it out as you inhale to the count of four. Take 10 deep breaths. Relax your jaw by opening your mouth widely a couple of times to take the tension out of the joint, signalling your body to relax. This process, called 'managing your state', will quieten the panic response that can aggravate pain.

3. Do a pain inventory. Move just a little by leaning forward a few centimetres, then back. Bend to the left side, to the right, then rotate from the waist just a little. What you feel will help you determine a course of action. If the pain is severe or if you experience any unusual symptoms other than pain, such as numbness or loss of function, stop immediately. You need professional attention. If you have full function and the pain is not severe, then proceed to step 4.

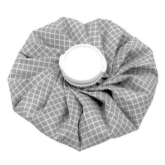

4. Get out the ice. We know how wonderful it feels to sink an aching back into a hot bath, but, in fact, that's the limit of the benefit. External heat can certainly be comforting and relaxing, but when you're trying to throw the brakes on a back spasm and facilitate muscle and tissue recovery, you are going to need a little more assistance.

Cold reduces swelling and initially restricts blood flow, providing a natural compress on the microscopic tears in the tissue that are leaking blood into the traumatised area and causing the spasm. Shortly, the body will recruit new blood to the cold area (notice how the skin always turns a little red?), which will help to flush out metabolic wastes created by damaged cells.

If you have a localised 'sore spot', you can treat it with a home-made ice pack. Fill a paper cup with water and keep it in the freezer. Peel down the rim to expose the surface of the ice. The paper cup will help to keep your fingers warm and dry. Gently rub or swirl the ice surface on your injured or traumatised body part. Keep it moving and apply as much pressure as you can stand. In the first minute, it will feel uncomfortable, but this will ease. Treat yourself for between 5 and 10 minutes. Keep watch on your skin to make certain that it doesn't turn white, signalling frostbite.

If the area you are treating is a little larger and harder to reach, a bag of frozen peas acts as a wonderfully pliable ice pack that can be refrozen frequently and reused for a long time. Lie down on top of it. Or press it between your back and the wall to hold it in place. If the cold is uncomfortable, wrap yourself in a blanket.

For a full-scale treatment (such as for post-marathon backache) you can fill a bathtub with cold water and add five to ten 2kg bags of ice. Grit your teeth and sink into it for up to 10 minutes – the initial shock will soon wear off. *Please note:* This is not suitable for people with heart conditions or high blood pressure.

Do not rely on topical creams and ointments. They feel warm and tingly, but they are not going to help a back spasm. The only exception might be a cream that contains capsaicin, the chemical 'heat' extracted from hot peppers.

5. Stretch. Once you have calmed the inflammation and pain with ice, it's time to move, if only a little.

Remember the principles of the Active-Isolated Stretching programme? When your back hurts, you want to relax it,

which means you'll be firing muscles in your chest and abdomen to allow your back to let go. Go to the section of the workout programme that outlines back stretches (pages 48 to 65), grab your stretch rope or strap and get to work.

Ideally, you'd be able to do the full stretch routine because it unlocks joints and relaxes muscles in a sequence that would really help your spasm. But we're realistic. If you're desperate, go for the back stretches.

Now more than ever, it's important to stretch correctly, allowing the muscles in the front of your body to do all the work, while the muscles in your back enjoy gentle stretching. At first you might be able to move only a few centimetres or so, but as the back relaxes, you'll see some progress. Do only a few repetitions in small, deliberate, careful movements and remember to breathe. If the stretches cause acute pain or any other new symptom, stop immediately and see your doctor.

6. Ice again. When you've stretched your back for a few minutes, return to icing for 5 to 10 minutes.

7. Stretch again. Return to the back stretches and see if you can get a little further on each stretch or do a few more repeats. You may be pleasantly surprised at your progress.

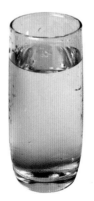

8. Drink plenty of water. Although you might be tempted to anaesthetise yourself with a six-pack of beer, alcohol will only dehydrate you. Instead, consume at least a litre of water within the next four hours. Without adequate hydration, your body can't heal properly.

9. Have a light meal. Injury takes a tremendous amount of energy. If you're in pain, you're burning extra calories, even when you're standing still. You need fuel, but just a little. If you put too much food into your stomach, your body will divert blood away from your muscles and into all matters digestive. The idea is to keep your blood flowing easily, so it can bring in healing oxygen and take away all the metabolic waste that has accumulated from those injured and exhausted cells.

10. Get a good night's sleep. When your back is injured, you become mentally, physically and emotionally exhausted by the effort to get out of pain. You need, and deserve, lots of rest.

You need rest, but your back also needs a break. Lie on your back; physiologists confirm that the forces on your spine are at a minimum when you're lying flat. A small pillow is all right to use if it feels okay. If you turn over onto your side, the forces on your body are nearly doubled. Definitely avoid sleeping while sitting in a chair. The forces are then nearly four times as great as when you're lying down flat.

Not only does sleep's relaxation of body and mind assist healing, a good night's rest will help you emotionally. Pain-management experts tell us that sleep deprivation or disruption is almost worse than the injury – it can unravel even the strongest person.

When you awaken, get up slowly. Roll over on your side, swing your legs over the side of the bed, and use your arms to push your torso vertically until you are seated. Do a quick inventory. If you feel all right, put your feet on the floor shoulder-width apart and lean forwards very slightly. Keep your back straight and stand. Repeat the routines of aspirin or NSAIDs, ice and stretch. If things aren't better, consider seeing your doctor.

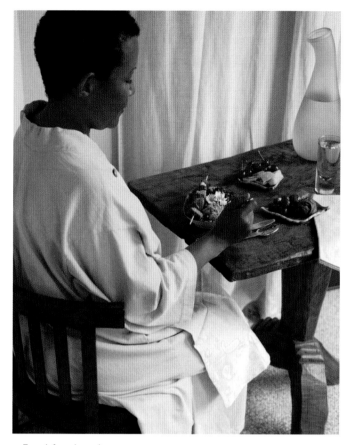

▲ Food for thought
When the body is in pain it burns more calories – even when still. A light meal will help to refuel the body without diverting healing blood and oxygen from an injured back.

What Next?

How long your back spasm lasts depends on the severity of your injury and how successful your intervention has been. A mild injury can be gone in a day, but sometimes progress can take longer to manifest itself – you could be sore for a couple of weeks.

Don't let that stop you from working out. You can, and should, continue to stretch, even from the moment of the onset of pain. Do make sure, however, that you avoid lifting and heavy work; sports are also inadvisable until you are completely symptom-free.

A Crick in the Neck

We have yet to understand the exact pathology of a crick, nor can we positively identify the muscles, tendons and ligaments involved. Next to the common cold, the crick might just be the most common malady to affect humans. The good news is that it's easy to fix.

You know the scenario: during the day, your back becomes fatigued from overuse or sitting in one position for too long. By the end of the day, the muscles in your back have tightened up so that you start to feel stiff or sore. No big deal in itself, as you are looking forward to sleep. But you are tired, so when you climb into bed, you sleep so soundly that, instead of redistributing weight and pressure on your body all through the night as you usually do, you don't change positions at all.

If you weren't contorted with your neck at an odd angle, held there by the weight of your head all night, this might not be a problem – but unfortunately, this time, it is not the case. You awaken with a painful crick and you are unable to move your neck. (We see this commonly among people who sleep sitting up on aeroplanes and trains, or in the passenger seats of cars.)

Actually the crick is a simple but painful spasm of neck muscles, easily stretched out into relaxation. All you need is some blood flow. Let's get started.

I

Semi-circumduction of the Neck

Active Muscles You Contract: None (This is a warm-up to increase the circulation of the neck.)

Isolated Muscles You Stretch: None (This is a warm-up to increase the circulation of the neck.)

Hold Each Stretch: This is just a relaxed roll **Reps:** Back and forth 10 times

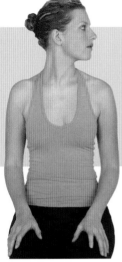

I Sit on the edge of a bed with hands on your thighs. Face forwards, then turn your head to the side until facing over one shoulder.

2 Relax the neck and let your head roll towards the midline of the body until the chin is against your chest. Continue the roll until your head is facing over the opposite shoulder. Allow your head to fall forwards again and roll back the other way.

2

Neck Extensors

Active Muscles You Contract: Muscles in the front of your neck

Isolated Muscles You Stretch: Muscles in the back of your neck and the top of your back

Hold Each Stretch: 2 seconds **Reps:** 10

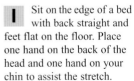

I Sit on the edge of a bed with back straight and feet flat on the floor. Place one hand on the back of the head and one hand on your chin to assist the stretch.

2 Tuck in your chin and roll your head forwards until your chin meets your chest. You can gently assist the end of the movement with your hand at the back of your head. Keep your shoulders down.

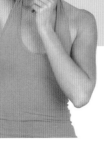

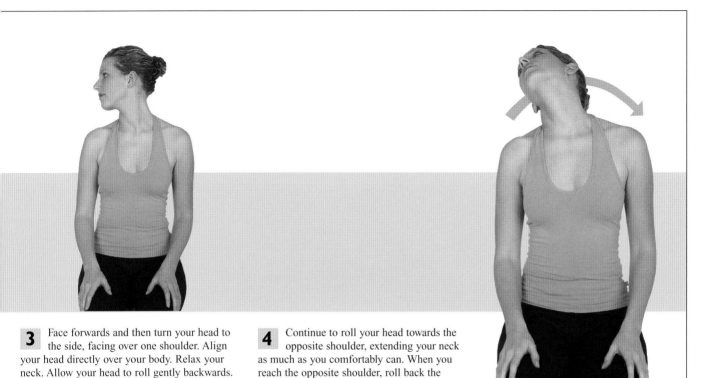

3 Face forwards and then turn your head to the side, facing over one shoulder. Align your head directly over your body. Relax your neck. Allow your head to roll gently backwards.

4 Continue to roll your head towards the opposite shoulder, extending your neck as much as you comfortably can. When you reach the opposite shoulder, roll back the other way. Do this a few times, gently.

3

Neck Flexors

Active Muscles You Contract: Muscles in the back of your neck and the top of your back between your shoulders

Isolated Muscles You Stretch: Muscles in the front of your neck

Hold Each Stretch: 2 seconds **Reps:** 10

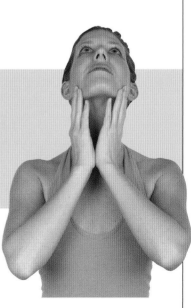

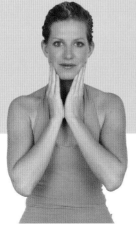

1 Sit on a bed with your back straight and feet flat on the floor. Align your head over your body. Place your fingertips along your jawline just under your chin.

2 Roll your head backwards very gently. You can assist the end of the movement with your fingertips. Keep your shoulders down.

4

Neck Lateral Flexors

Active Muscles You Contract: Muscles in the side of your neck

Isolated Muscles You Stretch: Muscles in the opposite side of your neck

Hold Each Stretch: 2 seconds **Reps:** 10 right, 10 left

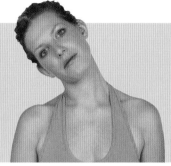

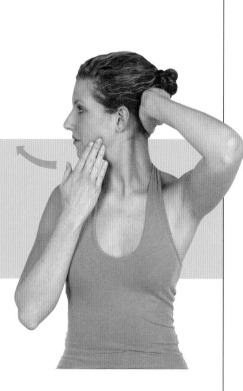

1 Sit on the edge of a bed with your back straight and your feet flat on the floor. Look straight ahead. Cock your head to one side, lowering your ear straight down towards your shoulder.

2 Reach up over the top of your head with the hand that is on the same side as the shoulder, gently place your fingertips on your temple, as shown, and press very gently down to assist the end of the movement. Keep your shoulders down and keep your body still.

5

Neck Rotators

Active Muscles You Contract: Muscles on the opposite side of your neck

Isolated Muscles You Stretch: Muscles in the side of your neck

Hold Each Stretch: 2 seconds **Reps:** 10 right, 10 left

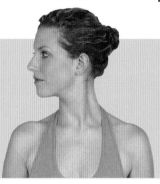

1 Sit on the edge of a bed with your back straight and your feet flat on the floor. Look straight ahead. Turn your head to the right, until your chin is over your shoulder.

2 Place your left hand behind your head at the base of the skull. Take your right hand and place your fingertips along your left jawline, and press very gently to guide. Be certain to keep your shoulders down and your body still.

6

Neck Oblique Extensors

Active Muscles You Contract: Muscles in the front of your neck

Isolated Muscles You Stretch: Muscles in your upper shoulders to the side of the base of your neck

Hold Each Stretch: 2 seconds **Reps:** 10 right, 10 left

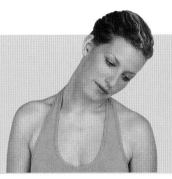

1 Sit on the edge of a bed with your back straight and your feet flat on the floor. Turn your head left to a 45-degree angle. Maintaining the angle, drop your head forwards with your ear towards your chest.

2 Place your left hand on top of your head, as shown, and gently press down to assist the end of the movement. Be certain to keep your shoulders down and your body still.

7

Neck Oblique Flexors

Active Muscles You Contract: Muscles in the base of your neck and upper back

Isolated Muscles You Stretch: Muscles in your neck and upper chest

Hold Each Stretch: 2 seconds **Reps:** 10 right, 10 left

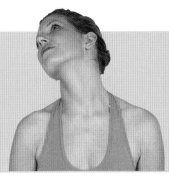

1 Sit on the edge of a bed with your back straight and your feet flat on the floor. Turn your head right to a 45-degree angle. Still at the angle, drop your head backwards with your ear over your shoulder.

2 Place your right hand on your forehead, as shown, and gently press back to assist the end of the movement. Be certain to keep your shoulders down and your body still.

WHAT YOUR DOCTOR CAN DO FOR PAIN

In the 18th century, Voltaire said, 'The purpose of a doctor is to entertain the patient until the disease takes its course.' Doctors today still sometimes 'entertain' and wait, because about 85 per cent of patients who suffer from lower-back pain can't be precisely diagnosed. The source of the pain remains vague until it eventually goes away. Some studies indicate that time heals as often as intervention. Unless something is horribly wrong, you'll probably be all right, in time.

That doesn't mean you should avoid the doctor and tough it out. In fact, we always advise that when in doubt, seek help as quickly as possible. (See chapter 6 for advice on doctors.) Even if your doctor can't 'fix' the injury, much can be done to keep you comfortable and out of pain. Let's look at the different ways your doctor can help you manage the pain.

Prescription Medicines

Although over-the-counter medications can certainly do a lot to ease the pain of an aching back, they also have limitations. Your doctor can widen the selection of medications with prescription drugs.

Non-steroidal anti-inflammatory drugs. NSAIDs work to reduce inflammation and are often compared in results to aspirin. The difference is that NSAIDs have fewer side-effects. They are most effective when taken continuously rather than taken only when the patient experiences pain. Many of these are available over the counter, but if you would like to try a new class of NSAIDs called COX-2 inhibitors, your doctor will have to prescribe them. Sold under the names rofecoxib (Vioxx) and celecoxib, these medications selectively inhibit the chemical reaction that causes inflammation, but do a better job of protecting the stomach lining from ulcers.

Neuroleptic medications. These medications, such as gabapentin, help to stop or inhibit seizures. They're also sometimes prescribed for patients with nerve pain or

▼ Getting a prescription from your doctor
If you are suffering from a painful back injury or condition, don't be afraid to ask your doctor to prescribe medication to help reduce the pain. Your doctor may also suggest a course of ultrasound or electric stimulation.

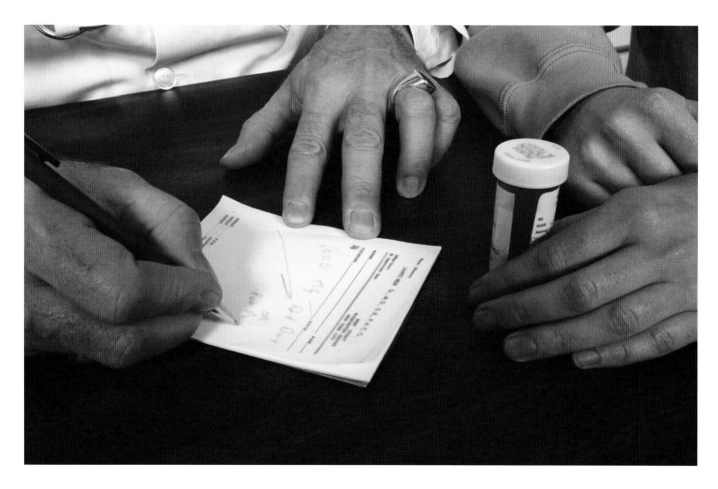

degeneration. They are most often used when treating post-surgical leg pain, but they also may be used for back pain. They are not addictive and can be taken over a long period of time.

Antidepressants. Back pain can be both a cause and an effect of depression. Recognising this, doctors often prescribe both a pain medication and an antidepressant at the same time. Antidepressants that elevate mood and reduce anxiety, called tricyclics, are prescribed in low doses as sedatives to help a patient sleep, and, although no one is quite sure why, they also diminish pain. They are not addictive. Examples are amitriptyline (Elavil), nortriptyline, and imipramine (Tofranil). Other drugs used to treat depression are selective serotonin reuptake inhibitors, or SSRIs. Serotonin is a neurotransmitter in the brain that governs a person's mood. Enhancing levels seems to make a mood better. Probably the most well-known of these is fluoxetine (Prozac).

Non-narcotic medications. These drugs, like tramadol (Zamadol), act on the central nervous system to block pain, but have no value as an anti-inflammatory. They're stronger than aspirin but not as strong as narcotics. They're not usually addictive.

Steroids. With names such as methylprednisolone, these are anti-inflammatory medications that can quiet a raging backache and reduce swelling. They are only intended for use over a short period. Also, once a patient starts a course of steroids, he or she must taper off rather than simply stop taking the pills. Side-effects can be weight gain, excessive thirst and ulcers.

Muscle relaxants. This group of drugs, which includes carisoprodol, cyclobenzaprine and diazepam (Valium), sedates and relaxes the body. They act on the central nervous system, so they tend to quiet the entire body. Used in fighting spasm, they are generally prescribed for the short term.

Narcotics. When pain is severe, narcotics are used. They don't block pain, but work to disassociate the patient from it. As it is easy to build up a tolerance to narcotics, the medication becomes less effective during the course of treatment. They are usually prescribed for short periods of time in order to avoid developing an addiction to them. Probably the most well-known narcotic is oxycodone.

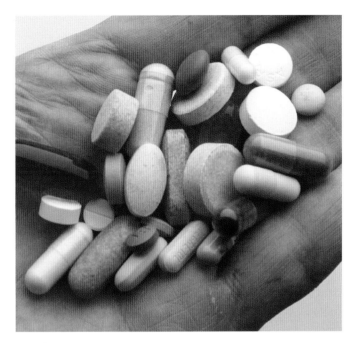

▲ Medication
Prescription medicines come in many different forms. Common types used to treat back pain include antidepressants, muscle relaxants, neuroleptics and steroids.

Stimulation

Your doctor or therapist might be able to reduce pain and inflammation by introducing electric stimulation to the injury site. Additionally, steroids can be administered the same way. These treatments are done in the surgery.

TENS. This low-voltage electric stimulation is also known by its longer name: transcutaneous electrical nerve stimulation. The impulses from TENS interact with nerves to disrupt and override pain signals. The therapist holds the device in place, over the site of your injury.

It's also possible for your doctor to surgically implant a peripheral nerve stimulator that works similarly to TENS for more consistent nerve disruption.

Ultrasound. This involves the use of deep heating generated by sound waves. The therapist glides the device over the site of your injury to penetrate into soft tissue. This treatment might relieve acute, spasmodic episodes and recruits healing blood flow to the area.

Iontophoresis. In this treatment, a steroid is applied to the skin over the injury, then an electrical current is applied to send the steroid through the skin to the injury. Steroids are anti-inflammatories that reduce swelling and pain.

Injections

Injections are an intermediate measure used after a course of medications, physical therapy or both have failed to solve the problem and before surgery is considered. Injections are more effective than oral medications, because they can zero in on the spot that is causing trouble and deliver pain relief directly and quickly. Injections are also sometimes useful as diagnostic tools. The doctor can inject a numbing medication directly into an area suspected of being problematic. If the pain goes away, you've spotted the problem. If it doesn't, it lets the doctor know that it's time to look elsewhere for the source of the pain.

Facet joint block. Each vertebra of the spine has facets, or flat surfaces, that make contact with each other where the vertebrae fit together. Facets are paired with cartilage between them, and these points of contact are called facet joints. Injuries from twisting or degeneration of cartilage can cause a facet joint to become irritated and inflamed. At this point, a steroid (anti-inflammatory) and lignocaine (painkiller) can be injected directly into the joint to relieve the pain. The doctor will use fluoroscopy, or a real-time X-ray, to make sure the injection is positioned in exactly the right place.

Facet rhizotomy. If a few facet blocks are effective but can't sustain the relief, your doctor may determine that the temporary results can be made permanent with a facet rhizotomy. A needle with a probe is inserted just outside the facet joint. The probe emits heat through radio waves to permanently disable the nerve. Once the nerve is deadened, it is unable to transmit pain messages to the brain.

Trigger point injections. A trigger point – a painful knot of muscle fibres in your back – is formed when small strains and microscopic tears in the muscle fibres fail to realign properly as they heal. They stick together in a wad called an adhesion, like scar tissue. Medication can be injected directly into the knot to deaden the pain, so a patient can stretch the muscle and break up this adhesion.

Lumbar epidural injection. This is the most common of all spinal injections. A steroid is injected into the dura, the sac around nerve roots that contains cerebrospinal

▼ Injections

Injections are often used if oral medication has failed to remedy a back problem. They may be administered once only or in a cycle over one year to promote mobility and healing in the back.

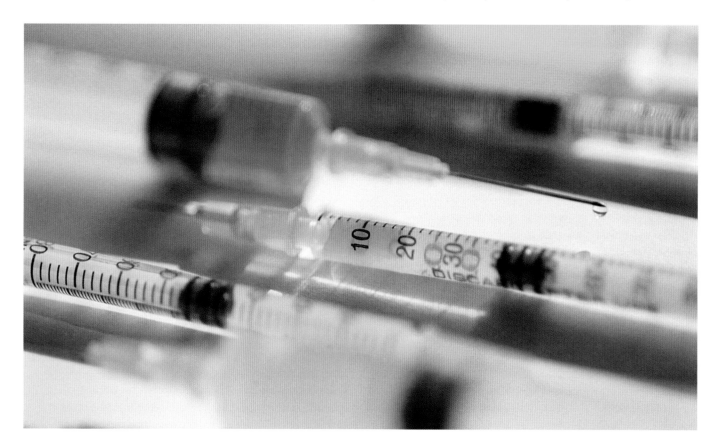

fluid in the lumbar spine, to relieve pain and reduce inflammation. The injection won't actually stop the pain, but it will help to relieve it enough to break the cycle for a time, so a patient can get increased mobility. Moving recruits blood supply, assists the relaxation of muscles and reduces spasms.

The pain relief might take a day or two to kick in, and the injection works in only 50 per cent of people who try it. The effects are temporary – from a week to a year. These injections are sometimes given in a series of three per year to keep a patient comfortable. Sometimes lumbar epidural injections are used to diagnose an injury by giving the doctor a way to pinpoint the location more precisely. By injecting a specific dura, the doctor can observe the effect of the medication. If you experience relief, you're right on target. If you don't, it's time to look elsewhere for the culprit.

Selective nerve root block. When a nerve root is blocked, impinged or inflamed, the pain can radiate through the back and legs. Your doctor will try to determine which nerve root is in trouble with an imaging study, but sometimes they're hard to see. For this reason, a selective nerve root block can be useful as a diagnostic tool, helping to identify the source of your pain. A steroid and lignocaine are injected directly into the nerve where it exits the space between your vertebrae. The doctor uses fluoroscopy to make sure he is on target.

Sacroiliac joint block. The sacroiliac joint is the connection between the pelvis and the base of the spine called the sacrum. A steroid and lignocaine are injected directly into the joint. The doctor uses fluoroscopy to make sure he is on target. Once the pain is deadened, the patient *must* get moving to improve range of motion. This block can be repeated three times a year.

Braces

When a lumbar spine has been fractured or fused, it's like any other broken bone in the body: you need a period of time during which the bone can be immobilised so that it can remodel and knit back together. It also hurts, so keeping everything still can help a person feel better while the healing process begins.

Rigid brace. This is a sort of removable body cast. Limiting spinal movement up to 50 per cent, it's used when the doctor wants a patient to keep still. Rigid braces are fitted to the individual torso and can be removed when the patient is lying down.

Corset. A corset is a fitted brace that keeps a patient from bending forwards from the waist. They are most often used after lumbar fusion surgery, especially if the fusion was done without the use of appliances or stabilising materials and the patient must rely on mending bones to heal. A corset can be removed when the patient is lying down.

Surgery

Depending on the diagnosis, surgery may be considered after prescription drugs and injections have failed to improve a patient's condition. There are as many surgical procedures as there are injuries, conditions and diseases. Your doctor will know when and if it's time to consider this. See chapter 6 for a comprehensive look at selecting the right doctor and getting the most out of your relationship.

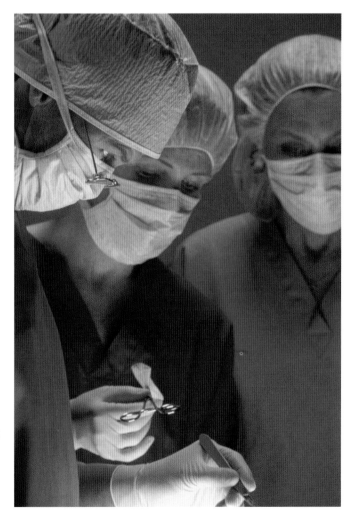

▲ Surgery
Your doctor may refer you to a surgeon if a back injury or condition fails to respond to medication. Surgery may also be recommended when treating certain specific diseases.

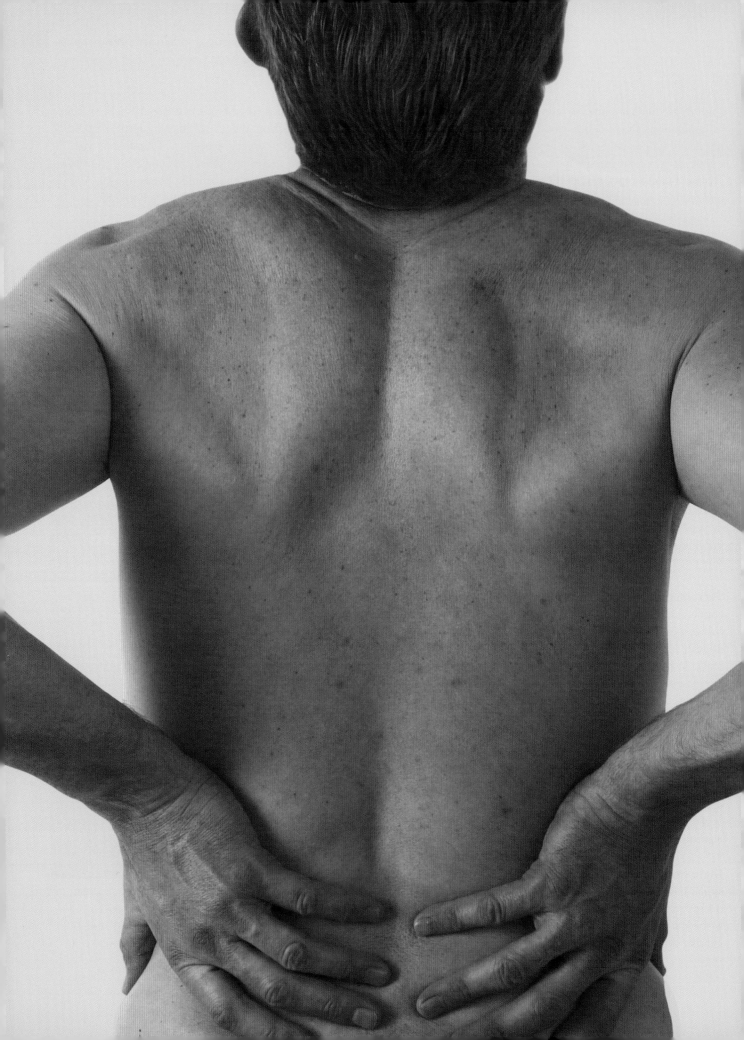

CHAPTER 6

WHEN IT'S TIME TO SEEK HELP: A GUIDE TO BACK DOCTORS

When you have a back problem, getting well might *begin when you visit a healthcare professional who specialises in diagnosing – discovering what's wrong so that you'll be able to make the right decisions about treatment. It's human nature to try a few things on your own first... and you will. But without an accurate diagnosis, at best you'll be taking a hit-or-miss approach to treatment and wasting valuable time.*

In a worst case scenario, you'll be risking further injury, which can precipitate a nightmarish cascade of other medical problems. Promise us that you'll seek professional help – the best you can find. And promise us that you'll do it immediately, under any of the following circumstances:

- if the pain is severe and persists for more than a day
- if the pain impedes your ability to move
- if you also have a fever and chills
- if the site of the pain feels hot or is swollen or reddened
- if the pain starts at your back but radiates down through your buttocks to your leg – especially below your knee
- if the pain is linked to an injury, such as a fall or a trauma
- if one or both of your legs feels numb or weak
- if the pain is keeping you from enjoying your life or sleeping well
- if you have sudden bowel and/or bladder incontinence
- if you have tried several remedies yourself without any success
- if you have a history of cancer with sudden weight loss

DOCTORS WHO CAN GET YOU STARTED

When your back hurts, we suggest that you start with the basics. Although your instinct will be to run to the office of someone who you think can make the pain go away, you should try and stay focused on discovering *why* you're in pain.

Remember that back pain can generate from many sources, both subtle and surprising, so you need someone who can examine you from a broad, comprehensive perspective. We recommend that your first appointment is with your doctor.

General Practitioners

Even though a GP might refer you to a more specialised practitioner, we advise you to make sure that all your medical records are copied and sent back to your primary-care doctor for safe keeping. Why? Medicine today is complicated. You might be consulting several doctors simultaneously, and it can be tricky for one doctor who sees you infrequently to know what treatments you're receiving from everyone else. Medications prescribed from several sources might interact with each other, so it's advisable to have one person who has all your medical information.

Osteopaths

Osteopaths study disciplines including anatomy, physiology, pathology, biochemistry and neurology, as well as osteopathic diagnosis and treatment. A feature of the training is the development of great sensitivity of the hands.

Practitioners who have completed a formal training will be members of a medically recognised organisation, and may also have other professional qualifications.

SURGICAL SPECIALISTS

The spine is a complex amalgamation of bone, spinal cord, soft and connective tissue, and nerves. Diagnosis and treatment are matters of understanding all the systems involved. The two types of surgeons who are uniquely qualified to handle back injuries and disease are neurosurgeons and orthopaedic surgeons.

As spinal surgery has advanced, a hybrid doctor has emerged in each of the two professions: neurosurgeons who can handle the bone, and orthopaedic surgeons who can handle the spinal cord and nerves. Make sure that the surgeon you're consulting has expertise in both skills.

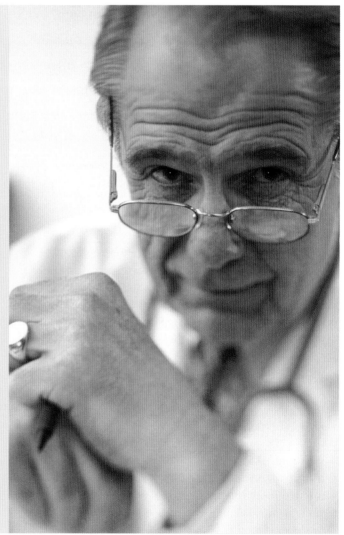

How Your Doctor Decides on Treatment

When you arrive at the surgery, your doctor moves through a very systematic method of evaluating your back pain.

1. Determine if the condition is urgent. Your doctor may refer you for diagnostics or an appointment with a specialist if you have had a major trauma, recent bacterial infection or history of cancer. He may also refer you to a specialist if you are experiencing any of the following symptoms:

- focal spine tenderness (it hurts in a specific place);
- fever;
- very severe pain;
- numbing or paralysis; or
- new bladder dysfunction.

2. Determine if it is 'garden-variety' back pain.
Doctors treat some back pain without extensive diagnostics or intervention by specialists. This might apply to conditions such as sciatica (a pain that radiates from the buttocks down the leg) and generalised lower-back pain (once known as lumbago).

3. Determine if you can be helped by a chiropractor.
When serious neurologic and orthopaedic problems have been ruled out, your doctor may refer you to a chiropractor.

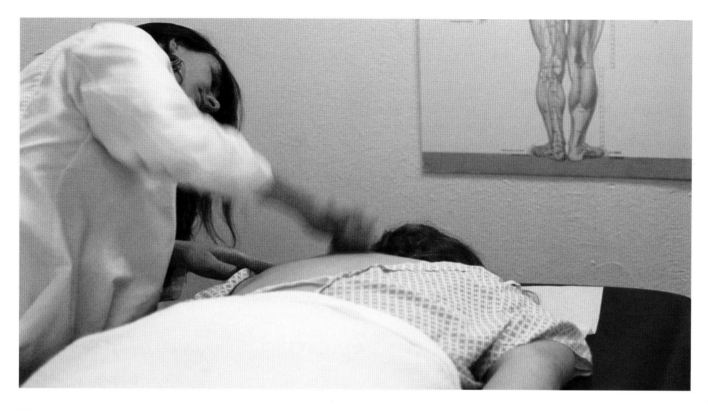

Neurosurgeons

Many neurosurgeons aren't just 'brain surgeons', but are also experts in surgery of the spine, including the mechanics of bone.

These doctors are trained in the diagnosis and treatment of disorders, injuries and diseases of the brain and spine, and the nervous systems and blood supplies that serve and complement them.

Orthopaedic Surgeons (Orthopaedists)

If you are referred to an orthopaedic surgeon, the source of your pain is probably in the bones of your spine.

These doctors are trained in the diagnosis and treatment of skeletal disorders and injury and disease of bones.

NON-SURGICAL SPECIALISTS

While surgeons can provide skilled diagnostics that might or might not include surgery, other doctors can evaluate back problems and treat many of them without surgery.

Chiropractors

Chiropractors are trained in the diagnosis and treatment of skeletal dysfunction, particularly that of the spine.

Practitioners are hands-on care providers who treat without surgery or drugs. Although they can recommend

▲ Chiropractors
Once viewed as 'alternative' practitioners, chiropractors have recently been welcomed into mainstream medicine. Treatment is based on the manipulation and realignment of the body.

nutritional supplements, they cannot write prescriptions for medications. Their practices are centred on diagnosis of imbalance and misalignment, non-invasive corrective procedures such as manipulation or adjustment, and therapies to promote healing, such as ultrasound or massage. If you have bone disease, bone cancer, sciatica, rheumatoid arthritis, osteoporosis or fractures, or if you are pregnant, consult your medical doctor before you undergo chiropractic treatment. Alternatively, contact a national organisation (see 'Further Resources' on page 276).

Neurologists

These doctors are trained in the diagnosis and treatment of disorders, injuries and diseases of the brain and spine, spinal cord, muscles, nerves and all systems and functions involved. They do not perform surgery.

Neurologists are brilliant at diagnosis of back problems, because their clinical knowledge is broad and their access to diagnostic procedures and equipment is vast. Some serve as consultants to other physicians, but many maintain long-term management of patients with chronic disorders.

Rheumatologists

If your back pain is caused by a disease, you'll probably be referred to a rheumatologist. These doctors are trained in the diagnosis and treatment of arthritis and other chronic diseases of bone, connective tissue and muscle such as osteoporosis and fibromyalgia. They do not perform surgery.

Anaesthesiologists

Anaesthesiologists don't just put patients to sleep and wake them up again after surgery. They are also trained in pain management. Your back pain may be treated by an anaesthesiologist in a pain-management clinic or a multidisciplinary integrated care centre.

YOUR REHABILITATION TEAM

When the doctor has made the diagnosis, treatment might include physical therapy – professional training to bring the body back into physical strength and balance. Rehabilitation not only helps to heal, it also teaches ways to prevent injury.

Physiotherapists

Rehabilitation of your back after injury or surgery will often involve physiotherapy. A physiotherapist can help prevent or slow down the progress of debilitating conditions. Physiotherapists can help with back and neck injuries, strains, fractures, arthritis and many other conditions.

Physiotherapists are experts in movement and function. They use exercise and training as their basic tools, but they also do hands-on assistance with joint range of motion, massage, heat and ice, and ultrasound.

These doctors are particular favourites among athletes because of their unique knowledge of biomechanics. If your back injury has been caused by an imbalance in your body or a dysfunction in the way you move, a physiotherapist will spot it. Trained in physical medicine and rehabilitation, they diagnose and treat problems in muscle, bone, connective tissue and nerve conduction. They do not perform surgery.

Occupational Therapists

Occupational therapists help people who have injuries or disabilities that make independent living difficult. Practitioners work across office and home environments. They will evaluate how you move, how you handle tools and implements, how you sleep in bed and how you drive, then help you to make adjustments and train you (and everyone in your environment) to be more effective.

ALTERNATIVE MEDICINE

We work all over the world, so we've seen all sorts of medical practices. Some were as ineffective as we thought they might be. Some worked like charms. All were well intended. These experiences pretty much sum up our opinion of complementary and alternative practices: some are ineffective, some work. And it's all well intended when practised by honourable people.

About a third of us use an alternative therapy at least once a year and the number of us visiting alternative practitioners is growing all the time. Many doctors have also become increasingly open-minded about the patient benefits of alternative treatments.

A word to the wise: don't delay seeking medical attention because you're exploring alternative treatments – you could be wasting valuable time as your back problem deteriorates. When investigating these therapies, make sure you do your homework regarding safety, effectiveness, risks, side-effects, results you can expect and length of treatment. Keep asking questions.

Acupuncture

Channels of vital life energy (chi or qi) run throughout your body. In order for a person to be healthy mentally, physically, emotionally and spiritually, the channels must be clear and free flowing. When chi does not flow properly, it causes imbalance and disease.

The purpose of acupuncture is to examine your channels, discover disruptions and impediments to the flow of chi, and clear the obstruction to restore free flow. It's done through the insertion of small needles or pressure. Sometimes the practitioner heats the needles or uses them to conduct small currents of electrical stimulation.

It is important that you find a reputable and fully qualified acupuncturist. Do not rely on friends or advertisements for a practitioner; instead, contact a national organisation (see 'Further Resources' on page 276). If you are treated by an unqualified acupuncturist, you will almost certainly gain no benefit from the treatment and may be harmed. It is advisable to ask a practitioner about the length of his or her training. All reputable acupuncturists should have trained for at least four years.

Applied Kinesiology

When the musculature of your body and back is out of balance or badly toned, organs and glands do not function properly. These imbalances are caused by poor posture, allergies, stress and injury. In order to make a diagnosis in applied kinesiology, the practitioner will apply force to a muscle, and the patient will resist. If the resistance is successful, the muscle is then determined to be strong and balanced and the related organs and glands healthy. If the patient can't resist the applied force, the muscle is then determined to be weak and the related organs and glands unhealthy.

Allergies and food sensitivities are diagnosed similarly. The applied kinesiologist gives the patient a substance and tests muscular resistance. If the muscle is weak and the patient can't resist the applied force, the substance could be a source of sensitivity and allergy. By applying acupressure to reflex points on a muscle and chiropractic manipulation, the practitioner balances the muscles and improves well-being. Dietary change may also be recommended.

A reputable kinesiologist should have trained for at least two years and undertaken at least 200 hours of kinesiology. Information can be obtained from all major kinesiology organisations (see 'Further Resources' on page 276).

Ayurvedic Medicine

For more than 5,000 years, Ayurvedic medicine has been the cornerstone of patient care in India. It promotes good health not by treating a single symptom, such as a pain in your back, but by treating you as a whole person in body, mind and spirit.

Treatments includes herbal medicine, dietary counselling, massage, yoga, exercise, lifestyle counselling, meditation, aromatherapy, colour therapy, chanting, cleansing and other body work. Because of the extensive, comprehensive nature of diagnosis and treatment, Ayurvedic medicine is sometimes practised in retreats or residential clinics, where a patient can expect to spend at least a few days.

There are only a limited number of Ayurvedic practitioners in the West. Consult only those with an officially recognised degree and beware of charlatans. Contact a national organisation for a list of qualified practitioners (see 'Further Resources' on page 276).

Traditional Chinese Medicine (TCM)

Treatment generally centres on acupuncture, massage, qigong, and the use of herbs to regulate your vital life forces, the chi. Rather than treat symptoms of your back pain or dysfunction, the practitioner brings you into total balance so that pain or dysfunction simply cannot thrive.

If you are considering TCM therapy, first you need to choose from acupressure, acupuncture, Chinese herbal

▼ Chinese medicine
The broad disciplines of Chinese medicine have been practised for thousands of years and often involve acupucture, massage, qigong and the use of herbs.

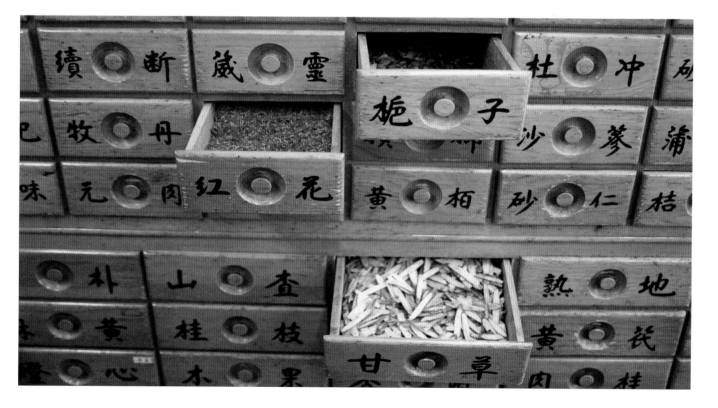

medicine, qigong, shiatsu and tai chi, each of which has its own method of treatment. For further information on these disciplines, consult a national organisation (see 'Further Resources' on page 276).

Faith Healing

When your back is in pain, a faith healer may call upon a god or spirit to intervene and restore health. The healing can take place in a face-to-face meeting between you and the healer, or it can be invoked by thought, ritual and prayer with you and the healer remote from one another.

While the act of faith healing has not been validated by scientific study, prayer is supported and even encouraged by most doctors. Studies indicate that meditation or prayer lowers blood pressure, heart rate, respiration and metabolism. The result is deep relaxation – good for a tight back. Additionally, belonging to a church or spiritual organisation often provides a patient with a strong support base.

Faith healers are not trained, regulated or licensed. There are no requirements except intention and faith. Faith healers may be ministers, preachers, exorcists, spiritualists, lay clerics, priests, evangelists, shamans or witch doctors affiliated with an organised faith. For more information on healing, contact an officially recognised organisation (see 'Further Resources' on page 276).

Homeopathic Medicine

Homeopathic doctors evaluate you as an entire person and then select therapeutic substances to match your symptoms. This can activate the body's healing capacity, triggering a cure. The principle is known as 'like cures like' and also states that the smaller the amount of the remedy, the greater the effect. Homeopathic remedies are available in low dilutions over the counter for self-treatment.

Homeopathic doctors are naturopathic physicians who have undergone formal training and have certification, but the availability of the substances and courses for laypeople make it easy for untrained enthusiasts to set up practice. Contact a national organisation for further information (see 'Further Resources' on page 276).

Hypnosis

In hypnosis, a trained therapist leads you into deep relaxation and concentration. In this focused state, you can be coached to modify behaviours and control pain, anxiety and other chronic conditions that are often exacerbated by tension in your back.

▼ Hands-on healing

Massage promotes feelings of well-being and can be a useful treatment when dealing with muscular tension in the back.

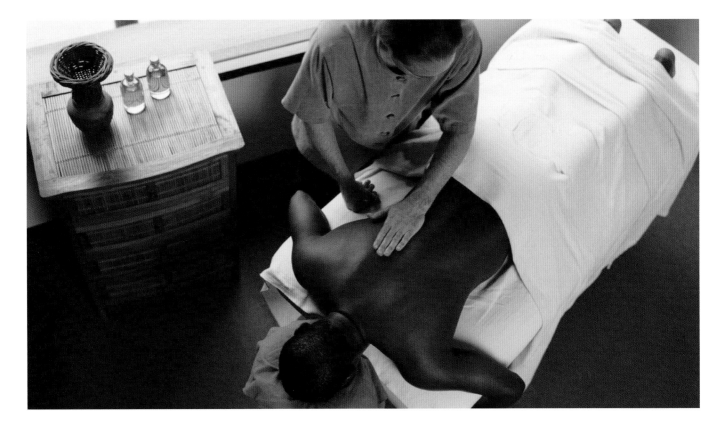

Hypnotists are trained in classes or in apprenticeships. As a profession, they are not regulated, but many are licensed counsellors, psychologists and therapists. To find a registered therapist with a guaranteed level of excellence, contact a national organisation (see 'Further Resources' on page 276).

Massage

A good choice for a tired, aching back, massage is touch work, in which a trained therapist manipulates tissue. Nearly 150 recognised hands-on techniques are designed to improve health and well-being by loosening tightened and knotted muscles, relieving pain, easing tension, inducing relaxation, restoring movement, redirecting energy and improving circulation.

Your doctor may be able to provide you with the name of a qualified practitioner. Alternatively, contact a national organisation (see 'Further Resources' on page 276).

Naturopathic Medicine

Whenever possible, medical intervention should work in harmony with, and support, your body's natural ability. Naturopathic medicine works on the assumption that your body contains a powerful, innate healing ability. The practice centres on finding causes for problems rather than treating symptoms of your back pain: eliminate the cause, and you will heal.

Treatment may focus on dietary adjustment, nutritional supplements, homeopathic remedies, hydrotherapy or herbal medicines. Some practitioners have a specific approach, while others draw on a wide range of techniques. To find a fully qualified therapist, contact a national naturopathic organisation (see 'Further Resources' on page 276).

Qigong

Qigong is an ancient Chinese practice of curing disease and promoting health through the manipulation of energy, by either meditation and visualisation or physical movement. Most visible among the qigong disciplines in the West is tai chi, the slow dance of postures and positions that restore balance, build strength, remove disruptions in energy flow and stimulate the flow of chi throughout the body.

Practitioners are more teachers than clinicians. Contact a national organisation for more information (see 'Further Resources' on page 276).

Reiki

This practice probably originated in Tibet, but it has been passed from master to master in a Japanese lineage that only found its way to the Western world in the 20th century. In

Reiki, the practitioner acts as a passive conduit by drawing energy from the God-consciousness and the life force and then passing it through to your body, focusing on areas of disrupted energy. This influx of energy charges your own life forces, until the negative energies and disruptions are overcome and fall away.

Choose a therapist who has trained with a Reiki master or contact a national organisation for further information on practitioners (see 'Further Resources' on page 276).

Yoga

Yoga is an ancient Hindu spiritual practice with a number of disciplines. All have three components in common: breathing, exercise and meditation. Breathing increases oxygenation, helping you feel alert and focused. Yoga exercise can raise the heart rate, which, when combined with increased oxygenation, helps to remove metabolic waste from the body, promoting healing. And meditation, the last component, can help calm the mind of a stressed person.

Instructors are neither licensed nor regulated. Contact a national organisation to find a qualified practitioner (see 'Further Resources' on page 276).

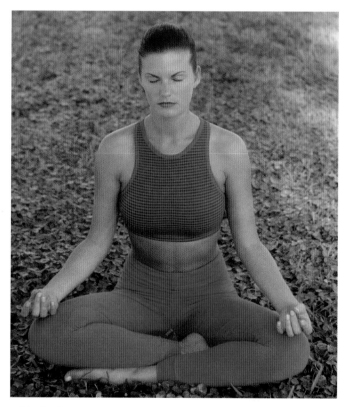

▲ Meditation
Yoga postures are particularly well-known for promoting calmness, balance, flexibility and strength.

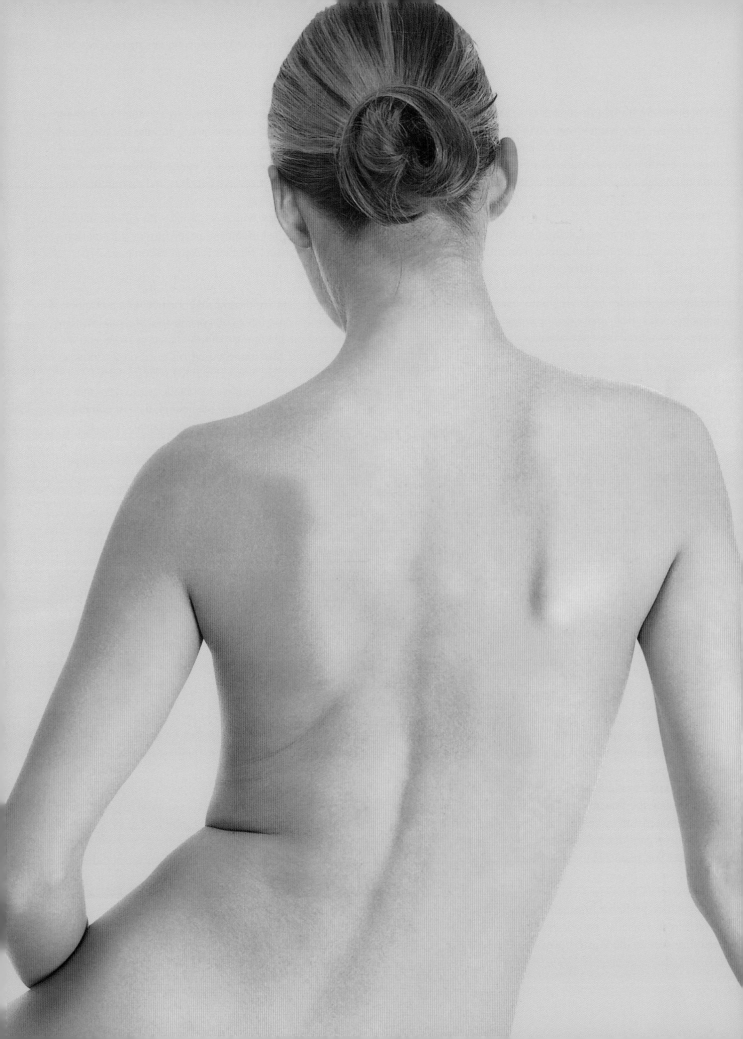

CHAPTER 7

AFTER THE DIAGNOSIS: GETTING OUT OF PAIN QUICKLY

Hopefully, your back will remain so healthy, strong *and flexible that you'll never have a problem requiring medical intervention. But if you do, and your doctor takes you out of commission, we want to prepare you to be a good partner to your health-care team. Although medical people can do a tremendous amount to help you get well, the ultimate responsibility is yours. It's your back.*

We have listed some of the most common diagnoses for back disorders and explained each one in simple terms. Of course, your doctor will give you much more detail. Following the description of the diagnosis, we've made suggestions about getting into action, taking responsibility for getting out of pain, and restoring flexibility, strength and balance to your body in general and your back specifically. If you were to come into our clinic with a particular malady, we would use the routines listed here to help ease your pain, relax your raging muscles, restore your circulation and increase your ability to move. You would feel progress from the first minute.

The stretches and strengthening exercises in this section are also in chapter 4. Please refer to the listings of individual exercises for explicit instructions – we've included thumbnail photos for you here as a quick, at-a-glance guide to the most critical poses for each condition.

Keep in mind that getting well is usually not a matter of performing miracles. Sometimes, recovery takes perseverance and patience. We battle on. If we can make even a slight improvement, our client will feel better. We want full recovery for you. But if this can't happen, we want you to be able to recover as much comfort and function as you can.

Before you begin these or any exercises after a diagnosis of a back disorder, it is critically important that your doctor knows in advance exactly what you would like to do and gives your plan his blessing. Take this book to your next appointment and study the suggestions together. Follow your doctor's instructions to the letter. If you get the green light, begin immediately. If he wants you to modify a move, do it. If he denies you permission to work out, then take a break. When you're well and strong again, hopefully you'll be cleared to rejoin us. We'll wait for you.

Please note that we may repeat some of our general recommendations, with slight modifications for each condition. Often, you'll want to begin by drinking plenty of water, taking a mild non-steroidal anti-inflammatory (unless otherwise directed by your doctor), and alternating stretching with icing the affected area. We'll modify this advice as necessary below.

In offering suggestions for short-term relief or for kick-starting recovery, we aren't implying that a full fitness programme is no longer necessary. In fact, as soon as you are able, we urge you to return to the complete programme for flexibility, strength and cardio work. You need a well-rounded, lifelong workout plan of action to keep you fit and healthy, and to make sure that back problems are things of the past.

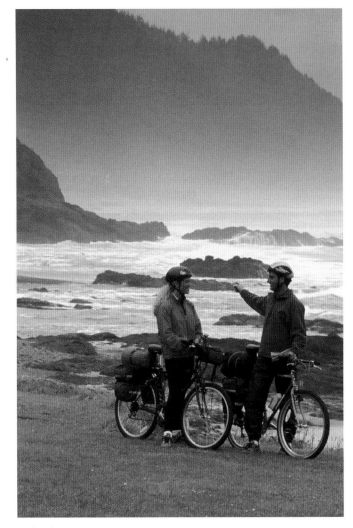

▲ Fresh air and exercise
Regular gentle exercise such as cycling and walking will speed your recovery and help prevent problems from recurring.

DIAGNOSIS: ANKYLOSING SPONDYLITIS

Ankylosing spondylitis (AS) is a chronic, painful, rheumatic inflammatory disease that fuses the vertebrae in your spine from top to bottom. It can also appear in other joints, organs, connective tissues and the chest wall. It's a form of inflammatory arthritis that's also called rheumatoid spondylitis or Marie-Strümpell disease. Ankylosing spondylitis usually presents itself in people between the ages of 20 and 40, attacking more men than women by a ratio of three to one. No one knows the cause, but genetics appear to play an important role in predicting the likelihood of contracting the disease.

Because the joints between the vertebrae fuse, the patient will 'lock up', frozen into position. The disease is painful and debilitating, with flare-ups and progressive difficulties. Sometimes ankylosing spondylitis will trigger the vertebrae to generate bone spurs, protective coarsening of bone, like scarring. These spurs can compress and irritate the spinal cord and nerve roots, causing even more pain, numbness, weakness and lack of coordination.

What You Can Do

While there is nothing you can do to stop an inflammatory disease, you can relax and restore circulation to the muscles and soft tissues surrounding your spine and take some of the compression off inflamed nerve roots. You can also slow down and possibly reverse this fusing phenomenon with stretching. You must get moving – the sooner the better.

Drink plenty of water to make sure you're always hydrated. Take a mild non-steroidal anti-inflammatory (such as ibuprofen or naproxen) to get pain under control so that movement and subsequent relaxation are easier.

Stretch through the entire routine given on pages 50 to 65. Do 10 repetitions of each. Move slowly and very gently, and within the smallest ranges of motion. At no time should a movement hurt. Ice your back for 10 minutes to soothe the area. Then stretch again. You can repeat the stretch-ice-stretch sequence several times, or until the pain eases and you feel that you've restored range of motion to the smallest extent.

You must keep everything moving so that muscles are kept flexible and strong to support your back, circulation is restored and maintained, and the neurological patterns and connections between nerve roots and extremities remain sharp. And you have to fight the fusion of your vertebrae. When you're ready, add the strengthening routines. Be patient, move slowly, and keep the weights light and the movements very small.

Bone spurs are the biggest impediment to doing these exercises. Do the best you can. Work within the ranges of your own mobility and tolerance for discomfort, but don't push it. At no time should a movement hurt.

DIAGNOSIS: BACK SPASM

Back spasm is a painful, involuntary seizure of the muscles in your back. It is literally a cramp. The spasm can last for a few minutes or several hours; it can even come and go. It might be caused by injury to – or inflammation in – muscles, ligaments, tendons, the bones of your spine or the discs between vertebrae. The spasm is your body's way of immobilising the area around the injury or inflammation. Locking up muscles creates a natural splint so that you can't move and cause more damage.

What You Can Do

Your mission is to relax the muscles to calm the spasm. Drink plenty of water to stay hydrated. Relaxing a spasm is very tough when you're dehydrated because the cells of your muscles are depleted. Take a mild non-steroidal anti-inflammatory (such as ibuprofen or naproxen) to help with the pain so that movement and relaxation are easier.

TWO EXERCISES FOR SPASM IN THE MID-BACK

1. Trunk Extensors

See complete instructions for this two-step exercise on page 55.

2. Thoracic-lumbar Rotators

See complete instructions for this four-step exercise on page 56.

TWO EXERCISES FOR SPASM IN THE LOWER BACK

1. Single-leg Pelvic Tilts

See complete instructions for this two-step exercise on page 50.

2. Double-leg Pelvic Tilts

See complete instructions for this two-step exercise on page 50.

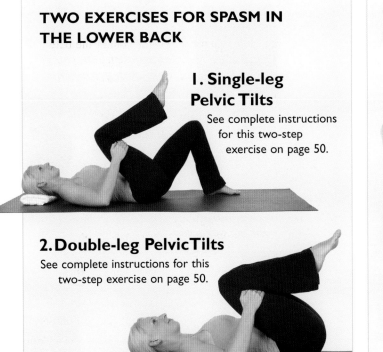

TWO EXERCISES FOR SPASM IN THE UPPER BACK

1. Rotator Cuff 1

See complete instructions for this two-step exercise on page 63.

2. Neck Extensors

See complete instructions for this three-step exercise on page 65.

DIAGNOSIS: BRUISE

Deep-muscle bruising is a well-known injury among those who play contact sports, but is uncommon among the rest of us. The bruise is usually caused by either by a strain that rips tissue, or a direct blow or repeated blows to the body that crush the blood vessels, muscle fibres, and underlying connective tissue, but don't break the skin. When blood vessels are damaged or broken, blood leaks out of the damaged vessel and into deep tissue, forming a raised, swollen bump that is bluish. This is called a haematoma. When the blood leaks out to the top layers of the skin, the bruise is a flat, purple mark called an ecchymosis.

The bruise is not an injury – it's only a leak. It's a sign the body uses to point the way to an injury. How easily a person bruises depends on many factors that have to do with the fragility of blood vessels and the clotting capacity of blood. When the back is bruised, the doctor will be less interested in the bruise and more interested in the damage caused by the blow or rip.

What You Can Do

You need to relax and restore circulation to the muscles and soft tissues that surround the bruise. Drink plenty of water and take a mild non-steroidal anti-inflammatory (such as ibuprofen or naproxen) for the pain. Until you can do a full stretch routine, choose from the four groups of stretches opposite and overleaf. Do 10 repetitions of each stretch, or as many as you can without discomfort. Move gently and within the smallest ranges of motion. Ice your back for 10 minutes to calm the area. Then stretch again. You can repeat the stretch-ice-stretch sequence several times, or until the pain eases and you feel that you've restored range of motion to the smallest extent.

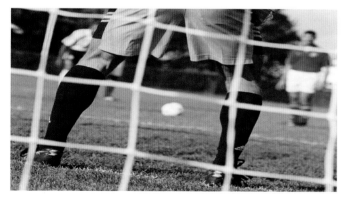

▲ Rough and tumble
People who play contact sports are continually prone to deep-muscle bruising through frequent heavy blows to the body.

NINE EXERCISES FOR BRUISE TENSION IN THE UPPER BACK

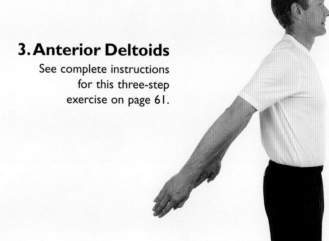

1. Shoulder Circumduction
See complete instructions for this three-step exercise on page 60.

2. Pectoralis Majors
See complete instructions for this two-step exercise on page 60.

3. Anterior Deltoids
See complete instructions for this three-step exercise on page 61.

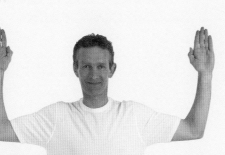

4. Shoulder Internal Rotators

See complete instructions for this three-step exercise on page 62.

7. Rotator Cuff 2

See complete instructions for this three-step exercise on page 63.

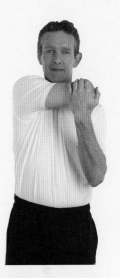

5. Shoulder External Rotators

See complete instructions for this three-step exercise on page 62.

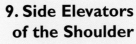

8. Forward Elevators of the Shoulder

See complete instructions for this three-step exercise on page 64.

6. Rotator Cuff 1

See complete instructions for this two-step exercise on page 63.

9. Side Elevators of the Shoulder

See complete instructions for this two-step exercise on page 64.

TWO EXERCISES TO RESTORE CIRCULATION TO A BRUISED HIGHER BACK

1. Thoracic-lumbar Rotators

See complete instructions for this four-step exercise on page 56.

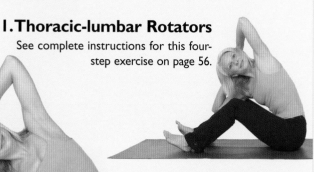

2. Trunk Lateral Flexors

See complete instructions for this three-step exercise on page 56.

TWO EXERCISES TO RESTORE CIRCULATION TO A BRUISED LOWER BACK

1. Single-leg Pelvic Tilts

See complete instructions for this two-step exercise on page 50.

2. Double-leg Pelvic Tilts

See complete instructions for this two-step exercise on page 50.

TEN EXERCISES FOR BRUISE TENSION IN THE LOWER BACK

1. Bent-leg Hamstrings

See complete instructions for this three-step exercise on page 51.

2. Straight-leg Hamstrings

See complete instructions for this two-step exercise on page 51.

3. Hip Adductors

See complete instructions for this two-step exercise on page 52.

4. Hip Abductors

See complete instructions for this two-step exercise on page 52.

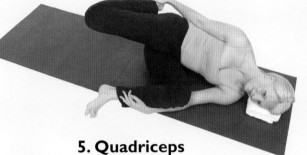

5. Quadriceps

See complete instructions for this three-step exercise on page 53.

8. Trunk Extensors

See complete instructions for this two-step exercise on page 55.

6. Gluteals

See complete instructions for this two-step exercise on page 54.

9. Thoracic-lumbar Rotators

See complete instructions for this four-step exercise on page 56.

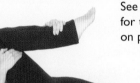

7. Piriformis

See complete instructions for this four-step exercise on page 54.

10. Trunk Lateral Flexors

See complete instructions for this three-step exercise on page 56.

DIAGNOSIS: CAUDA EQUINA SYNDROME

A small bundle of nerve roots at the base of the lower lumbar spine is called the cauda equina. These nerve roots are the transmitters of information from your brain through your spinal cord to your pelvic organs (including the bladder and bowel) and lower extremities, and back again the other way. When the cauda equina bundle is compressed or damaged, a lot can go wrong.

Cauda equina syndrome can cause permanent paralysis, dysfunction of the bladder and bowel, and pain and loss of sensation in one or both sides of your legs, buttocks, inner thighs, backs of legs, feet or heels. The syndrome can be caused by herniated disc, tumour, infection, stenosis of the spinal canal, fracture or trauma. If it's not corrected quickly, impairment can be permanent.

What You Can Do

The treatment of cauda equina syndrome depends on its cause. This condition can be so serious that we urge you to rely on your doctor if you have this condition.

DIAGNOSIS: DEGENERATIVE DISC DISEASE

Degenerative disc disease is associated with the natural process of ageing. Throughout life, vertebrae are cushioned from one another by soft, gel-like discs between them. The discs assist the flexion, extension and rotation of the spine – just enough, but not too much. They help stabilise the spine, absorb shock and distribute the ever-changing forces on your body.

When a disc is compromised by normal ageing, injury from trauma, repetitive stress, instability or inflammation, pain and weakness can step in. Interestingly, it's possible to have degenerative disc disease and have no symptoms at all. Still, it's good to know whether or not you have it because a measure of caution can go a long way in protecting a fragile back from injury. If you have degenerative disc disease and are bothered by it, your doctor might suggest replacing the disc or fusing the spine to stabilise it. But he might also allow trying a few things first to strengthen the supporting muscles and connective tissues surrounding the disc.

What You Can Do

While there is nothing you can do to regenerate a disc, you can do a little to relax and restore circulation to the muscles and soft tissues that surround the degenerated disc. Drink plenty of water to make sure you're hydrated. Take a mild

NINE EXERCISES FOR DEGENERATIVE DISC DISEASE

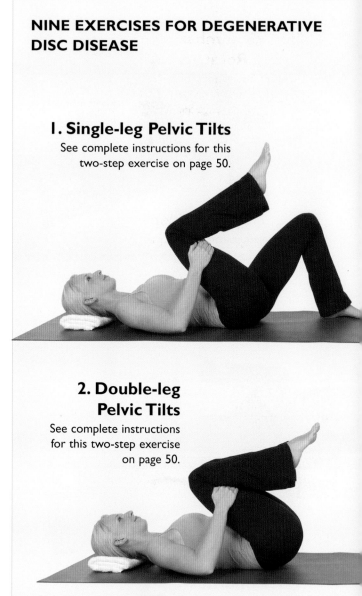

1. Single-leg Pelvic Tilts
See complete instructions for this two-step exercise on page 50.

2. Double-leg Pelvic Tilts
See complete instructions for this two-step exercise on page 50.

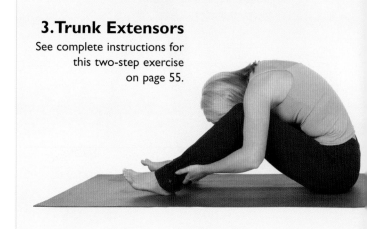

3. Trunk Extensors
See complete instructions for this two-step exercise on page 55.

4. Thoracic-lumbar Rotators

See complete instructions for this four-step exercise on page 56.

5. Upper Abdominals

See complete instructions for this two-step exercise on page 75.

6. Oblique Abdominals

See complete instructions for this three-step exercise on page 76.

7. Lower Abdominals

See complete instructions for this three-step exercise on page 76.

8. Trapezius

See complete instructions for this two-step exercise on page 85.

9. Rhomboids

See complete instructions for this two-step exercise on page 86.

non-steroidal anti-inflammatory (such as ibuprofen or naproxen) to get pain under control so that movement and relaxation are easier.

Stretch with the exercises on pages 126–127, moving very slowly and gently. Do 10 repetitions of each. Small movements add up fast, so be patient. At no time should a movement hurt. When the stretching is completed, you need to strengthen the muscles that support your back to take the pressure off the disc. This workout routine has a little stretching and strengthening.

After completing one set of each exercise, ice your back for 10 minutes to soothe the area. Then stretch again. You can repeat the stretch-ice-strengthen sequence several times or until the pain eases and you feel that you've restored range of motion to the smallest extent. When you have finished stretching and strengthening, lie down flat on your back for a little while with a rolled towel at the base of your neck and another at your lower back.

DIAGNOSIS: DISLOCATION

There are two types of dislocation. In everyday life, *partial* dislocations, called subluxations, of the vertebrae are common reasons for visits to the chiropractor. The vertebrae are no longer perfectly 'stacked' and in alignment. The ligaments behind your spine keep everything together and stable, but the misalignment and strain cause pain and a possible degree of weakness and numbness in your arms and hands. Also, muscles surrounding the subluxation are pulled out of alignment when the vertebrae are torqued, and eventually those muscles fatigue in their efforts to keep the back in balance.

When the articulating joints between the vertebrae are no longer making any contact and the ligaments behind the spine are torn and can no longer support the spine, this is *true* dislocation. The vertebrae are out of whack, and it can be extremely painful.

What You Can Do

If ligaments are not torn, your main strategy is to get strong and flexible enough to support your spine during the healing process. You have to work to relax and restore circulation to the muscles and soft tissues that surround the dislocation. If this doesn't happen, tension in those muscles keeps the dislocation under pressure and will slow the healing process.

Drink plenty of water to make sure you're hydrated. Take a mild non-steroidal anti-inflammatory (such as ibuprofen or naproxen) to help lessen the pain so that movement and subsequent relaxation are easier.

▼ Dislocated vertebrae
The commonest form of dislocation in the spine is when the vertebrae become misaligned or poorly 'stacked' – also known as partial dislocation. This condition ususally warrants a visit to a chiropractor. 'True' dislocation is, fortunately, a lot rarer.

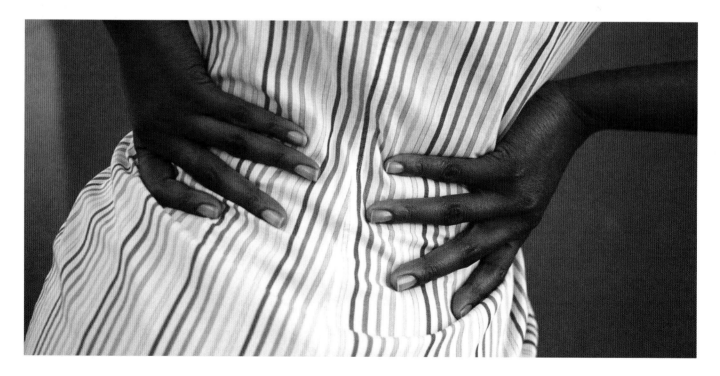

Doing a full stretch routine is best (see the 24 exercises starting on page 50). Go very slowly and work very gently. Nothing should ever hurt. If the smallest movement is all you can manage, go for it. Small movements add up quickly.

If your diagnosis is dislocation *with* torn ligaments, you should do nothing except listen to your doctor. You'll have to stabilise and immobilise the site of the tear so it can heal and your spine can stay aligned. You can resume working out later. Until then, keep the rest of your body moving – as long as you place no strain on the dislocation.

DIAGNOSIS: EXERCISE-INDUCED MUSCLE SORENESS

Many people who start physical exercise after a break of some years experience discomfort as the body engages for the first time in a long time. And although we preach 'No pain', sometimes an athlete overdoes it and feels sore. There may be no injury but the athlete still feels exercise-induced muscle soreness.

Sometimes the pain manifests itself immediately following the activity, as a function of simple fatigue. When the muscles are pushed, they can't flush the build-up of metabolic waste fast enough, so that accumulation of waste stays in the muscle, causing pain and weakness. Rest and a good stretch routine will flush the painful area, and the muscle will feel better.

Another, more confusing, exercise-induced muscle soreness is delayed-onset muscle soreness (DOMS). DOMS doesn't show up immediately after the activity that caused it, but appears 24 to 48 hours later. Sometimes the delay is so lengthy and the pain so severe that the person can't link the pain to the event and, in confusion, seeks medical attention. Muscles are stiff, sore and weak. When a muscle is worked too hard, the muscle fibres tear very slightly as they strain. In addition to the tearing, the fibres swell, increasing pressure on surrounding tissue. For reasons not quite understood, DOMS is most common following activities where muscles contract while they are lengthening in braking actions, such as walking down stairs, running down hills, or lowering weights.

Although exercise-induced muscle soreness is usually not serious, only your doctor can evaluate the magnitude of the damage that may accompany the pain and swelling.

What You Can Do

It's important to relax to restore circulation to the muscles and soft tissues that surround the area of pain in your back.

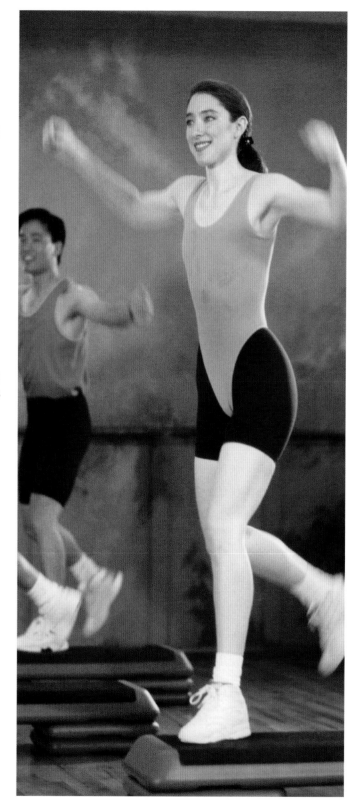

▲ **Don't over-stretch yourself**
It's easy to get carried away when you resume exercise after a break – resist the temptation or your muscles will pay the price.

Drink plenty of water to make sure you're always hydrated; this will speed up your recovery. Take a mild non-steroidal anti-inflammatory (such as ibuprofen or naproxen) to keep pain down to tolerable levels so that movement and relaxation are more bearable.

Start with the stretches for the upper back (see below and opposite) and for the lower back (see page 132), and do 10 repetitions of each. Soreness, unfortunately, can be accompanied by slight swelling, which can impede range of motion and make working out uncomfortable. Move slowly and very gently and in the smallest ranges of motion. At no time should a movement hurt.

Ice your back for 10 minutes to soothe the area. Then stretch again. You can repeat the stretch-ice-stretch sequence several times, or until the pain eases and you feel that you've restored range of motion to the smallest extent. When you've finished stretching, lie down flat on your back for a little while with a towel roll at the base of your neck, and another at your lower back, one under the backs of your knees and another under your heels. Try to position your legs a little higher than your head.

If the soreness is high on your back, restore circulation with the two stretches below. Don't forget to drink three or four glasses of water to facilitate the healing process.

NINE EXERCISES FOR UPPER BACK TENSION

1. Shoulder Circumduction
See complete instructions for this three-step exercise on page 60.

2. Pectoralis Majors
See complete instructions for this two-step exercise on page 60.

3. Anterior Deltoids
See complete instructions for this three-step exercise on page 61.

TWO EXERCISES FOR UPPER-BACK SORENESS

1. Thoracic-lumbar Rotators
See complete instructions for this four-step exercise on page 56.

2. Trunk Lateral Flexors
See complete instructions for this three-step exercise on page 56.

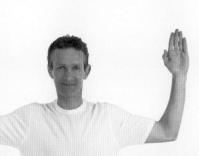

4. Shoulder Internal Rotators

See complete instructions for this three-step exercise on page 62.

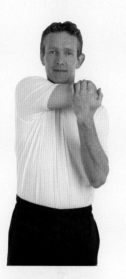

7. Rotator Cuff 2

See complete instructions for this three-step exercise on page 63.

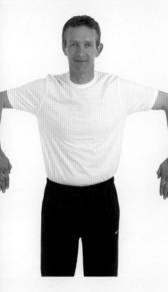

5. Shoulder External Rotators

See complete instructions for this three-step exercise on page 62.

8. Forward Elevators of the Shoulder

See complete instructions for this three-step exercise on page 64.

6. Rotator Cuff 1

See complete instructions for this two-step exercise on page 63.

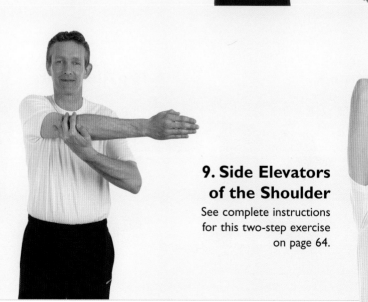

9. Side Elevators of the Shoulder

See complete instructions for this two-step exercise on page 64.

TWELVE EXERCISES FOR LOWER-BACK SORENESS

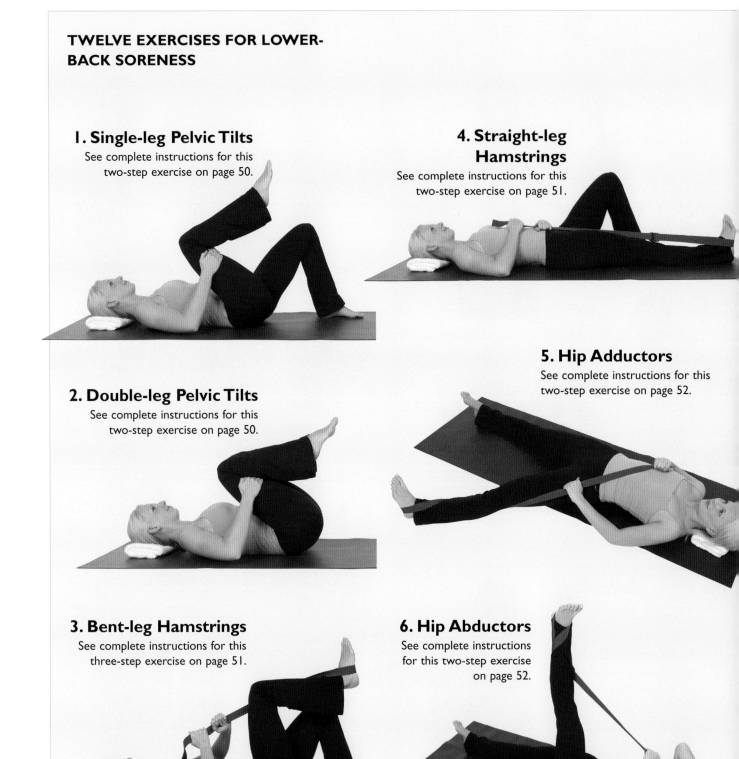

I. Single-leg Pelvic Tilts
See complete instructions for this two-step exercise on page 50.

2. Double-leg Pelvic Tilts
See complete instructions for this two-step exercise on page 50.

3. Bent-leg Hamstrings
See complete instructions for this three-step exercise on page 51.

4. Straight-leg Hamstrings
See complete instructions for this two-step exercise on page 51.

5. Hip Adductors
See complete instructions for this two-step exercise on page 52.

6. Hip Abductors
See complete instructions for this two-step exercise on page 52.

7. Quadriceps
See complete instructions for this three-step exercise on page 53.

8. Gluteals
See complete instructions for this two-step exercise on page 54.

9. Piriformis
See complete instructions for this four-step exercise on page 54.

10. Trunk Extensors
See complete instructions for this two-step exercise on page 55.

11. Thoracic-lumbar Rotators
See complete instructions for this four-step exercise on page 56.

12. Trunk Lateral Flexors
See complete instructions for this three-step exercise on page 56.

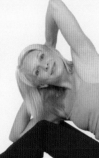

DIAGNOSIS: FRACTURE

When vertebrae crack, it literally means that bones in your back have broken. Usually fractures occur with trauma, but when bones are weakened by disease, such as osteoporosis, these can also happen spontaneously.

In trauma, the type of fracture depends on the force of the blow, the location of the fracture in the spine, and the spatial orientation of the break. With a stable fracture, ligaments behind the vertebrae have not been disturbed, so the body still has a natural splint to support the spine. With an unstable fracture, the ligaments have been torn, so the spine is without support and the break is serious. In a simple compression fracture, the break appears to be minimal and is towards the midline of the vertebra. A vertical compression is like a simple compression, but the force of the break was more damaging. A comminuted cervical vertebral body fracture (a teardrop fracture) is caused by maximum force that causes explosive failure of the vertebral body – like a shatter.

▼ Fractured vertebrae
Any kind of bone fracture in the spine can be serious. A specialist will have to determine the type of fracture and its severity before recommending how best to immobilise and heal the injury.

When the vertebra shatters, the spinal cord can be in serious trouble. Bone fragments can potentially penetrate or sever the cord, or the complete failure of the vertebra can cause serious compression of the cord.

Of all the bones in the body to be broken, a fractured vertebra has the most potential for disaster. No matter how large or small the fracture, an unstable vertebra can compress, damage or sever a spinal cord. Unfortunately, with a vertebral fracture, it's impossible to isolate the broken bone and immobilise it in a cast. The entire area has to be immobilised to allow healing and, more importantly, protect the spinal cord from injury.

What You Can Do

If your diagnosis is fracture, you should do nothing except listen to your doctor. You have to stabilise and immobilise the site of the break to allow the bones to knit back together. You can resume working out later. Until then, keep the rest of your body moving – as long as you place no strain on the break.

DIAGNOSIS: HERNIATED DISC

Also called a ruptured disc or a slipped disc, a herniated disc happens when the outer band of the disc bursts,

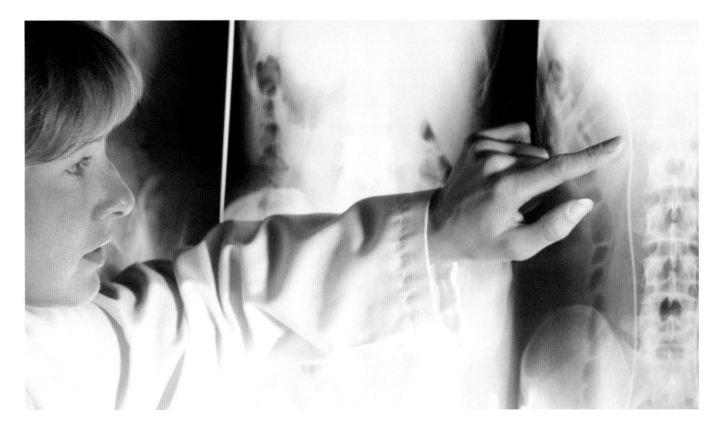

allowing the soft, gel-like inner pulp to bulge out. The medical term for this is *herniated nucleus pulposus*.

The discs between each vertebra absorb shock and help hold the bones together in a stable, yet flexible way so that the back can move. When the outer band of a disc is herniated and the inner pulp bulges, that pulp can press against the spinal cord, causing extreme pain, nerve disruption and coordination problems. In less severe cases, the escaped pulp can compress nerve roots, causing pain.

When the herniation or rupture is in the cervical spine, you can also feel pain and numbness in the neck, shoulders, arms and hands. You can make the pain lesser or greater by positioning the neck to manipulate the bulge of pulp through the herniation.

Interestingly, it is possible to have a herniated disc without showing any symptoms at all. A herniation can take place quite suddenly or develop over a long period of time as the outer band deteriorates. Lack of regular exercise, poor nutrition, ageing, normal wear and tear, dehydration and bad posture can all contribute to the chance of developing a herniation.

What You Can Do

While there is nothing you can do to restore the integrity of a herniated, ruptured or slipped disc, you can relax and restore circulation to the muscles and soft tissues that surround your spine, to take some of the compression off inflamed nerve roots.

Stay hydrated and take a mild non-steroidal anti-inflammatory (such as ibuprofen or naproxen) to control pain and promote movement. Stretch through the whole routine on pages 50 to 65. Do 10 repetitions of each exercise, moving slowly in the smallest ranges of motion. At no time should a movement hurt. Ice your back for 10 minutes to soothe the area. Then stretch again. You can repeat the stretch-ice-stretch sequence several times, or until the pain eases and you feel that you've restored range of motion to the smallest extent. When you've finished stretching, lie down flat on your back for a little while with a towel roll at the base of your neck and another at your lower back.

You have to keep everything moving so that muscles are kept flexible and strong to support your back, circulation is restored and maintained, and the neurological connections between nerve roots and extremities are kept sharp.

When you're ready, add the strengthening routines. Be very careful, be patient, move slowly, keep the weights light, and keep the movements very small. It can't be repeated enough: at no time should a movement hurt.

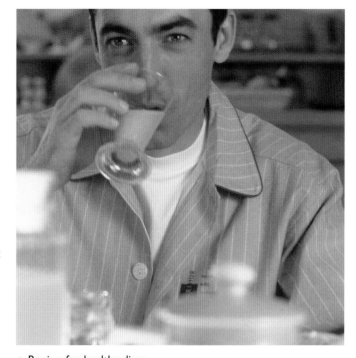

▲ Recipe for healthy discs
A balanced diet, lots of exercise and good posture can lessen the chances of a herniated disc.

Diagnosis: Juvenile Rheumatoid Arthritis

Juvenile rheumatoid arthritis (JRA) is an inflammatory arthritis that begins during childhood and comes in three different forms. The monoarticular form attacks only one joint, the polyarticular form attacks many joints, and the systemic form attacks several joints and organs of the body, causing not only arthritis symptoms but also high fevers and rashes.

The systemic and polyarticular forms commonly attack the cervical spine. At first, these forms of JRA cause pain and stiffness; later, they can interfere with the normal formation of the vertebrae and cause a fusion of the facet joints between the vertebrae.

In addition, ligaments that support the spine can be damaged by inflammation. When the ligaments are damaged and weakened, the vertebrae can't stay in alignment. When the vertebrae slip out of formation, the spinal cord and nerve roots become compressed, resulting in pain, weakness, numbness and, often, a lack of coordination.

What You Can Do

Your mission is to get strong to support the spine so that no fusion can take place. Your first task is to relax, so you can restore circulation to the muscles and soft tissues that surround your spine and take some of the compression off inflamed nerve roots. At the same time, it's imperative that you strengthen muscles to support the spine.

Drink plenty of water to make sure you're hydrated. Take a mild non-steroidal anti-inflammatory (such as ibuprofen or naproxen) to get pain under control so that movement and subsequent relaxation are tolerable.

We've designed a strengthening sequence to help with JRA symptoms (see right). Do 10 repetitions of each exercise, moving slowly and very gently. Small movements add up fast. Be patient. At no time should a movement hurt. Make sure you ice your back for 10 minutes to soothe the area after your workout. If you're an adult dealing with JRA, you may use light weights during the exercises. If you're a young person, start with no weights at all and gradually progress to the lightest weights you can find. You'll discover that movement and the resistance of your own body weight are sufficient to make big changes in your fitness level. These exercises can and should be fun. Why not play some music while you are working out or how about recruiting an exercise partner?

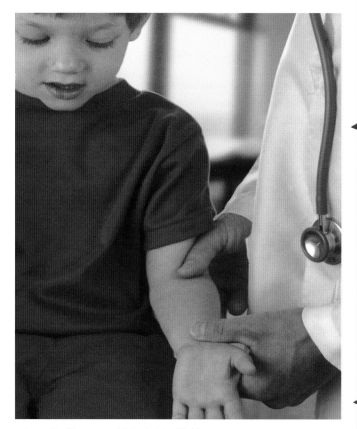

▲ Juvenile Rheumatoid Arthritis (JRA)
Diagnosing JRA in a child usually involves a non-painful physical examination to rule out other possible causes.

TEN EXERCISES FOR JUVENILE RHEUMATOID ARTHRITIS (JRA)

1. Deltoids
See complete instructions for this four-step exercise on page 82.

2. Pectoralis Majors
See complete instructions for this two-step exercise on page 82.

3. Triceps – Supine Position
See complete instructions for this two-step exercise on page 83.

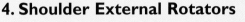

4. Shoulder External Rotators

See complete instructions for this two-step exercise on page 84.

5. Shoulder Internal Rotators

See complete instructions for this two-step exercise on page 84.

6. Triceps – Prone Position

See complete instructions for this two-step exercise on page 85.

7. Trapezius

See complete instructions for this two-step exercise on page 85.

8. Rhomboids

See complete instructions for this two-step exercise on page 86.

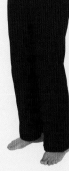

9. Biceps

See complete instructions for this three-step exercise on page 86.

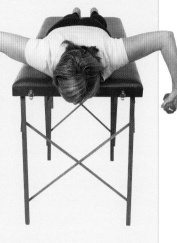

10. Shoulders (The Roll)

See complete instructions for this two-step exercise on page 87.

DIAGNOSIS: KYPHOSIS

Kyphosis – a term used to describe an abnormal hunching or curving of the thoracic or cervical spine – describes any spinal curve over 45 degrees. There are several types.

Postural kyphosis. Kyphosis is 'hunchback'. It's a rounded upper back that could be caused by something as simple as bad posture and slouching. When the abdominals are weak and a child slouches, this can stretch the ligaments in the spine – the connective tissue that connects vertebra to vertebra. That stretching can become significant and increase the natural curve of the spine. (This is why parents are always yelling, 'Stand up straight!')

Kyphosis usually shows up in teen years and is more common among females. Some young women might be sensitive to calling attention to developing breasts, so they slouch to allow clothing to hang loosely from their shoulders. Or, perhaps it is merely the increase in weight on the chest as breasts develop. The posture can become a permanent habit, and the curve can be forever. It is rarely painful, but like any curvature that is unnatural, it can become problematic as the child develops into adulthood. Most children grow out of it and stand tall.

Weak abdominal muscles and tight hamstrings (the muscles in the back of the thighs) contribute to the slouch. When the child is able to strengthen the abs to support the back and get the hamstrings to let go and elongate, the situation improves immeasurably. By the way, weak abs and tight hamstrings are the signature problems of sitting too much. These problems are identical to those found with people who are deskbound most of the day.

So what happens as a sloucher grows up? Because the natural curve of the thoracic spine is forwards anyway, any weakness of the muscles or soft tissue in the back will draw it further down. And an overdeveloped chest will do the same thing. A damaged or diseased vertebra will deteriorate and collapse its forward edge first (the edge towards the chest), so that will further pronounce the curve. (Hyperkyphosis is an exaggerated form of kyphosis characterised by rounded shoulders and a sunken chest.) But even if none of this happens, postural kyphosis in an adult may produce headaches, backaches and joint pain.

Congenital kyphosis. In some infants, the spine never develops properly. The bones may not form correctly or a bone bar might develop between two vertebrae and cause a progressive hunch as the child grows up. If it's present from birth, it gets worse as the child matures. Children with disorders such as spina bifida can have severe kyphosis. The only treatment is a medical or surgical option. Intervention will normally take place by the time a child reaches the age of five.

Scheuermann's kyphosis. In this form of kyphosis, three or more vertebrae are irregular and wedged at five degrees each. Like postural kyphosis, it becomes obvious during teen years – however, it affects more males than females. Scheuermann's kyphosis isn't usually painful, but it is an obvious cosmetic deformity that is disturbing to many people, and it can progress and become painful and cause neurological symptoms. The only way to distinguish it for sure from postural kyphosis is with an X-ray. It can be treated with bracing that permits restricted remodelling of the bone in the vertebrae.

Kyphosis from compression fracture. The dowager's hump is a classic example of kyphosis that results from a compression fracture. It's caused when the vertebrae collapse because of osteoporosis (as is the case of dowager's hump), tumour or infection. As with all fractures, and the accompanying soft-tissue damage and strain of deformity, this is painful. It can also lead to neurologic deficits. (Preventing osteoporosis *is* possible. See chapter 10 for more information.)

What You Can Do

For postural kyphosis, you can do a lot to correct a rounded back. Remember that muscles work in pairs, so if the back is weak and extending into a slouch, then the chest is constricting and flexing to pull it forwards.

Stability of the back is highly reliant on strong abdominals. When the abs are weak and the hamstrings are tight from sitting, then the back has no support. It tries to do all the work itself and shorts out. Over it goes.

When kyphosis is caused by compression fracture stemming from osteoporosis, there's only so much one can do to relieve the imbalances – fractures aren't so easy to fix. But osteoporosis can be prevented with calcium and load-bearing exercise; there are also other medications that help fortify bone so that it won't become porous and collapse. If osteoporosis has already set in, its progression can be slowed. If the spine is already fractured, surgical stabilisation may be possible, and the rest of the body can certainly be conditioned with strength and flexibility.

Until you're able to do a full workout, we suggest that you start with four stretches (see right). Do your workout on a soft surface such as your bed or an exercise mat.

FOUR EXERCISES FOR POSTURAL KYPHOSIS

1. Single-leg Pelvic Tilts

See complete instructions for this two-step exercise on page 50.

2. Double-leg Pelvic Tilts

See complete instructions for this two-step exercise on page 50.

3. Pectoralis Majors

See complete instructions for this two-step exercise on page 60.

4. Anterior Deltoids

See complete instructions for this three-step exercise on page 61.

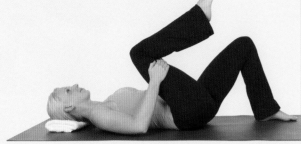

DIAGNOSIS: LORDOSIS

Lordosis (or swayback) refers to a severely arched back. The spine is naturally lordotic between the cervical and lumbar spine, but lordosis describes a curve that is excessive. As kyphosis describes a forward hunch, lordosis describes exactly the opposite – it's a swayback just above the buttocks, making the buttocks appear pronounced.

In fact, the prominence of the buttocks is the major clinical feature of lordosis. If you lay a child with lordosis on its back on a flat surface, there will be visible air space between the lower back and the surface. If the child can flatten the back to the surface or if the lordotic curve is flexible and corrects when he bends forward, then lordosis is of little medical significance.

Lordosis can be a simple matter of poor posture. Or it can be present from birth or result from infection, injury, neurological and muscular problems, or back surgery. Symptoms vary, especially if there are accompanying defects such as muscular dystrophy. Sometimes lordosis is associated with bowel and bladder problems and pain in the back and down the legs. If it's anything other than postural lordosis, the only intervention should be medical and surgical options.

Hyperlordosis. Of particular interest to us are gymnasts and dancers, who assume a lordotic posture in many of their biomechanics. Studies suggest that although the initial postures are deliberate, they can become permanent. Hyperlordosis is an exaggerated curvature of the lumbar spine between L5 and S1 (lumbar 5 and sacral 1), which handles the greatest loads and stresses of the spine. It's also called hyperextension of the back. Although it produces a graceful line, it contributes to the majority of dance-related injuries.

Hyperlordosis often occurs when there is a pelvic tilt caused by weak abdominals, tight psoas, weak inner thigh muscles, hyperextended knees (that appear to bend backwards), a bow in the tibia that forces weight distribution back, tight hamstrings, weakness in the feet, and shoulders carried too far back, causing the upper torso to lean back and the chin to protrude. Where these imbalances are present without hyperlordosis, they often precede the onset of the condition. This disorder can lead to pain and stress fractures of the spine. If the dancer is male, lifting with hyperlordosis is dangerous for himself and the partner he'll drop when his spine collapses. The younger the dancer or gymnast who develops these bad habits, the greater the risk of injury.

Prenatal lordosis. As the weight of your unborn child puts pressure on your spine and unbalances your body, the natural tendency to arch your back for comfort takes over. Experts tell us that it will do no harm, nor will problems remain when returning to your former posture after your child is born and the weight is gone.

What You Can Do

Because lordosis is a swayback, we can assume that the abdominals are weak, the abductors are weak, the hamstrings are tight, and the lumbar spine is compensating with contraction. Because these muscles work in pairs, straightening up the spine is a matter of tightening up the loose stuff and loosening up the tight stuff. As we said earlier, stability of the back is highly reliant on strong abdominals. When the abs are weak and the hamstrings are tight, then the back has no support. In the case of lordosis, it is pulled forwards as the pelvis tilts.

The answer is simple: loosen up the pelvis and strengthen the back. Loosen up the hamstrings and strengthen the abdominals. By following the complete programme of Active-Isolated Stretching and Strengthening, you'll reverse the roles of the muscles in the pairs, and they'll balance. The result? The sway will go away.

DIAGNOSIS: LOWER-BACK PAIN

In light of all the possible diagnoses that might explain a back problem, hearing a diagnosis of lower-back pain might sound odd, but, in fact, it's a very real phenomenon. Lower-back pain is non-specific discomfort in the lumbar and sacral regions – the area between the waist and the middle of the buttocks. This condition can become problematic when the pain is so intense that it begins to restrict movement, disturbs sleep, or radiates through the buttocks to the legs.

Lower-back pain has many causes. Sometimes the source of the problem can be traced to muscle strain, overuse, ligament sprains, poor posture, spasm, injury, arthritis, weakness or postural mistakes. Sometimes the source is more elusive and will require diagnostic imaging to rule out more serious conditions.

What You Can Do

You need to relax the muscles and begin to restore circulation and movement. Drink plenty of water, so you'll stay hydrated. It's very tough to relax a muscle and restore circulation to an inflamed area when you're dehydrated, because the cells of your muscles are depleted. Take a mild

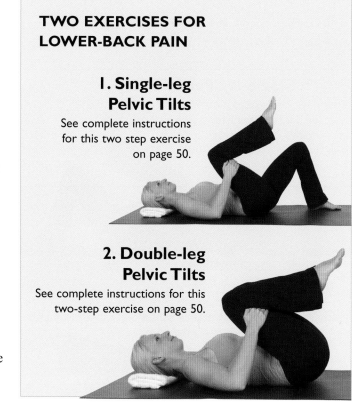

TWO EXERCISES FOR LOWER-BACK PAIN

1. Single-leg Pelvic Tilts
See complete instructions for this two step exercise on page 50.

2. Double-leg Pelvic Tilts
See complete instructions for this two-step exercise on page 50.

non-steroidal anti-inflammatory (such as ibuprofen or naproxen) to get pain under control so that movement and relaxation are easier.

When the pain gets especially acute, try the two suggested stretches (see above). Do 10 repetitions of each, but go very gently and settle for the smallest movements. Ice the site of pain for 10 minutes to soothe the area. Then do the two stretches again.

You can repeat the stretch-ice-stretch sequence several times, or until the pain eases. When you have finished stretching, lie down flat on your back for a little while with a towel roll placed at the base of your neck and another positioned under your lower back.

DIAGNOSIS: LUMBAR SPINAL STENOSIS

The word 'stenosis' comes from the Greek word *stenos*, meaning 'narrow'. As we age, degenerative changes occur in our vertebrae, causing stenosis – a narrowing of the central spinal canal, through which the spinal cord runs. This narrowing can strangle nerve roots that run from the spinal cord through the vertebrae and branch out into the body. The net effect is pain, numbness or weakness that can radiate down through the buttocks, thighs and legs.

Occasionally, the pain can begin in lower legs and radiate up. The discomfort can sometimes abate with rest and flexibility that increases the area of the canal and decompresses the nerves.

The narrowing of the spinal canal is caused by a thickening and coarsening of the ligamentum flavum, a large connective band that runs along the inside of the spinal canal and holds everything together. In addition, extra bony, protective growths called osteophytes form within the canal at sites of little traumas and irritations, narrowing the spinal canal.

Researchers are not sure why, but not everyone develops spinal stenosis as they age. They suggest that there might be a genetic predisposition to the condition.

What You Can Do

Although there is nothing you can do to widen a narrowed spinal canal, you can take steps to relax and restore circulation to the muscles and soft tissues that surround your spine and take some of the compression off those inflamed nerve roots.

Make sure you drink plenty of water, so you'll stay hydrated. Take a mild non-steroidal anti-inflammatory (such as ibuprofen or naproxen) to help reduce the pain so that movement and relaxation start to become easier. Then stretch. Do 10 repetitions of each exercise shown opposite, moving slowly and very gently. As you know, small movements add up fast, so be patient. At no time should a movement hurt. Ice your back for 10 minutes to soothe the area. Then stretch again. You can repeat the stretch-ice-stretch sequence several times, or until the point the pain eases and you feel that you've restored range of motion to the smallest extent. When you've finished stretching, lie down flat on your back for a little while and put a rolled towel at the base of your neck and another underneath your lower back.

These stretches will help your back, but stenosis is tricky because the pain radiates to and from sites that are not injured at all. Therefore it's very important that you work out your entire body – even those areas that hurt. One of the real dangers in dealing with stenosis is that a particular area of the body can become immobilised due to a person's perception of pain. Before you know it, a perfectly healthy set of muscles and connective tissues begins to deteriorate needlessly. It's vital that you make sure you're not pampering an area that needs no pampering or protection. You can easily compound the damage of the stenosis and render your body more debilitated than it ever needed to be.

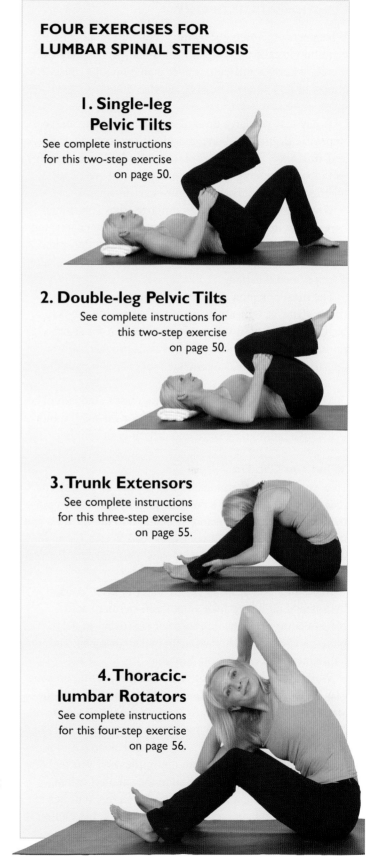

FOUR EXERCISES FOR LUMBAR SPINAL STENOSIS

1. Single-leg Pelvic Tilts
See complete instructions for this two-step exercise on page 50.

2. Double-leg Pelvic Tilts
See complete instructions for this two-step exercise on page 50.

3. Trunk Extensors
See complete instructions for this three-step exercise on page 55.

4. Thoracic-lumbar Rotators
See complete instructions for this four-step exercise on page 56.

DIAGNOSIS: MYELOPATHY

Whenever something goes wrong with the spinal cord, the condition is called myelopathy. This nonspecific diagnosis merely describes difficulty rather than pinpoints cause. It's almost always accompanied by another diagnosis that is much more specific.

To say that you have myelopathy is to say that you have a specific disorder of bone, muscle or connective tissue… and, of course, the spinal cord is involved. Most commonly, myelopathy presents itself in the elderly and is a result of other degenerative diseases of the cervical spine.

When degenerative diseases progress, they can trigger bone spurs, in which the bone gets a protective coarsening similar to a scar. These spurs can press against the spinal cord or compress nerve roots, causing pain, numbness and a lack of coordination.

The most common cause of myelopathy, however, is spinal stenosis, the narrowing of the spinal column (see pages 140–141 for a full description). When the space through which the spinal cord travels is progressively constricted, function is disrupted. Not only is it painful, it could lead to problems with walking.

Myelopathy begins slowly and progresses gradually. The first symptoms are neck pain, difficulty with small motor skills, like buttoning a shirt, and difficulty in walking.

What You Can Do

How you deal with myelopathy will depend on your doctor's diagnosis and advice. It's possible to get your back to relax to some extent and to restore circulation to the muscles and soft tissues that surround your spine and to take some of the compression off inflamed nerve roots that emanate from an irritated cord.

Make sure you drink plenty of water to keep yourself hydrated at all times. Take a mild non-steroidal anti-inflammatory (such as ibuprofen or naproxen) to get pain under control. This will help make movement and subsequent relaxation more bearable.

Work through the entire stretch routine (starting on page 50). Do 10 reps of each exercise. Move slowly and in the smallest ranges of motion. At no time should a movement hurt. Ice your back for 10 minutes to soothe the area. Then stretch again. You can repeat the stretch-ice-stretch routine several times, or until the pain diminishes and you feel that you've restored range of motion to the smallest extent.

You have to keep everything moving so that muscles are kept flexible and strong to support your back, circulation is restored and maintained, and the neurological connections and patterns between nerve roots and extremities are kept sharp. Whatever you can move, move.

When you're ready, add the strengthening routine (starting on page 68). Be patient, move slowly, keep the weights light, and keep the movements very small. Remember, pain is a signal that you should stop.

Bone spurs can be a real problem when you work out with myelopathy. Not only are they excruciatingly painful, they can also impede movement. Actually, they present quite an obstacle. Our only advice is to do the best you can. Work within the ranges of your own mobility and tolerance for discomfort, but don't push it.

DIAGNOSIS: OSTEOARTHRITIS

Osteoarthritis is the most common of all joint diseases and it affects men and women in equal proportion. In men, the onset is generally before age 45 and manifests most commonly in the hips, knees and spine. In women, the onset is generally after age 55 and manifests most commonly in hands and knees. This disease attacks bone and also cartilage – the specialised, dense connective tissue that forms part of the skeleton and covers the ends of bones in a joint.

Almost all people over age 65 have some of the bone and cartilage changes associated with osteoarthritis, but researchers tell us that it's not an inevitable part of ageing. Many older people have the physical changes but no

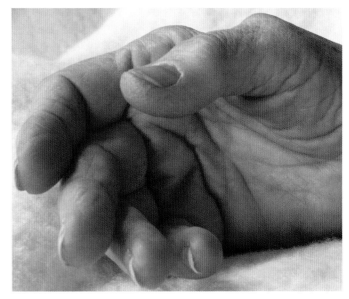

▲ Osteoarthritis
Osteoarthritis affects the hands, hips, spine and knees, causing pain and inflammation in the joints and cartilage.

symptoms, such as pain or debilitation. The way people move and use their joints into their later years greatly affects the severity of symptoms.

Osteoarthritis is a low-grade inflammatory disease, like rheumatoid arthritis, that causes debilitating pits and cracks in cartilage. As the cartilage degrades, small bits may break and float into the liquid spaces that surround joints (the synovium), and bone is gradually exposed. Unprotected by cartilage, the action of bone on bone grates and irritates. Although the bone continually remodels to protect itself, the surface of the bone forms osteophytes, or bone spurs, 'scars' that mark a site of injury or stress on the bone.

These uneven surfaces and spurs make joints less efficient and eventually cause deformities. Before long, the tissues surrounding the joint and connecting key parts struggle to compensate for biomechanical inefficiency. Inflammation engulfs the area and pain sets in.

At first, osteoarthritis is characterised by pain and stiffness when a person has 'overdone it'. As cartilage erodes, soft tissue surrounding the area inflames. The joint may eventually enlarge. When osteoarthritis strikes the lower spine, radiating pain to the buttocks and legs is often the result. When it sets into the hips, pain radiates to the buttocks, groin, inside the thigh and knee. When it sets into the cervical spine, pain radiates to the shoulders and arms.

What You Can Do

While there is nothing you can do to restore the integrity of damaged cartilage and bone, you can relax and restore circulation to the muscles and soft tissues that surround your spine, to take some of the compression off inflamed nerve roots. Drink more water to make sure you're always hydrated. Take a mild non-steroidal anti-inflammatory (such as ibuprofen or naproxen) to help with the pain and make movement and subsequent relaxation easier. You have to keep everything moving so your muscles can remain flexible and strong to support your back, circulation can be restored and maintained, and the neurological connections between nerve roots and extremities are kept sharp.

Stretch through the entire routine (starting on page 50). Do 10 repetitions of each exercise. Move slowly and very gently and in the smallest ranges of motion; at no time should a movement hurt. Ice your back for 10 minutes to soothe the area, then stretch again. Repeat the stretch-ice-stretch sequence several times, or until the pain eases and you feel that you've restored range of motion to the smallest extent. When you've finished stretching, lie down flat on your back with a towel roll at the base of your neck and another at your lower back, and rest for a little while.

When you're ready, add the strengthening routine (starting on page 68). Again, be patient: move slowly, keep the weights light, and keep the movements very small. At no time should a movement hurt.

The real problem in working out with osteoarthritis is the bone spurs, which not only are excruciatingly painful but also can impede movement. Frankly, they can be a difficult hindrance. Our only advice is to do the best you can. Work within the ranges of your own mobility and tolerance for discomfort, but don't push it.

DIAGNOSIS: OSTEOPOROSIS

In some older people, bones become porous as a result of slowed bone remodelling and diminished calcium content. These fragile bones are more likely to fracture. In the spine, it's possible for a fracture or collapse of one or more vertebrae to occur without impact or apparent reason. Sometimes severe and disabling, this pain can affect not only the back but also the extremities when the nerve roots are involved. See chapter 10 for a more complete discussion of this disease.

DIAGNOSIS: RADICULOPATHY

The word 'radiculopathy' is used to describe pain, numbness, weakness or tingling in arms and hands or legs and feet that is caused by an injury or disruption to nerve roots in your spine.

The nerve roots are the communication conduits between your spinal cord and the rest of your body. When a nerve root is injured or disrupted, communications can become unclear and problems begin. The injury or disruption can be caused by compression or inflammation of the spinal cord and the nerve roots – often the result of a herniated disc or a degenerative disease.

Sensory problems, such as pain, are more common than motor problems, such as weakness. In fact, if motor problems are present, it's a clue that the nerve root compression or inflammation might be more serious.

What You Can Do

Treatment depends on the cause of the radiculopathy. If your doctor gives you the green light, get to work relaxing and restoring circulation to the muscles and soft tissues that surround your spine and taking some of the compression off inflamed nerve roots.

Drink lots of water to make sure you're hydrated. Take a mild non-steroidal anti-inflammatory (such as ibuprofen or naproxen) to control the pain so that movement will be easier.

Do 10 repetitions of each stretch below, making sure that you move slowly and very gently at all times. Small movements add up fast. Be patient. At no time should a movement hurt you or cause pain. Afterwards, ice your back for 10 minutes to soothe the area. Then do the stretch again. You can repeat the stretch-ice-stretch sequence several times, or until the pain diminishes and you feel that you've restored range of motion to the smallest extent. When you've finished the stretching exercises, lie down flat on your back for a little while with a rolled towel at the base of your neck and another underneath your lower back.

These stretches will help your back, but radiculopathy is tricky because the pain radiates to and from sites that are not injured at all. It's very important that you work out your entire body – even those areas that hurt. One of the real dangers in dealing with this condition is that an area of the body can become immobilised due to the perception of pain. Before you know it, a perfectly healthy set of muscles and connective tissues begins to deteriorate needlessly. You have to make sure that you're not pampering an area that needs no pampering. You can compound the damage of the original injury and render your body more debilitated than it ever needed to be.

FOUR EXERCISES FOR PAIN RADIATING TO THE BUTTOCKS AND LEGS

1. Single-leg Pelvic Tilts
See complete instructions for this two-step exercise on page 50.

2. Double-leg Pelvic Tilts
See complete instructions for this two-step exercise on page 50.

3. Gluteals
See complete instructions for this three-step exercise on page 54.

4. Piriformis
See complete instructions for this three-step exercise on page 54.

TWO EXERCISES FOR PAIN RADIATING TO THE ARM, WRIST, ELBOW OR HAND

1. Rotator Cuff 1
See complete instructions for this two-step exercise on page 63.

2. Rotator Cuff 2
See complete instructions for this three-step exercise on page 63.

DIAGNOSIS: RHEUMATOID ARTHRITIS

Rheumatoid arthritis is an inflammatory, degenerative condition of the synovial membrane – the tissue that lines the joints. This condition usually presents itself between the ages of 20 and 50, and women are three times more susceptible to it than men.

Although the disease attacks the entire body, including hands and fingers, feet and toes, and hips, the back is in danger. The vertebrae in the neck just below the head – the atlas and the axis (see page 16) – are especially susceptible to damage, particularly in people who have had rheumatoid arthritis for more than 10 years.

When the atlas and axis are attacked and begin to degenerate, too much movement between the vertebrae makes the cervical spine unstable. As the disease progresses, the tip of the atlas might protrude up into the base of the skull, compressing the brain stem and causing difficulty in balance and coordination.

Finally, rheumatoid arthritis can cause the lower vertebrae in the cervical spine to slip forwards, forcing a thrusting posture of the head and a hunch forwards of the neck. If you have been diagnosed with rheumatoid arthritis, there is a 60 per cent chance that it will eventually progress into your spine. Being vigilant about monitoring and treating the condition is very important.

What You Can Do

The mission here is to get circulation back into inflamed joints. You need to get the blood flowing in order to carry oxygen in and remove waste products to keep the bone remodelling and the tissues healthy. You also have to restore range of motion.

While there is nothing you can do to stop rheumatoid arthritis by yourself, you can do a few things to restore circulation to the muscles and soft tissues that surround the attacked vertebrae. Drink plenty of water to stay hydrated. Take a mild non-steroidal anti-inflammatory (such as ibuprofen or naproxen) to help with the pain – movement and subsequent relaxation will be more bearable.

Do 10 repetitions of each stretch (see above right), moving slowly and very gently. Small movements add up fast. Be patient. At no time should a movement hurt. Ice your cervical spine for 10 minutes to soothe the area. Then stretch again. You can repeat the stretch-ice-stretch sequence several times, or until the pain eases and you feel that you've restored range of motion, even to the smallest extent.

If you feel your cervical spine tightening, do these two stretches frequently throughout the day.

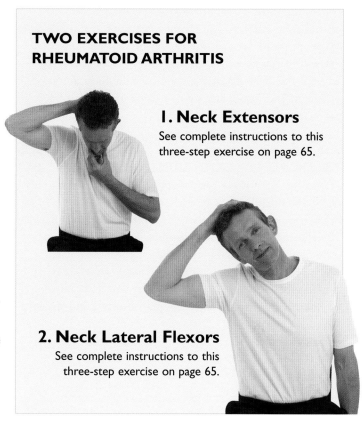

TWO EXERCISES FOR RHEUMATOID ARTHRITIS

1. Neck Extensors
See complete instructions to this three-step exercise on page 65.

2. Neck Lateral Flexors
See complete instructions to this three-step exercise on page 65.

DIAGNOSIS: SCIATICA (OR PIRIFORMIS SYNDROME)

The largest nerve in your body, the sciatic nerve is as wide as your thumb and runs from your lower back through your buttocks and into the backs of your thighs, all the way down to your feet. When that nerve is compressed or strained in your lower back in some way, the nerve becomes irritated. Instead of transmitting messages for movement from your spinal cord to your legs, it transmits messages of pain. This condition is called sciatica.

Many things can cause the compression: arthritis, a tumour, a herniated disc, an infection in the spine or an injury. The pain is generally on one side only and most often starts in the buttocks. Occasionally, it manifests as numbness or weakness in the leg and foot, which makes walking difficult. Patients generally complain of a deep pain in the buttocks that becomes excruciating when sitting, climbing stairs or squatting. Studies in Finland reveal that the predisposition to back problems in general, and sciatica in particular, is mainly genetic. Researchers have identified a genetic mutation that damages the protein charged with helping the body maintain the integrity of cartilage between the discs. If your parents suffered from sciatica, research suggests that you have to be extra vigilant.

One of the most common causes of sciatic pain is piriformis syndrome. The piriformis muscle is the external rotator muscle in the centre of your pelvis that runs right through the buttock over to the greater trochanter of the femur – the large, protruding bump on the outside top of the thigh. The sciatic nerve passes right underneath the piriformis muscle.

In about 15 per cent of the population, however, that nerve runs right through the fibres of the piriformis muscle. When the muscle is contracted and compresses the sciatic nerve, the piriformis strangles it, causing irritation and all the symptoms of sciatica listed above.

Intense repetitive activity that hammers the lower back, buttocks and hip can cause this muscle to swell. Sitting on something that puts pressure directly on the muscle will do it – like sitting on a wallet. Being out of shape can do it, too. Weakness in the hip muscles and gluteals in your buttocks will tighten up the piriformis and strangle the sciatic nerve.

What You Can Do

It's important to relax and restore circulation to the muscles and soft tissues that surround your lower back and to get the piriformis to relax and let loose its stranglehold on the sciatic nerve.

Drink plenty of water to make sure you're always hydrated. Take a mild non-steroidal anti-inflammatory (such as ibuprofen or naproxen) to control pain so that movement and subsequent relaxation are easier.

Start with stretching (see right). Do 10 repetitions of each. Soreness can be accompanied by slight swelling that can impede range of motion and make working out uncomfortable. Move slowly and very gently and in the smallest ranges of motion. At no time should a movement hurt. Ice your back for 10 minutes to soothe the area. Then stretch again. You can repeat the stretch-ice-stretch sequence several times, or until the pain eases and you feel that you've restored range of motion to the smallest extent.

Take a look at your lifestyle and see what you're doing to cause this impingement. Are you overweight? Do you carry your wallet in your back pocket? Do you do one activity repeatedly, without giving your body a rest? Pay attention to this signal, and think of a way to give your overtaxed sciatic nerve a break.

This stretching sequence is designed in a specific order to relax muscles that surround the piriformis and then sneak up on it. One day of work will not alleviate the problem, but patience will prevail. Stop all stretches if you are feeling any kind of pain.

TEN EXERCISES FOR SCIATICA

1. Single-leg Pelvic Tilts

See complete instructions for this two-step exercise on page 50.

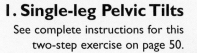

2. Double-leg Pelvic Tilts

See complete instructions for this two-step exercise on page 50.

3. Bent-leg Hamstrings

See complete instructions for this three-step exercise on page 51.

4. Straight-leg Hamstrings

See complete instructions for this two-step exercise on page 51.

5. Hip Adductors

See complete instructions for this two-step exercise on page 52.

8. Quadriceps

See complete instructions for this three-step exercise on page 53.

6. Hip Abductors

See complete instructions for this two-step exercise on page 52.

9. Gluteals

See complete instructions for this three-step exercise on page 54.

10. Piriformis

See complete instructions for this three-step exercise on page 54.

7. Psoas

See complete instructions for this two-step exercise on page 53.

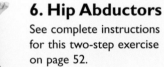

DIAGNOSIS: SCOLIOSIS

If you take an X-ray of a healthy spine from the back, it appears to be a straight line up and down. But if that line looks more like the sideways curve of the letter C, or worse, the letter S, then you're looking at scoliosis.

Paediatricians are always on the lookout for scoliosis, as are school nurses. Scoliosis can be caused by spinal deformities from birth, genetic disorders, neuromuscular disorders, atrophy of muscles surrounding the spine, leg-length discrepancies, spina bifida, cerebral palsy and tumours, but more than 80 per cent of scoliosis cases have no explanation or origin. This idiopathic scoliosis 'just happens'. Most of the time, it presents itself in childhood between ages 10 and 15, but it can develop as we grow older. Or it can go undetected in childhood and then become obvious and problematic as we grow older.

Scoliosis runs in families, and it occurs equally in males and females. Nonetheless, females are seven to nine times more likely to have a severe curve that progresses more aggressively and that will require some sort of intervention. No one is really certain why this happens.

Several types of scoliosis can develop.

The C-shaped curves. Scoliosis, if serious and untreated, can pull the rib cage out of its normal position, compressing and crowding the ribs on the inside of the curve and pulling apart the ribs on the outside of the curve. If the C-shaped right thoracic curve shifts the ribs on the right side, it can constrict the heart and lungs. Breathing is difficult. Or if the C-shape is lower – in the lumbar region – it can distort the hips. Extreme curves can certainly make some activities difficult and most others painful.

The S-shaped curves. The most common S-shaped curve is a double curve – a combination of major curves. One will distort the thoracic spine and the chest, and the other, going the other way, will distort the lumbar spine and hips. Although this sounds horrendous – and it can be – generally the two curves in opposition sort of balance each other out and cause less deformity.

The rotation phenomenon. Another problem with serious, uncorrected scoliosis is that as the spine grows and develops, the forces of the scoliosis cause it to rotate on its own axis. This rotation eventually pulls the rib cage around so that one side of the rib cage appears higher than the other in the back. While that's going on, the ribs on the

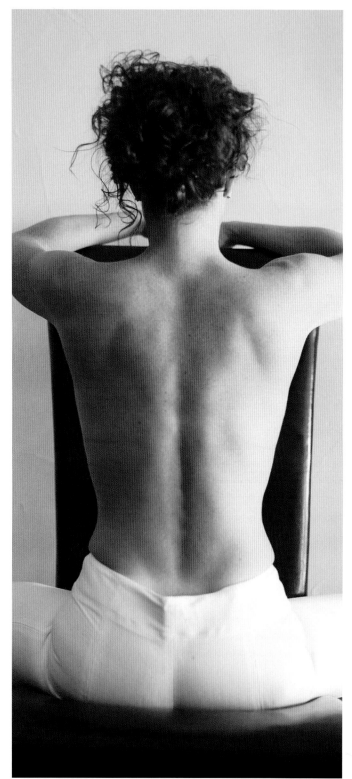

▲ The spine
A healthy spine like this appears to be a straight line up and down, but curvature of the spine probably indicates scoliosis, which can be confirmed by an X-ray.

inward side of the rotation are bunched together and the ribs on the outward side are spread. Ultimately, this can contribute to respiratory difficulty and cardiac problems later in life.

Neuromuscular scoliosis. When scoliosis is present in children with other neuromuscular disorders (these may include spina bifida, muscular dystrophies, spinal cord injuries), the scoliosis is called neuromuscular scoliosis. As children with this condition grow and their trunks become weaker, the scoliosis worsens from progressive deformity and collapse of the spine. Neuromuscular scoliosis always requires medical and surgical intervention.

Congenital scoliosis. If a child is born with scoliosis, the culprit is a malformation of the vertebrae. This form of scoliosis is frequently accompanied by other physical abnormalities in systems that develop in the foetus at about the same time the spinal column is forming, such as urinary anamolies. It's also possible that a birth defect may cause an imbalance in the way the spine grows, causing it to become crooked as the child matures.

Under these circumstances, scoliosis can be a serious matter. Treatment options in these cases are strictly medical and surgical.

In most cases of scoliosis, the curve tends to be minimal and causes no real problems, and rarely is it painful. But the condition should be handled when your child is young, because the curve can become more pronounced in adulthood and cause all sorts of problems. (If you notice any pain or loss of function, the condition warrants serious and immediate attention.)

Once the scoliosis is confirmed by X-ray, it's often appropriate to take a 'wait and see' approach, especially if the angle of the curve is not severe (less than 20 degrees). Some curves never progress beyond a few degrees, while others increase rapidly. Researchers have not been able to determine why these differences exist.

Whether or not your child's doctor will advise treatment will also depend on the child's developmental stage of growth. An 18-year-old girl whose doctor discovers scoliosis during a physical is already mature skeletally. Major changes in the curve are not likely to happen. If she has been symptom-free, the doctor will probably not recommend intervention. On the other hand, a five-year-old girl who has not yet reached peak maturity might be a candidate for intervention.

What You Can Do

Before you panic about your child, first go through this checklist of early-warning signs of the condition:

- Shoulders are of different heights.
- One shoulder blade appears more prominent than the other.
- Hipbones or waistline are uneven.
- Bottoms of each sides of the rib cage don't line up.
- Body leans to one side.
- Head appears to be off centre with the pelvis.
- One arm appears longer than the other.
- Hemlines of skirts and trousers are uneven.
- When the child bends over, ribs form a hump on one side.
- Head appears to be tilted.

Another option is to do a home version of the nurse's office test, officially called 'Adam's Forward-Bend Test'. Have your child wear a tight T-shirt or no shirt at all, and stand directly behind him. Have him put his feet together, and with his back straight, have him bend from the waist 90 degrees. His torso will be parallel with the floor. Look straight over his back, and you'll be able to see if it's even and symmetrical. If it's not, then you might suspect scoliosis.

In our clinic, we've frequently found scoliosis to be nothing more than the result of a compensation by the body to bring itself back into balance when one side of the back is weaker than the other. When the doctor has ruled out neuromuscular scoliosis or congenital scoliosis, we take over. As long as most doctors take a 'wait and see' attitude with scoliosis, why not try a few things?

When the body is out of balance, one side is weak, and the other side is constricted from trying to bring the body into alignment and balance. Muscles work in pairs. When one flexes, the other elongates. Scoliosis can be a battle of muscle pairs. By strengthening weak muscles and relaxing and elongating constricted ones, we are frequently able to correct scoliosis.

By the time scoliosis has set in, the child may have a lot of muscular and connective tissue imbalances and weaknesses, so correction is not instantaneous. Old habits are hard to break – even at the cellular level. Use the complete Active-Isolated programme to restore structural integrity, and build new neural patterns so that the body will know how it's supposed to align. Then make sure everything is strong and flexible enough to sustain the new positions. Small results are nearly immediate, but full correction does take time.

DIAGNOSIS: SPONDYLOLISTHESIS

In some people, the architecture of the individual vertebra is defective. When the bone on the back of a vertebra is deformed, it's possible for the vertebra to move forwards out of alignment. This migrating vertebra may tease the vertebrae above it out of alignment as well, setting off a cascade of discomfort.

Spondylolisthesis can result in sciatica, lower-back pain that travels through the hips and buttocks to the thighs. Athletes who bear weight and torque in their backs – such as American football players, weight lifters and javelin throwers – appear to be prone to this condition. Degenerative spondylolisthesis is deformation of the architecture of the vertebrae due to wear and tear that erodes the facet joints between the bones. At particular risk are people with diabetes, who are four times more likely to develop degenerative spondylolisthesis than the average person. Among our patients, it's not uncommon for a person to have spondylolisthesis and scoliosis (curvature of the spine) at the same time.

What You Can Do

Because spondylolisthesis deforms the spine and is sometimes accompanied by scoliosis, it's important for you to begin stretching out your body immediately. You need to relax and restore circulation to the muscles and soft tissues that surround your lower back, and generally to strengthen your body and bring it back into balance.

Drink plenty of water to make sure you're always hydrated. Take a mild non-steroidal anti-inflammatory (such as ibuprofen or naproxen) to get the pain under control so that movement is tolerable.

Start with stretching. Do 10 repetitions of each described opposite. Soreness, unfortunately, can be accompanied by slight swelling that can impede range of motion and make working out uncomfortable. Move slowly and very gently and in the smallest ranges of motion. At no time should a movement hurt. Ice your back for 10 minutes to soothe the area. Then stretch again. You can repeat the stretch-ice-stretch sequence several times or until the pain eases and you feel that you've restored range of motion, even to the smallest extent.

Also, take a moment to examine the repetitive movements you make, to see if they may be contributing to your problem. If diabetes is the root cause of your spondylolisthesis, we trust you have a lot of reasons to try to control your weight and manage your condition – consider the relief of your back pain to be another incentive.

TEN EXERCISES FOR SPONDYLOLISTHESIS

1. Single-leg Pelvic Tilts
See complete instructions for this two-step exercise on page 50.

2. Double-leg Pelvic Tilts
See complete instructions for this two-step exercise on page 50.

3. Bent-leg Hamstrings
See complete instructions for this three-step exercise on page 51.

4. Straight-leg Hamstrings
See complete instructions for this two-step exercise on page 51.

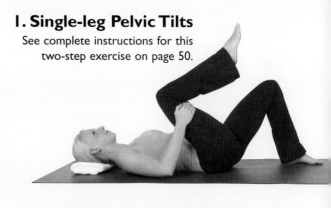

5. Hip Adductors

See complete instructions for this two-step exercise on page 52.

8. Quadriceps

See complete instructions for this three-step exercise on page 53.

6. Hip Abductors

See complete instructions for this two-step exercise on page 52.

9. Gluteals

See complete instructions for this two-step exercise on page 54.

10. Piriformis

See complete instructions for this four-step exercise on page 54.

7. Psoas

See complete instructions for this two-step exercise on page 53.

DIAGNOSIS: SPONDYLOSIS

Spondylosis is a common degenerative disease of the spine, most likely caused by age-related changes in intervertebral discs. Also called spinal osteoarthritis, the disease may attack the cervical, thoracic or lumbar spine, or a combination of all three.

As we age, the structures of the discs change. The collagen content and water content of the anulus fibrosus (the bands of collagen that encase the gel-like interior of the disc) diminish. The disc actually decreases in height. Without the stability and spongy shock absorption of the anulus fibrosus, the vertebrae become less secure. Also, each vertebra has four facet joints, or hinges, that allow the spine to bend forwards and backwards, rotate, and do all of these in combination. Each of these facet joints is covered with cartilage that allows the bones to glide over each other without grating. Spondylosis causes degradation of cartilage where the vertebrae lay down osteophytes – extra mineralisation in places they perceive to be injured.

These osteophytes – also known as bone spurs – are nasty. Not only do they hurt, they can impede the blood supply to the vertebrae and irritate nerve roots from the spinal cord to the body. As if this isn't bad enough, the ligaments that hold the spine in position, and yet allow it to move, degenerate or thicken and weaken and are no longer able to hold the spine in alignment.

When spondylosis attacks the cervical spine, it's painful. The bone spurs can cause nerve root compression and consequent weakness from your shoulders down through your arms and hands (otherwise known as radiating pain and weakness). In extreme cases, bone spurs at the front of the cervical spine can even interfere with the neural signals that the brain sends to swallow. When spondylosis attacks the thoracic and lumbar spine, it causes pain when you move to bend forwards or backwards. Additionally, the stress and pressure of sitting can cause compression of the lumbar spine, no longer able to absorb and dissipate the forces of your body's weight.

What You Can Do

Although you cannot stop the disease, you can do a lot to make yourself more comfortable. Restore circulation to the muscles and soft tissues that surround your spine and take some of the compression off inflamed nerve roots. It is especially hard to restore circulation to the ligaments, so you must concentrate on restoring circulation to everything that surrounds them. To restore balance to your muscles is going to take time. You have to be diligent and patient.

TEN EXERCISES FOR SPONDYLOSIS

1. Single-leg Pelvic Tilts
See complete instructions for this two-step exercise on page 50.

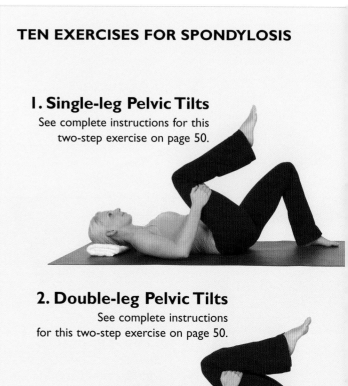

2. Double-leg Pelvic Tilts
See complete instructions for this two-step exercise on page 50.

3. Bent-leg Hamstrings
See complete instructions for this three-step exercise on page 51.

4. Straight-leg Hamstrings
See complete instructions for this two-step exercise on page 51.

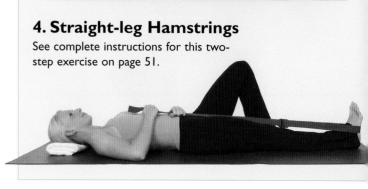

5. Hip Adductors

See complete instructions for this two-step exercise on page 52.

8. Quadriceps

See complete instructions for this three-step exercise on page 53.

6. Hip Abductors

See complete instructions for this two-step exercise on page 52.

9. Gluteals

See complete instructions for this two-step exercise on page 54.

10. Piriformis

See complete instructions for this four-step exercise on page 54.

7. Psoas

See complete instructions for this two-step exercise on page 53.

Drink plenty of water to make sure you're always hydrated. Take a mild non-steroidal anti-inflammatory (such as ibuprofen or naproxen) to ease the pain and make movement and subsequent relaxation easier.

Start with the stretches on pages 152–153. Do 10 repetitions of each. Unfortunately, soreness can be accompanied by slight swelling that can impede range of motion and make exercising uncomfortable. Move slowly and very gently, and in the smallest ranges of motion. At no time should a movement hurt. Ice your back for 10 minutes to soothe the area. Then stretch again. You can repeat the stretch-ice-stretch sequence several times, or until the pain eases and you feel that you've restored range of motion, even to the smallest extent.

The real problem in working out with spondylosis is the bone spurs. They are not only excruciatingly painful, they can impede movement. Actually, they can be a formidable impediment. Our only advice is to do the best you can. Work within the ranges of your own mobility and tolerance for discomfort, but don't push it.

DIAGNOSIS: SPRAIN

Ligaments are cord-like bands in a fibrous sheath that connect bone to bone in your joints. They hold the skeleton together so that joints can move, but ligaments also restrict movement so that joints don't move too much and drop you into a heap on the ground like a rag doll.

When a ligament is injured, the joint it serves is also injured, and its structural integrity and function are compromised. This is called a sprain. The bad news is that if trauma is severe enough to damage a ligament, there is a good chance that the surrounding soft tissue is also damaged.

Sprains can be difficult to heal. Ligaments are connectors; they are fairly free of blood and therefore fairly isolated from the healing powers of circulating blood that brings in oxygen and carries away metabolic waste generated by the injury.

When your back is sprained, the ligaments that hold your vertebrae in alignment are damaged, and pain and dysfunction are the result. As in a strain, doctors view a sprain as possibly overlying more serious injuries, so it's always treated carefully.

What You Can Do

Relax to restore circulation to the muscles and soft tissues that surround your spine and take some of the compression off inflamed nerve roots. It's hard to restore circulation to the ligaments, so you must concentrate on restoring circulation to everything that surrounds them. You have to be diligent and patient.

FOUR EXERCISES FOR LOOSENING A BACK SPRAIN

1. Single-leg Pelvic Tilts
See complete instructions for this two-step exercise on page 50.

2. Double-leg Pelvic Tilts
See complete instructions for this two-step exercise on page 50.

3. Trunk Extensors
See complete instructions for this two-step exercise on page 55.

4. Thoracic-lumbar Rotators
See complete instructions for this four-step exercise on page 56.

Drink plenty of water to make sure you're always hydrated. Take a mild non-steroidal anti-inflammatory (such as ibuprofen or naproxen) to get pain under control so that movement and subsequent relaxation are easier.

We would like to direct you to the entire stretch routine (starting on page 50), but if you can't tackle all of it, start with the few stretches shown opposite to get things moving. Do 10 repetitions of each. Move slowly, gently and in the smallest ranges of motion. At no time should a movement hurt. Ice your back for 10 minutes to soothe the area, then stretch again. You can repeat the stretch-ice-stretch sequence several times, or until the pain eases and you feel that you've restored range of motion, even to the smallest extent.

When you've finished stretching, lie down flat on your back with a towel roll placed at the base of your neck, at your lower back, under the backs of your knees, and under your heels. Position your legs a little higher than your head.

DIAGNOSIS: STRAIN

Strain usually occurs in the lower back in the lumbar region. A strain is an injury characterised by overstretching or tearing of the muscles, tendons or ligaments. You can strain your back by overuse, such as when you rake leaves all day when you're out of shape, or by trauma, such as when you lift something too heavy.

Your back muscles are among the largest in the body, and the erector spinae muscle group runs from the bottom of your lower lumbar spine all the way to the base of your head. This muscle group works in perfect concert to keep you standing upright and allows you to bend forwards and backwards, and rotate. To keep the erector spinae from fatiguing (because it's always on duty), the individual components of the group trade off functions, firing in sequence to keep you upright and moving seamlessly.

When the erector spinae is strained, the group can't function properly, and nearly every move can be painful. The erector spinae isn't the only vulnerable muscle group. Another is the psoas, which runs through the pelvis. If it's strained, its dysfunction places incredible exertion on the lumbar spine. Your doctor knows that a strain sometimes overlies a more serious injury, such as a disc injury that's not yet evident, so caution is always advised.

What You Can Do

Most strains heal completely. Focus on relaxing and restoring circulation to the muscles and soft tissues that surround your spine and taking some of the compression off inflamed nerve roots. Drink plenty of water to make sure you're hydrated. Take a mild non-steroidal anti-inflammatory (such as ibuprofen or naproxen) to control the pain and make movement and relaxation easier.

▼ Strain
Pulling on the same muscle repeatedly while lifting, pulling or playing sport can result in a lower back strain.

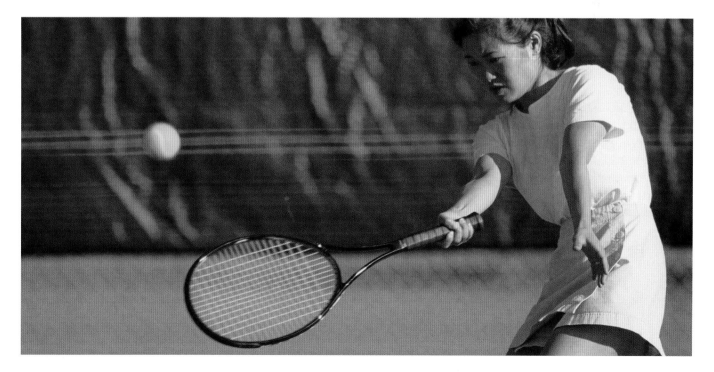

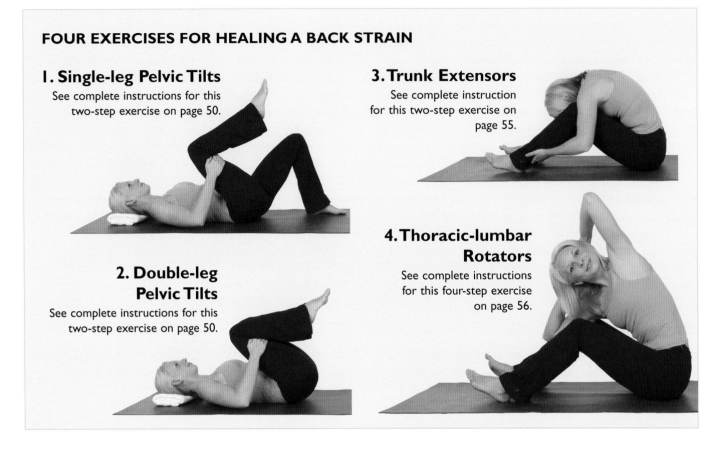

FOUR EXERCISES FOR HEALING A BACK STRAIN

1. Single-leg Pelvic Tilts
See complete instructions for this two-step exercise on page 50.

2. Double-leg Pelvic Tilts
See complete instructions for this two-step exercise on page 50.

3. Trunk Extensors
See complete instruction for this two-step exercise on page 55.

4. Thoracic-lumbar Rotators
See complete instructions for this four-step exercise on page 56.

Start with the stretches shown above, following the same advice given for Sprain on page 155 regarding repetitions and subsequent stretching.

DIAGNOSIS: STRESS FRACTURE

Normal bone is a dynamic organ that continuously remodels itself. As needed, it deposits minerals called osteoblasts, and reabsorbs minerals called osteoclasts. Bone reacts to stress by increasing density, or laying down osteoblasts to fortify the site of stress and make it stronger.

But there's a limit to how much deposit a bone can lay down. When stress (continued and repeated trauma to the same site on the bone) exceeds the bone's ability to regenerate, reabsorption occurs faster than the rebuilding. The results are microfractures of the trabecular layer of the bone, the inner layer. If the forces and stresses continue, eventually the fracture deepens to the cortical bone. When the cortical bone is cracked, it's called a stress fracture. If the stress continues, a full-blown fracture can occur.

Two types of stress fracture have been identified: *fatigue* fractures in which normal, healthy bone is exposed to continued stress (like distance running) until it cracks, and *insufficiency* fractures in which porous, unhealthy bone cracks under normal stress (like osteoporosis, bone cysts, osteoid osteoma or malignancies such as osteosarcoma).

The pelvis and sacrum are vulnerable sites for fatigue fractures in distance runners. A stress fracture, however, can be a big warning sign, an intermediate step between bone bruising (made up of multiple microfractures of the outer layer of the bone) and a full fracture. For example, an insufficiency fracture in a person with osteoporosis could be the precursor to compression fractures of the vertebrae, femoral neck fractures and fractures of the sacrum. Obviously, a stress fracture is a sign that your body is being taxed – be sure to get a bone scan to see where your particular problem may lie.

What You Can Do

A stress fracture is a break in the bone. It's important to let it heal with rest. Work around the injury site with stretching and strengthening so that your body doesn't deteriorate and you have plenty of circulation, but stay away from the stress fracture.

To help healing, start with drinking plenty of water to make sure you're hydrated. Take a mild non-steroidal anti-inflammatory (such as ibuprofen or naproxen) to lessen the pain so that movement and subsequent relaxation are easier.

Check with your doctor before doing any exercise. Show him the photos of the specific exercises you intend to do. If you do stretch, do so slowly and very gently. Small movements add up fast. Be patient. At no time should a movement hurt. Ice your back for 10 minutes to soothe the area. Then stretch again. You can repeat the stretch-ice-stretch sequence several times, or until the pain eases and you feel that you've restored range of motion to the smallest extent. Above all, stay off the stress fracture.

DIAGNOSIS: WHIPLASH

Whiplash is an injury often associated with car accidents. When a car is struck from behind, the passengers' heads in the front car are snapped forwards and backwards in an action very similar to that of a whip. Unfortunately, wearing a seat belt makes no difference.

The word whiplash (not actually an officially recognised medical diagnosis) describes a hyperextension-hyperflexion injury of the neck. When the head, which weighs about 8lb (3.6kg) in an adult, is suddenly jerked forwards and backwards beyond the limits of the neck's support, the neck muscles and connective tissues can be strained, sprained or torn. In extreme cases, the discs between the vertebrae can suddenly herniate (also called slipped disc or bulging disc).

Herniation occurs when the neck is snapped so explosively that the outer band of the disc bursts, allowing the soft, gel-like, inner pulp to escape. That pulp can press against the spinal cord, causing extreme pain, nerve disruption and coordination problems. In less severe cases, the escaped pulp can compress nerve roots. When the herniation or rupture is in the cervical spine, you will feel pain and numbness in the neck, shoulders, arms and hands. You might appear to be fine with no serious injury, but traumatised muscles can soon tighten up.

Either way, tightened muscles can cause huge problems, starting with headaches. Also common are back spasms of overtaxed muscles that are trying to compensate for a neck that appears to be out of balance. At its very worst, whiplash can cause a brain injury.

What You Can Do

When they're caused by whiplash, injuries of the neck can be tricky. The problem is that the jolt of impact shocks your entire body, and you have to relax it in sequence, working from the lower back up to the neck. If you unlock only your neck, the traumatised muscles and structures below will soon pull it back into misalignment. You need to relax and restore circulation to the muscles and soft tissues that surround your lower back and then work towards your neck.

Drink plenty of water to make sure you're always hydrated. Take a mild non-steroidal anti-inflammatory (such as ibuprofen or naproxen) to get pain under control so that movement and subsequent relaxation are easier.

Stretch, using the sequence on pages 158–159. Do 10 repetitions of each exercise. Move slowly, gently and in the smallest ranges of motion. At no time should a movement hurt. Ice your back for 10 minutes to soothe the area. Then stretch again. You can repeat the stretch-ice-stretch sequence several times, or until the pain eases and you feel that you've restored range of motion, even to the smallest extent.

The stretching sequence for whiplash is designed in a specific order to relax muscles in the lumbar region first, then the neck. One day of work will not alleviate the problem, but patience will rewarded. Stop all stretches short of pain.

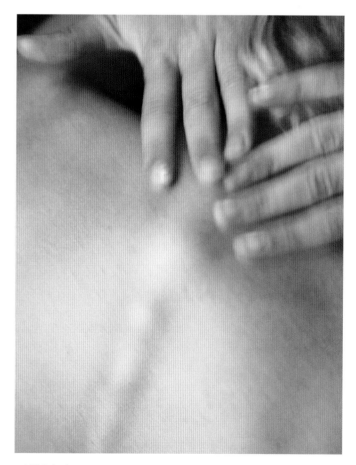

▲ Whiplash
This injury, caused by the head suddenly jerking forwards and backwards beyond the limit of the neck's support, is not only very painful but can cause headaches and back spasms.

NINE EXERCISES FOR WHIPLASH, STARTING FROM THE LOWER BACK

1. Single-leg Pelvic Tilts
See complete instructions for this two-step exercise on page 50.

2. Double-leg Pelvic Tilts
See complete instructions for this two-step exercise on page 50.

3. Bent-leg Hamstrings
See complete instructions for this three-step exercise on page 51.

4. Straight-leg Hamstrings
See complete instructions for this two-step exercise on page 51.

5. Hip Adductors
See complete instructions for this two-step exercise on page 52.

6. Hip Abductors
See complete instructions for this two-step exercise on page 52.

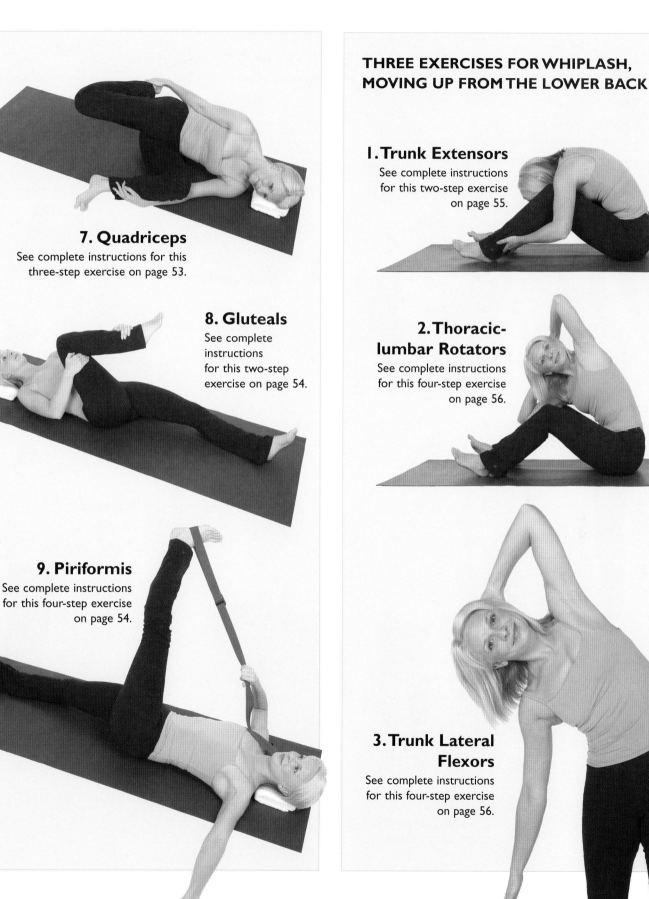

7. Quadriceps

See complete instructions for this three-step exercise on page 53.

8. Gluteals

See complete instructions for this two-step exercise on page 54.

9. Piriformis

See complete instructions for this four-step exercise on page 54.

THREE EXERCISES FOR WHIPLASH, MOVING UP FROM THE LOWER BACK

1. Trunk Extensors

See complete instructions for this two-step exercise on page 55.

2. Thoracic-lumbar Rotators

See complete instructions for this four-step exercise on page 56.

3. Trunk Lateral Flexors

See complete instructions for this four-step exercise on page 56.

NINE EXERCISES FOR WHIPLASH, MOVING TOWARDS THE NECK

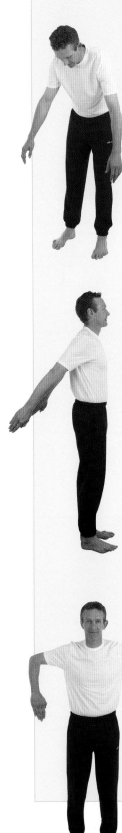

1. Shoulder Circumduction

See complete instructions for this three-step exercise on page 60.

2. Pectoralis Majors

See complete instructions for this two-step exercise on page 60.

3. Anterior Deltoids

See complete instructions for this three-step exercise on page 61.

4. Shoulder Internal Rotators

See complete instructions for this three-step exercise on page 62.

5. Shoulder External Rotators

See complete instructions for this three-step exercise on page 62.

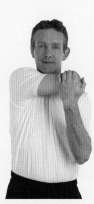

6. Rotator Cuff 1

See complete instructions for this two-step exercise on page 63.

7. Rotator Cuff 2

See complete instructions for this three-step exercise on page 63.

8. Forward Elevators of the Shoulder

See complete instructions for this three-step exercise on page 64.

9. Side Elevators of the Shoulder

See complete instructions for this two-step exercise on page 64.

TWO EXERCISES FOR WHIPLASH, FOCUSING ON THE NECK

1. Neck Extensors
See complete instructions for this three-step exercise on page 65.

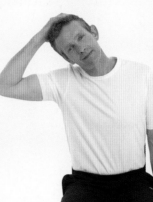

2. Neck Lateral Flexors
See complete instructions for this three-step exercise on page 65.

FOUR EXERCISES FOR WHIPLASH, KEEPING EVERYTHING LOOSE

1. Rotator Cuff 1
See complete instructions for this two-step exercise on page 63.

3. Neck Extensors
See complete instructions for this three-step exercise on page 65.

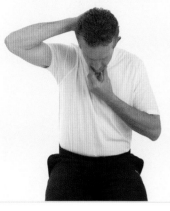

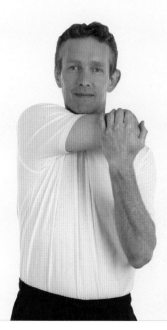

2. Rotator Cuff 2
See complete instructions for this three-step exercise on page 63.

4. Neck Lateral Flexors
See complete instructions for this three-step exercise on page 65.

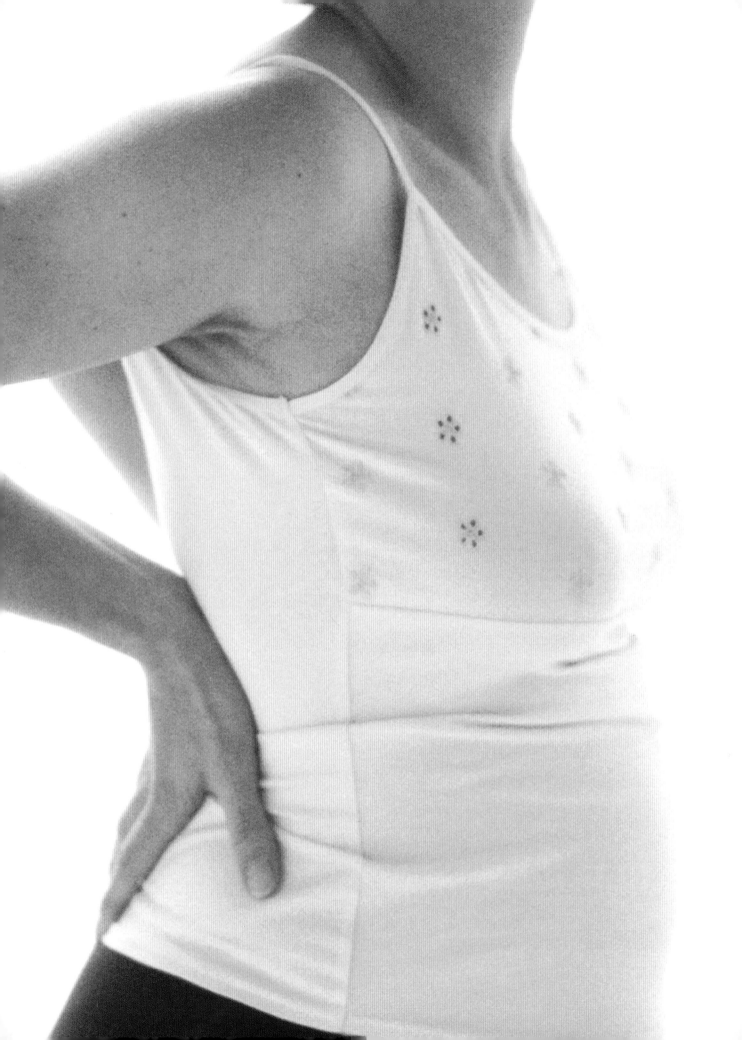

4

PROTECTING YOUR BACK THROUGH LIFE

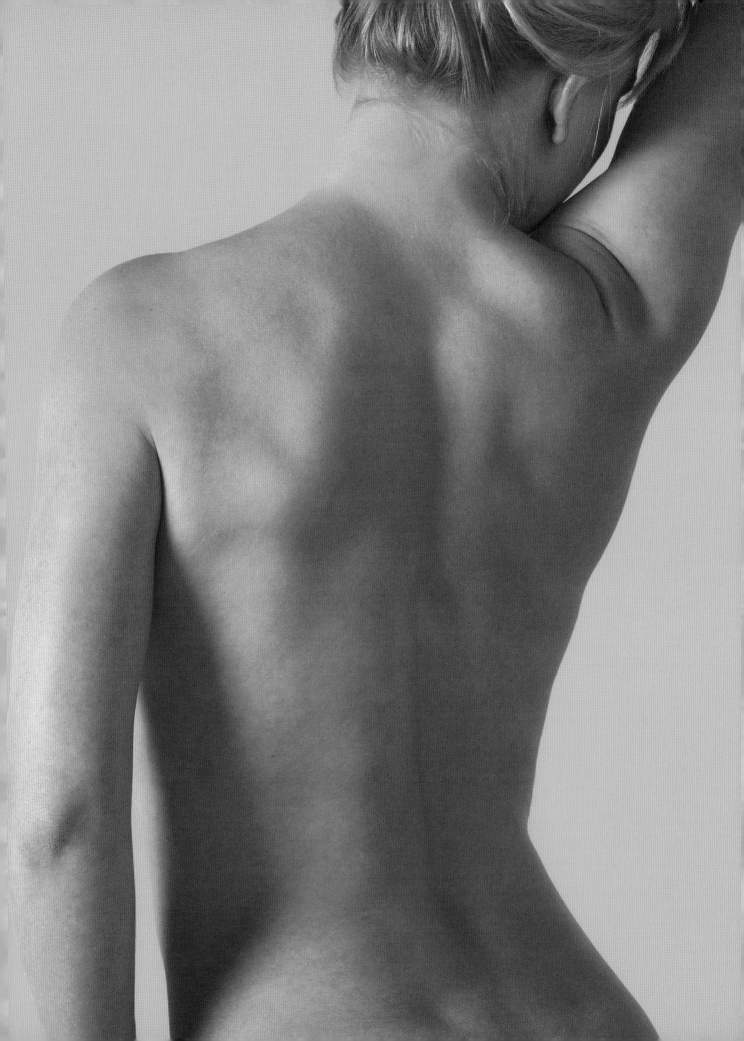

CHAPTER 8

TAKING OFF THE WEIGHT

Over the past two decades or so, obesity in the West *has risen dramatically and has been identified conclusively as a strong risk factor for some well-known killers, including cardiovascular disease, cancer, high blood pressure, strokes and endocrine disorders. What has not been as well-publicised is the link between excess weight and back pain – extra weight is really tough on the spine.*

In 2002, results of a study conducted by Dartmouth Medical School in New Hampshire, United States, conclusively linked obesity to back problems. Nearly 16,000 patients with spine disease were evaluated to determine the association between obesity and their health status. One theory suggested that the weight and bulk of the obese body placed abnormal mechanical loads on the spine. Another study looked at whether an initial injury to the spine leads to a sedentary lifestyle, which leads to obesity. The researchers concluded that while other factors may make spinal conditions worse, obesity is the only factor that can be changed relatively simply, either through diet, exercise and behaviour therapy, or, in more extreme cases, through surgery and medications. In fact, the Dartmouth researchers state, 'It is conceivable that as a patient's obesity improved, functioning and symptoms would also improve.'

In our experience, we can tell you that it is almost guaranteed.

Extra weight has to be supported by the spine. When you're too heavy, that weight puts extra compression on the discs in your spine. In addition, every time you bend or rotate, your spine has to help you support and balance against more weight than it was designed to handle. For example, if you have excess fat in your abdomen in the form of a potbelly, you're carrying too much weight forwards, forcing your back to sway to counterbalance to keep you upright. The strain can be enormous and can lead to muscular dysfunction as your body compensates for the overload. Some muscles will overdevelop. Some will weaken. The net effect is a body that can't work properly, and things start to go wrong over time. And it's not only the upper body that is affected: this compression caused by excess weight also has an effect lower down, with pressure put on the knees and ankles.

Being too heavy affects the arches of your feet. They can no longer work as shock absorbers to put spring into your step. When your arches are flattened under crushing weight with each foot fall, your ankles roll to the inside, throwing off the alignment of your knees. Shortly, the insides of your knees strain and weaken, transmitting the misalignment to your hips. The hips transmit it directly to your back.

Fat gets in the way of range of motion. Heavy and encased in bulky padding, it's hard to move. We have heavy clients who can't touch their knees when they first come to us. It's not that they have no flexibility. That might well be the case, but we'll not know that for a while because they have so much body fat that they can't reach around it. This immobilisation that creeps in as weight creeps up has a nasty double effect. The less you can move, the more sedentary you become. The more sedentary you are, the less able you are to burn calories – and the more easily you gain weight. Before you know it, you're in real trouble.

Being overweight puts your heart and lungs into constant overdrive. The additional weight gives your body extra tissue that still demands circulation and oxygen, which your heart and lungs must work extra hard to provide. One of the treadmill tests we use to determine cardiovascular fitness, the VO_2 max, is a sort of stress test to measure how much oxygen gets into the bloodstream. With heavy clients, we find that their VO_2 max is significantly lower than that of lean or fit people. Without sufficient oxygen making its way into tissues, and with a heart working far too hard to make up that deficit, the body tires easily. A tired body is a sedentary body. And once again, the more sedentary you are, the less able you are to burn calories and the more easily you gain weight. You're in a full-blown vicious cycle.

Being overweight can be very painful. When your body doesn't work properly, your back hurts. Joints are strained. Soft tissue is torn. Muscles are brutalised. Effort is agonising. Systems break down. Healing is difficult. Medical treatment is difficult. Therapy is difficult. Surgery is difficult, even dangerous. But almost more than all that, being overweight – even moderately so – can also be emotionally painful.

We want to help you get a grip on your love handles right now. The longer you wait, the harder it is to get control. Middle-age spread is one of the very real challenges of growing older. As we age, our metabolism – the rate at which our bodies burn calories – naturally slows.

As we get older, our metabolic rate starts to decrease by about two per cent per decade. By age 80, you're burning 200 fewer calories every day than you did when you were 30. It is therefore harder to lose weight the older we become. Regular exercise, along with a healthy diet, becomes increasingly important.

EXERCISE IS THE ANSWER

'I've put on weight! Time to go on a diet.'

These familiar-sounding words signal your best intentions and the primary reason for your downfall.

When you drop your calorie intake quickly or dramatically, your body is programmed to interpret your new diet as pending starvation and slows down to hang on to fat stores. The theory goes that each time you attempt a diet and drop your calorie count, your body gets even more efficient at triggering 'conservation mode', resulting in an uphill battle against a slower metabolism. You might gain that weight back quickly, and, even worse, gain back more than you lost.

So you try again. And again. It's this cycle of losing and gaining that we call yo-yo dieting. We have the secret that will help you succeed this time: exercise.

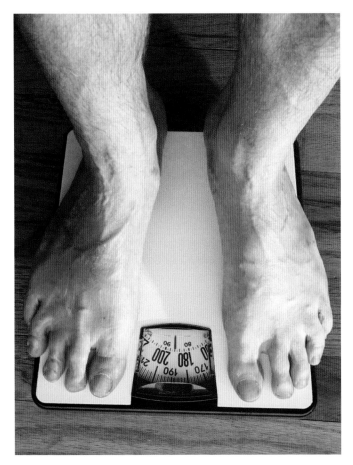

▲ Weight-watching
The more weight you put on, the more strain you will be putting on your back and joints. It is very important to keep exercising to avoid further weight gain and possible serious health problems.

How Does Exercise Control Weight?

Don't just take our word for it. Here are 10 proven ways in which exercise helps you shed weight and then keep it off. It is a more healthy and predictable method than cutting calories.

■ **Exercise burns the right kind of calories.** These calories come from two different sources: glycogen, made from converted sugars and stored in the muscles and the liver; and fat, stored in the fat cells.

During high-intensity exercise, you burn mostly glycogen; during low-intensity exercise, such as walking (suggested for the cardio portion of the Active-Isolated method), you burn mostly fat. A good rule of thumb is that if you can talk while you're exercising, you're burning more fat than glycogen. If you can't gasp out a word, you're burning more glycogen.

As you adapt to a training programme and you get stronger and fitter, the effort you exert drops. In other words, a previously tough workout gradually becomes easier. And – voilà! – your body goes back to burning fat as its primary fuel source. The workout programme that will work for you is in chapter 4.

■ **Exercise builds muscle.** Muscle cells are eight times more metabolically active than fat cells. The more lean muscle mass you have, the higher the demand for energy, the more efficiently you burn calories, and the faster you dip into and reduce fat stores. For every 1lb (455g) of muscle you add, you burn an average of 50 to 100 calories every day.

■ **Exercise increases fat-burning enzymes.** Muscles contain enzymes that burn only fat. Research has demonstrated that regular exercisers, as opposed to sedentary people, have developed muscles with more fat-burning enzymes. The more enzymes you have, the more fat you burn.

■ **Exercise helps build and maintain healthy bones, muscles and connective tissues.** When your body feels stronger, your body movements will be more fluid and seem more natural. Feeling great in your own skin is the best incentive to exercise – and once you make that connection, you'll understandably become more active and burn more calories.

■ **Exercise helps control blood pressure.** When your blood pressure is lower, you'll feel better able to be more active. As your activity level increases, you'll burn more calories, and your weight will drop even faster.

■ **Exercise helps regulate appetite.** Even though one might assume that a good workout would work up an appetite, the opposite is true. Exercise helps keep cravings and overeating in check.

■ **Exercise changes your body's fat-storing chemistry.** When the body is sedentary, it lowers its metabolism to conserve energy. Unfortunately, stored energy is fat. When the body is active, hormones signal a release of energy, so working out can help boost your fat-burning potential by improving the profiles of many hormones related to fat storage, such as insulin, adrenaline and cortisol.

■ **Exercise is physically addictive.** When exercise is intense, your body releases endorphins, chemicals that enhance a sense of well-being, and reduce stress. This encourages you to continue exercising.

■ **Exercise helps you sleep better.** When you're rested, you have more energy to be more active. When you're more active, you burn more calories.

■ **Exercise increases your motivation to eat well.** Once you've started to exercise and treat your body better, you'll be less likely to treat it poorly by polluting it with junk foods. Getting active brings great joy to your life. Once you've had a little taste of the fun of fitness, you're less likely to backslide.

THE 'SHED FAT, SPARE YOUR BACK' PLAN

We've sold you, right? You're ready to take responsibility for your back pain and start putting your body's health first.

First, it's time to set some goals. Read 'How Much Should I Weigh?' (see opposite) to learn more about your ultimate goal. Know that the most long-lasting, safest weight loss is an average of 1–2lb (455–910g) a week.

Then, work on getting your diet in line with your active lifestyle. Turn to page 170 and read 'Eating to Maximise Your Exercise'.

And finally, our favourite part – exercise. You already have the best plan for all of your needs: Active-Isolated Stretching to get your back out of immediate pain and increase your flexibility, Active-Isolated Strengthening to rebuild your muscles and prevent pain in the future, and cardio training to rev up that fat-burning engine to banish that extra weight forever. Turn to chapter 4 and get started today. (In order to get your calorie-burning activity ramped up right away, feel free to begin the cardio portion of the programme at the same time you begin Phase 1. Simply add one 20-minute walk three times a week. By the time

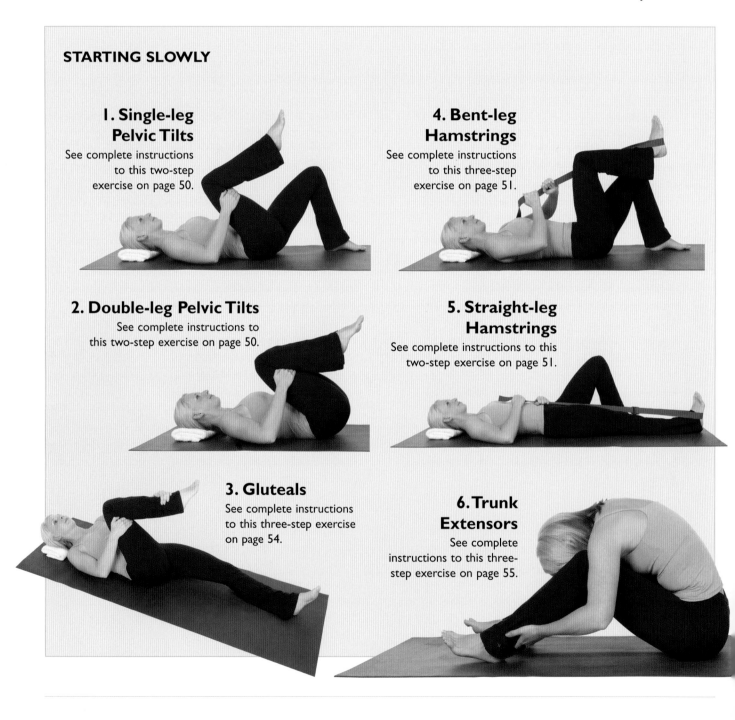

STARTING SLOWLY

1. Single-leg Pelvic Tilts
See complete instructions to this two-step exercise on page 50.

2. Double-leg Pelvic Tilts
See complete instructions to this two-step exercise on page 50.

3. Gluteals
See complete instructions to this three-step exercise on page 54.

4. Bent-leg Hamstrings
See complete instructions to this three-step exercise on page 51.

5. Straight-leg Hamstrings
See complete instructions to this two-step exercise on page 51.

6. Trunk Extensors
See complete instructions to this three-step exercise on page 55.

you get to the Advanced phase, you will be light years ahead of where you began, and you can step up your cardio training with confidence.) And, as always, check with your doctor before beginning any exercise programme.

In the beginning, we realise that any extra weight will put more strain on your lower back, hips, legs and feet. In that case, you may need to start with baby steps.

If you need to start slowly, try out the exercises on the opposite page for 30 days, or until you feel comfortable beginning the full programme.

How Much Should I Weigh?

We have a confession to make: what you weigh is unimportant. It's true. Keep your scales if you like, but pay very little attention to them on a daily basis.

The truth is that you need to be concerned with how much fat you're carrying in relation to your total weight. Determining your exact body composition will take the assistance of a health-care professional using skin-fold calipers or one of the high-tech electronic measuring devices, but you can get a general idea about whether you are fat or lean by calculating your body mass index

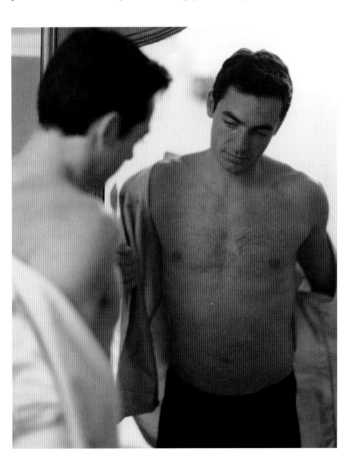

How to Find Your Body Mass Index

To calculate your body mass index (BMI), divide your weight in kilograms by your height in metres squared. So, for example, if you weigh 65kg and you are 1.7m tall, that will be 65 divided by 1.7, divided by 1.7, which equals a BMI of 22.5.

BMI	Risk
Below 19	Minimal
19–24.9	Low
25–29.9	Moderate
30–34.9	High
35–39.9	Very High
40 and above	Extremely High

(BMI), a ratio between your height and weight, with a formula that correlates with body fat (see above).

The higher the BMI, the greater the risk of cardiovascular diseases, cancer, high blood pressure, strokes, endocrine disorders and back pain. Having a low ratio is important for your health. It is generally recognised by the medical profession that adults with a BMI of over 25 should get their weight under control.

Where you carry your weight is important, too. 'Apple-shaped' people, who carry their weight around their waistlines, are at greater risk of weight-related disease than 'pear-shaped' people, who carry their weight on their hips, buttocks and thighs. This is because in pear-shaped people, their weight is not concentrated around the major internal organs, whereas in apple-shaped people, it is. Also, if your weight is in your abdomen, your back is more likely to be affected sooner than if the weight is distributed lower down your body. If you're a woman with a waist measurement over 35in (89cm) or a man with a waist measurement over 40in (102cm), you are at greater risk of back problems and other diseases associated with excess body fat. No matter where you fall in the fruit basket, if you're overweight, you need to deal with it. Now.

◀ It's your fat-to-weight ratio that counts
If you feel you are too heavy, you may not necessarily have a weight problem. It is how much weight you are carrying in relation to your height that is significant.

EATING TO MAXIMISE YOUR EXERCISE

We would never say that we're the ultimate authorities on diet (registered dietitians are your best bet there), but we have seen our athletes achieve medal-worthy bodies with some very simple strategies. Here are some of the best.

Keep a diary. A wise psychologist once told us, 'Obsession will be served'. If you eat some foods obsessively, when you try to cut them out or down, it is vital to replace them with foods that you will be able to keep eating – in other words, you have to replace the 'obsessions' with foods sufficiently enjoyable to fill the void. We have found that keeping a simple diary will help to keep your mind focused.

Write down everything you eat, recording at what time you ate and how you felt. If you're able to do so, use food labels and calorie counters to track your approximate calories. Several studies have found that keeping track of your daily food intake is the best predictor of success with an eating plan. Add that diary to your training log (see page 93), and you'll have a complete record of all your hard work – something to be very proud of.

Understanding what calories really mean. Technically, a calorie is the amount of heat needed to raise the temperature of one gram of water by one degree Celsius. This is hardly critical information, but it does lead us to the purpose of calories. Muscles are like furnaces. They convert calories into fuel to rev up those furnaces so that they can manufacture energy. So to describe calories in terms of heat is logical.

Not all foods deliver the same measure of calories. Simple carbohydrates (such as sugars) and complex carbohydrates (such as starches) have four calories per gram. Proteins (such as meat, milk and eggs) also have four calories per gram. And fat (such as lard) has nine calories per gram. And not all calories are equal. Some (such as spinach) deliver energy and are dense in nutrients. And others (such as beer) are 'empty' calories – they deliver the energy but have no nutritional value.

One pound (455g) of fat represents 3,500 calories of unused energy. If you consume 3,500 more calories than you need, you'll gain 1lb (455g) of fat. If you burn 3,500 more calories than you consume, you'll lose 1lb (455g) of fat. Food in, food out – it's that simple.

Know approximately how many calories you need. As we discussed earlier, consuming too few calories slows down your metabolism. When trying to lose weight, it's smarter to inch back on calories, but not too far. If you can keep your calories high enough to prevent your metabolism from dropping into 'starvation mode', you can burn through the calories you consume during your meal and then start depleting fat storage. And even better, you can kick up your metabolism with exercise to burn even more calories and deplete even more fat. Eating nutrient-rich foods gives you the energy to do that.

Know what food is – and what it is not. Food is fuel. Repeat after us: food is fuel. Food is *not* comfort, although it can be comforting. Food is *not* entertainment, although it

Daily Calorie Needs by Height, Weight and Activity Level for 30-Year-Old Adults

These dietary guidelines estimate daily energy requirements for people around age 30 of various sizes and levels of activity. Use this table as a loose guideline, as most of us are beyond age 30 and thus will burn fewer calories per day. You may be surprised just how few calories your body needs when you don't exercise, and, conversely, how much more you can eat when you do.

Height	Weight	Women Active	Sedentary	Men Active	Sedentary
5' 1"/1.54m	98–132lb/44–60kg	2,104–2,290 cals	1,688–1,834 cals	2,104–2,290 cals	1,919–2,167 cals
5' 5"/1.64m	Up to 150lb/68kg	2,267–2,477 cals	1,816–1,982 cals	2,490–2,842 cals	2,068–2,349 cals
5' 9"/1.74m	125–169lb/57–77kg	2,434–2,670 cals	1,948–2,134 cals	2,683–3,078 cals	2,222–2,538 cals
6' 1"/1.84m	139–188lb/63–85kg	2,605–2,869 cals	2,083–2,290 cals	2,883–3,325 cals	2,382–2,736 cals

To convert calories to kilojoules, see page 279.

can be entertaining. Food is *not* rest, although it can be rejuvenating. Food is *not* love, although it can evoke a loving memory. Food is fuel. Nothing more.

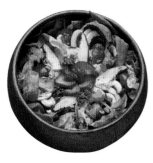

Fall in love with the salad bar. Experts such as dietitians tell us that vibrantly colourful fruits and vegetables are great for you. The brighter and deeper the colour of the fruit or vegetable, the more likely it is to be power-packed with phytochemicals – thousands of compounds that promote good health.

Another good reason to favour fruits and vegetables is that they are relatively low in calories and filled with fibre. Fibre helps control your appetite, aids digestion, and may even whisk a small number of calories out of your body before they can be absorbed.

When eaten in conjunction with other foods, such as whole grains, small amounts of lean protein and some unsaturated fats, it is the answer to a dieter's prayer.

Eat the right kind of fat. The experts recommend that you choose a diet moderate in all fat, but especially low in saturated fat and cholesterol. As odd as it may sound, we do need some fat in our diets. The trick, however, is to know which kind and how much, because not all fat is created equal. Here's a simple explanation.

Unsaturated fats, found mainly in cooking oils, nuts, avocados, salmon and olive oil, are good. They supply energy and essential fatty acids, and they help absorb some fat-soluble vitamins such as A, D, E and K. They don't increase cholesterol. Let's review: unsaturated fat – good.

Saturated fat, on the other hand, is not good. It increases cholesterol and the risk of cardiovascular diseases. This type of fat is found in fatty dairy products, fatty and processed meats, the skin and fat of poultry, lard, palm oil and coconut oil. Saturated fat – bad.

Cholesterol found in food tends to raise the blood level of cholesterol that naturally occurs in our bodies. An overabundance of cholesterol clogs arteries, which is not good. It's found in liver and other organ meats, egg yolks and dairy fats. Cholesterol – bad.

Trans fatty acids tend to raise blood cholesterol. The guilty foods are those high in partially hydrogenated vegetable oils like margarine and shortening, some commercial fried foods and baked foods. Trans fatty acids – bad.

Cleaner House, Trimmer Waist

Exercise doesn't have to be a chore, but a chore can be exercise. We're going to give you a simple system that will knock 15.5lb (7kg) off you in a year without your having to do anything but work around the house and garden.

Burning just 150 calories of extra energy a day will add up to 1,000 calories per week – and it will cut your risk of heart disease by 50 per cent and reduce your risk of high blood pressure, diabetes and colon cancer by 30 per cent. As a big bonus, you'll also help maintain healthy bones, muscles and joints; help control your weight by building lean muscle and reducing body fat; and take the strain of excess weight off your back.

Everyone is a little bit different and attacks a chore with different energy. If you do so with gusto, you'll burn more in an hour than someone who just goes through the motions. The chores we've listed below are designed for a woman who is 50 years old, 5 feet 6 inches (1.68m) tall, and of average weight (150lb/68kg). She is moderately fit, so she's going to fall somewhere in between high and low intensity. These are the times it will take to burn 150 calories for some common household tasks.

- **Chopping wood** 25 minutes
- **Gardening** 25 minutes
- **Heavy housework** 40 minutes
- **Heavy tool work** 20 minutes
- **Laying tile** 35 minutes
- **Light housework** 62 minutes
- **Mopping** 45 minutes
- **Mowing the lawn** 35 minutes
- **Plumbing** 50 minutes
- **Preparing a meal** 1 hour
- **Pushing a pram** 1 hour
- **Raking leaves** 35 minutes
- **Shopping** 1 hour
- **Shovelling snow** 25 minutes
- **Vacuuming** 45 minutes
- **Washing the car** 50 minutes
- **Watching TV** 2 hours, 30 minutes

Go sour on sugar. To most of us, sugar is a flavouring, but it's really a carbohydrate and a source of energy through calories. If you decide to eliminate sugar to save a few calories and substitute another form of sugar, like honey, it won't make any difference. The body can't distinguish between the sugar on your spoon and honey. For that matter, it can't tell the difference between your granulated sugar and the naturally occurring sugars in fruit and milk. It all looks the same chemically. Sugar has no nutritional benefit other than tasting great – and it adds empty calories. If you're wild for dessert, head for fruit.

Put aside your saltcellar. Sodium, the essential component of salt, is necessary for regulating fluid in your body and for maintaining blood pressure. Unfortunately, too much salt causes the body to retain fluid and raises blood pressure. Studies have also demonstrated that too much salt increases the amount of calcium excreted in urine and might increase the risk of osteoporosis. By checking salt labels on foods, you'll start to notice which foods go too far.

Chew your food 25 times before you swallow. Digestion begins in your mouth. Chewing 25 times allows you to mix your food with saliva, an important component in the chemical reactions that break down food, particularly starches. Chewing also slows you down, so that you become mindful of what you're eating, giving your brain and your fork time to catch up to each other. When your brain determines that you've had enough to eat and are full, it signals you to stop eating.

Consider vitamin and mineral supplements. One of the real challenges in cutting calories is to make sure that you still meet your need for nutrients. It's best to get all your nutrients from food, but if this is difficult, then you might want to consider vitamin and mineral supplements. (Read more about vitamin and mineral supplements on page 200.)

Break the caffeine habit. Caffeine is a powerful central nervous system stimulant found in hundreds of foods, beverages and drugs. Although you may be using it to

Case Study: **Bev Browning**

When we met our co-author Bev Browning in the early 1980s, she had just begun to search for a fitness programme that would fit into her busy lifestyle.

Bev had decided to run in a marathon taking place in a year's time. Although an ambitious goal, it was doable as there was the time to train up slowly. But Bev tried to do too much too soon, thinking that running would melt away her excess body fat. Her killer training programme launched without proper preparation meant she was soon hobbled by stress fractures in her shins and a pain in her left hip that translated right up into her lower back. Bev knew what was wrong and asked us to help her correct imbalances in strength and flexibility through a better training programme to prevent further injury and get her out of pain.

We explained to Bev that carrying excess weight (30 per cent body fat) was very hard on her body, but with hand-in-hand diet and exercise, we could lower her weight and increase her mileage.

We gave Bev a stretch rope and a programme for Active-Isolated Stretching with special emphasis on her back, hips and legs. Our dietitian put Bev on a healthy eating plan with reduced calories spread out over all the major food groups.

Bev started dropping weight at the same time she increased flexibility and circulation to her body. Injuries healed slowly but surely. As she became more healthy, she felt stronger in general.

She slept better. She had more energy and confidence.

We then re-evaluated her flexibility and the ranges of motion of her joints. She was lighter, leaner and looser. The pain in her back, hips, legs and feet had subsided almost entirely.

Gradually, we added in Active-Isolated Strengthening. As Bev built muscle, she burnt more body fat and lost more weight. Eventually, Bev returned to running with a tailor-made regimen. She reached 20 per cent body fat, two points below the average for her age and height, and ideal for a marathon runner. She completed that first marathon and now trains others to run them!

feel more alert when you crawl out of bed in the morning, you should consider cutting back. Caffeine makes it more difficult to fall asleep, decreases the time you stay asleep, and diminishes the quality of your sleep. It interferes with calcium absorption and, in doing so, increases the risk of osteoporosis. In addition, caffeine acts as a diuretic, causing dehydration.

Be smart with alcohol. Alcoholic beverages are packed with calories, but contain almost no nutrients. Empty calories, however, can be the least of your worries. Alcohol in excess impairs judgement and increases the risk of high blood pressure, stroke, certain types of cancers, birth defects, cirrhosis of the liver, inflammation of the pancreas and damage to the cardiovascular system and brain. If you're going to drink alcohol, do so moderately.

On a positive note, studies indicate that drinking in moderation might lower risk for coronary artery disease in men over age 45 and women over age 55.

Don't forget to drink. Your body's fluid is a miraculous balancing act between two components: sodium (salt) and water. If your blood is too high in sodium or too low in water, water leaches out of cells all over your body and into your blood to keep it in balance.

When the cells in your hypothalamus (a neural control centre in the brain) become dehydrated, they produce a natural antidiuretic that travels from your brain to your kidneys, telling them to hold on to as much water as they can. You'll be thirsty, and yet you'll retain water. Your hands and feet will swell. You'll be uncomfortable. You'll urinate very little, and the urine will be concentrated and dark in colour. Worst of all, your metabolism will begin to slow down.

Aim to drink 3.5 pints (2 litres) of water a day. Try to get more if you're exercising, living in a hot climate or flying on an aeroplane.

Speak with a dietitian. No amount of general advice could ever compare with the personalised, tailored advice you can get from a dietitian. These professionals can take all of your vital statistics – current weight, lifestyle, activity level, age, health conditions, even food preferences and eating styles – and turn them into a delicious nutrition plan that will help you achieve your goals quickly, easily and, most important, healthily. To find a dietitian in your area, ask your doctor for a referral, or contact the appropriate organisation in your country (see 'Further Resources' on page 276).

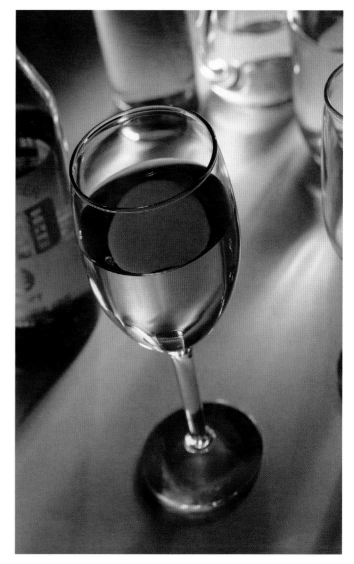

▲ A mixed blessing
Studies now suggest that moderate drinking might lower the risk for coronary heart disease, but drinking in excess increases the risk for many other complaints and is also very dehydrating.

YOUR NEW BODY IS BORN TODAY

Hey, athlete! Yes, you! A healthy body is an energetic body. Properly fuelled, you'll have enough petrol in the tank to get through even the toughest day and still have vigour to work out.

If you're overweight, and your doctor has ruled out medical reasons that are beyond your control as the cause, you now have the tools you need to put together a healthy diet and exercise plan that will get you on your way to a leaner, stronger, healthier body. Eat right, get fit, live long and be happy!

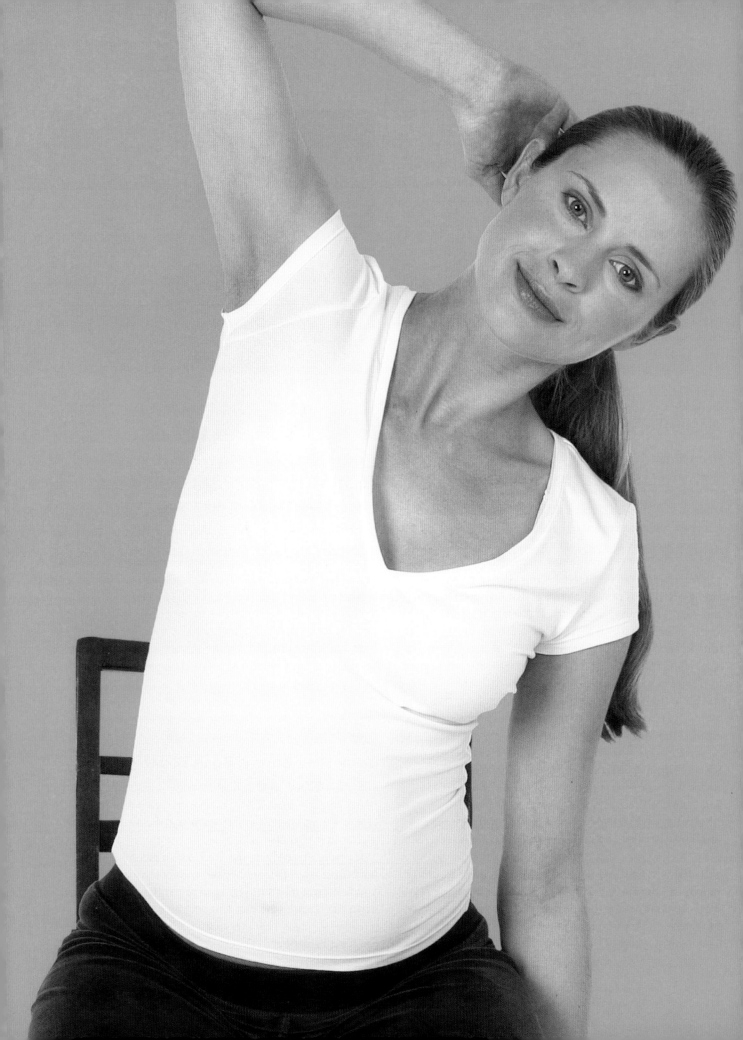

CHAPTER 9

ENJOYING A PAIN-FREE PREGNANCY

At one time, lower-back pain was considered part and *parcel of pregnancy, but today we know that lower-back pain, which can start just before the 12th week and last as long as six months after the baby is born, has specific causes and treatments. With an average weight gain of 25lb/11kg carried in front of the body, pregnancy requires strength and flexibilty to keep a mother-to-be's back healthy.*

We also know that if you had lower-back pain before the pregnancy, there is a pretty high chance that it will continue. Unfortunately, pregnancy isn't well known for making existing physical ailments improve or vanish altogther.

If you are suffering from lower-back pain, you're in good company. Just over half of all pregnant women experience it. Pregnancy is a complex, awe-inspiring miracle but it can be very difficult, so why is lower-back pain the problem? And, more importantly, how can we get you past it?

There are a number of causes. Sports medicine researchers tell us that lower-back pain falls into three categories, each with its own origin. In all cases, resist the urge to self-diagnose and consult your doctor instead.

1. Sacroiliac joint pain. This type of pain starts in the sacrum, where the spinal column joins the pelvis at the lower back. Levels of the hormone relaxin increase, signalling the pelvis to open up to cradle an expanding uterus and to allow safe, unobstructed passage of a child through skeletal structures. The ligaments relax to open the symphysis pubis, that little 'separation' in the front of the pelvic bone, by widening the sacrum.

By the 14th week, when relaxin peaks, there's a noticeable shift. Bones and connective tissue that are usually extremely stable are stretched, which can be painful. Although the pain appears to originate in the sacrum, it can shoot through the buttocks, down the thighs, and all the way down to the middle of the calves. Of all the lower-back problems, sacroiliac joint pain might last the longest and can even outlast the baby's delivery, continuing to plague mum for several months afterwards.

2. Lumbar pain. Non-specific pain in the lower back can have origins in bone, ligament, muscle and tendon; pain is often intensified when mum is lifting something or is seated for a long time. During pregnancy, it could have one of several causes: rapid weight gain; an expanded uterus that moves organs out of position and changes the centre of gravity; or tissues that are stretched to accommodate the expansion. The net effect is pain.

3. Nocturnal pain. This pain is often described as being like a cramp that mysteriously strikes mothers-to-be at night when they should be resting. Some women experience it with sacroiliac pain or lumbar pain; some women experience it exclusively. The source of this particular pain is not clearly understood, but a couple of theories exist. One theory is that nocturnal pain is the result of cumulative fatigue from a hard day of carrying a baby. We think this theory is probably on the mark. The supporting evidence is that a good night's sleep with rest and relaxation will eliminate the pain (until maybe the following evening).

The other theory is that nocturnal pain is caused by a bad positioning in bed. If an expectant mum lies flat on her back with her legs stretched out straight, the weight of the uterus can compress the vena cava – the large veins that run along the spine. In this case, the body will divert blood flow to other veins, increasing venous pressures, and this will cause discomfort. Doctors note that the compression is likely to be accompanied by nausea and dizziness that can be alleviated by shifting position to the side and getting the weight and pressure off the vena cava.

EXERCISE IS GOOD FOR MUM AND BABY

Research over the past 10 years on the physical responses of mothers and unborn children to exercise has significantly increased our understanding of the benefits and risks. Reassuring reports strongly suggest that exercise poses minimal risks for you and your baby and actually may make pregnancy and delivery a lot easier.

According to the Royal College of Obstetricians and Gynaecologists, exercise during pregnancy – within specific limits – can be very good for expectant mothers. Research has found that exercise helps you feel better; gives you

As tempting as it is to climb into a hot bath to relax your back, you should seek comfort elsewhere. Hot baths are dangerous for expectant mums. Overheating your body can be harmful to the well-being of your little one, and you run the risk of becoming dehydrated. It's easy to forget that your body is dissipating heat through sweat even when you're submerged in water. If you think warmth will help you feel better, consider a heating pad if you have your doctor's okay, or more layers of clothing.

energy; improves your mood and sense of well-being; eases some discomforts of pregnancy such as backaches, constipation, bloating, swelling and fatigue; prepares you for the rigours of labour and delivery; improves your sleep; and helps you recover from childbirth more quickly. (No bowl of pickles and ice-cream can do all that!)

But, please, don't use exercise to lose weight during pregnancy. Talk to your doctor about appropriate pregnancy weight parameters, based on your frame, activity level and weight prior to pregnancy.

MODIFYING YOUR WORKOUTS FOR PREGNANCY

As your body changes, you'll begin to notice different ways in which your workouts need to be adjusted. One thing that's working for two is your cardiovascular system. Your oxygen requirements will be higher, so you'll be huffing and puffing sooner than before you were pregnant. Also, remember that when you exercise, extra blood is deployed to your muscles and is less available elsewhere. You don't want to overdo it and end up light-headed.

Surprise! You're heavier and more cumbersome than you're accustomed to being. By the end of pregnancy, some women report gaining 30–50lb/13.5–22.5kg. This extra weight places greater stress on your joints and muscles. Your centre of gravity moves forwards, causing strain in your pelvis and lower back and challenging your balance. Your joints are lax, changing the way your body deals with a little extra tug or pull, and making you more prone to injury. And you may be struggling to overcome generalised fatigue. It's a tiring business. Face it, carrying a baby is hard work by day, and your sleep may well be interrupted at night.

Your body might feel awkward. You might have to compensate for confusing changes. You might not get the results you expect. But exercise – even under these conditions – is good for you. Your baby is floating, suspended in amniotic fluid, and is well-cushioned from your enthusiasm. All you have to do is make sure your workout is safe. Protect your baby and yourself from extreme heat, avoid impact and eat healthy foods in sufficient amounts to supply you and your little one with plenty of nutrients.

Drink as much water as you can. This last tip may seem particularly difficult to follow but it's also one of the most important. An expectant mother may experience difficulty when baby starts to get bigger and seems to be intent on taking over any space formerly enjoyed by the bladder. Additionally, mother's little angel likes to kick and has a canny knack for aiming straight for the bladder, especially when it's full. The effect is frequent and often urgent trips to the bathroom.

If this is happening to you, you might be tempted to reduce your intake of fluids. Not a good idea, especially if you're engaged in any sort of exercise programme. No matter how inconvenient, you must drink water, lots of it, and often. If you feel thirsty, you're already dehydrated.

We also urge you to cut back on caffeinated drinks like tea, coffee and some soft drinks. Caffeinated drinks are wet and may satisfy thirst, but they won't do the job for you and your baby because caffeine is a diuretic.

Your Back Bears the Brunt of the Changes

From the athlete's point of view, a first concern will be the extra weight that pregnancy brings – in a hurry. The average weight gain in pregnancy is 25lb/11kg. Not only is the weight gain a rapid one, it is carried in front of you. Your baby also displaces internal organs and puts pressure on places you didn't even know existed – it's the less glamorous side of pregnancy.

This weight in front of you places enormous stress on your back, particularly if your abdominal muscles are weak. In early pregnancy, your pelvis supports the baby's weight. But when the baby gets big enough to bulge out in front of your hips, the pull forward is significant if you're not strong enough to use your abdominal muscles to snug the baby back into that natural cradle of your pelvis. And furthermore, as the muscles are stretched to accommodate your increasing size, they are less able to do the work. Compensating for inability to support the weight causes that familiar swayback that we commonly and affectionately associate with pregnant women.

Stretch to Ease Your Back

Evidence suggests that flexibility gains made during pregnancy last beyond delivery, and women who are flexible during their first pregnancy have fewer problems with joint expansion in subsequent pregnancies. Active-Isolated Stretching just might be the perfect workout to ease an aching back and get a little gentle exercise.

Before you get started, here are a few tips to help lay the groundwork for stretching during pregnancy.

Start early in your pregnancy. As your pregnancy progresses and your body changes, even things that were simple in the beginning of your programme will become

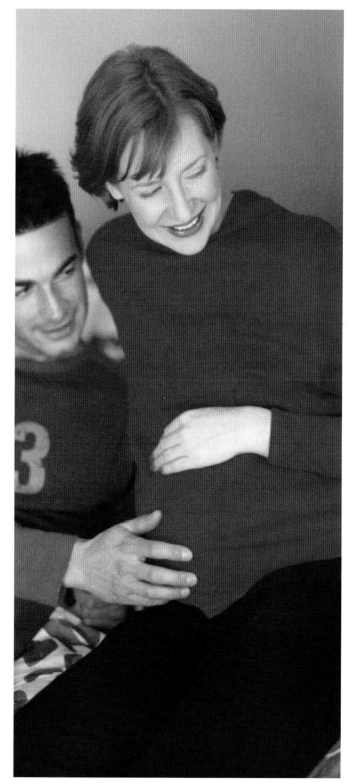

▲ Look after yourself during pregnancy
Rapid weight gain puts great strain on the back. The Whartons' Active-Isolated Stretching programme, along with some gentle exercise and plenty of rest, will protect you and your baby.

more difficult. Start your workout programme as early in the pregnancy as possible and make small adjustments as you progress. The longer you wait to get started, the more difficult everything will be and the less likely you will stick with the programme. Actually, compelling evidence suggests that it's best to start working out *before* you get pregnant.

Clear your programme with your doctor. Show him your planned workout, and get a blessing before you begin. Remember to discuss the specific stretches, the intensity, the frequency and the duration of your workouts. Each time you visit, follow up with a progress report. Make sure your doctor is advised of aches, pains and changes in ability, such as something you did well a month ago that now seems difficult. You might be advised to scale down your exercise programme or stop it completely if you have any of the following:

- High blood pressure
- Heart disease
- Pulmonary disease
- Pregnancy-induced high blood pressure
- Symptoms or a history of going into labour before the baby is due
- Vaginal bleeding or spotting
- Any compromise in the cervix, uterus or membrane

Protect your back. After the first trimester, avoid exercises that put you flat on your back with your legs straight and extended. In this position, your uterus might compress the vena cava, large veins that run along your spine. The result might be the pain, dizziness and nausea that accompany a spike in venous pressures. The later in your pregnancy you are and the larger your uterus and baby, the more at risk you are of this unpleasant experience. It's easily avoided.

Dress comfortably. How you dress will depend on where you stretch. Generally, we advise you to wear cool, lightweight, loose clothing that will allow you to move easily and comfortably. You should avoid tight or restricting seams or belts. Your shoes, as always, should be low-heeled, fit well, and be securely fastened. Make sure the soles of your shoes are slip-proof.

▶ **Keeping cool and comfortable**
Buying maternity clothing made from lightweight, natural fibres will keep you moving easily and comfortably. Also try to keep yourself hydrated with plenty of water, especially after exercising.

Choose a workout surface that is comfortable. We suggest a carpeted floor or a floor over which you have thrown a folded beach towel, mat or blanket. Even your bed will work, provided it's not too soft. Most of the stretches we designed for you require a chair. Just make sure the chair is comfortable, supports you without slipping, and allows you to place your feet flat on the floor without any sort of strain.

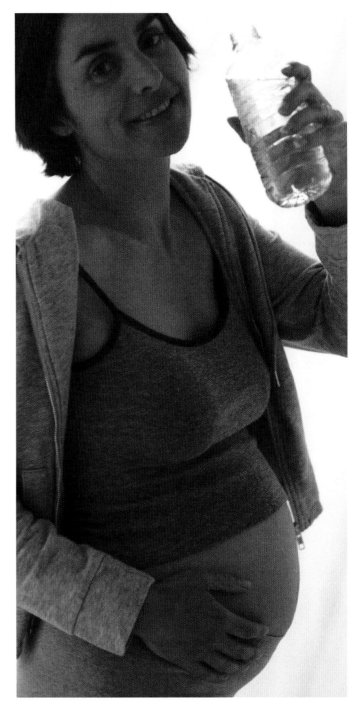

Regulate the temperature. Make certain that you set the thermostat to keep you warm enough to be relaxed and yet cool enough to protect your baby from difficulties that may arise from being overheated. Researchers caution that babies are generally safe when mum exercises – unless she is overheated. Stay out of the blazing sun, the sauna and the steam room.

Stay alert for signals that tell you enough is enough. Pay attention to these warning signs: pain, nausea, a persistent cramp, dizziness, ringing in your ears, a racing pulse that you can't explain, a feeling of 'fluttering' in your chest, breathlessness, tingling, numbness, sudden fatigue, headache, discharge of amniotic fluid or blood, a noticeable decrease in your baby's movement, or any potential symptom that your doctor may have suggested earlier as being a concern. If you experience anything unusual, stop working out immediately and phone your doctor or dial 999.

Expect to continuously adjust your programme. Although these stretches are designed just for you, as your body changes you might have to adjust or eliminate some stretches. As your abdominal muscles elongate over your expanding tummy, they eventually separate from top to bottom along the centre line of your navel. It's more difficult for you to contract them, if you can do it at all.

Additionally, later in your pregnancy, your enlarging tummy might get in the way of something you'll try to do. Continue to include a stretch only if you are comfortable. A little imagination and persistence go a long way. We urge you to keep at it.

Take 20 minutes a day for yourself. Take 20 consecutive minutes every day to stretch. Think of it not as an indulgence, but as your training – a necessary investment in the beginning of life with your new baby.

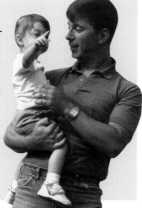

Back protection doesn't stop when your baby arrives. Remember to frequently switch the side on which you carry your child. Always cradling junior in your left arm will cause you to overdevelop your left side and create a muscular imbalance that will put strain on your back. As the baby increases in weight, the imbalance will become more pronounced. This warning goes for dads, too.

Getting the Pressure Off Your Back

Beyond exercise, there are a number of other things you can do to help ease back pain during pregnancy.

- Wear low-heeled (but not flat) shoes with good arch support.
- Always seek assistance when attempting to lift or move heavy objects.
- When standing for long periods, place one foot on a stool or box.
- If your bed is too soft, have someone help you place a board between the mattress and box spring.
- Don't bend over from the waist to pick things up. Squat with bent knees and a straight back.
- Sit in chairs with good back support, or use a small pillow behind the low part of your back.
- Try to sleep on your side with one or two pillows between your legs for support.
- Apply heat or cold to the painful area, with your doctor's permission, and massage it.

If Your Back Pain Continues

If you've tried the exercises and you're still feeling pain, there are two other options that may alleviate the symptoms. A pregnancy brace could help to support the abdominal weight and take some of the pressure off the back. Or you could try prescription painkillers that are safe for expectant mums, or bed rest and professional physical therapy.

If your back pain continues or worsens, not responding to simple attempts to get it under control, make sure you see your doctor immediately. Back pain can also be caused by premature labour or other problems unrelated to pregnancy that need immediate attention.

A STRETCHING AND STRENGTHENING WORKOUT GUARANTEED TO EASE MUM'S BACK

We'd love to see you do the full Active-Isolated Stretching and Strengthening programme (see chapter 4), but a changing body needs special attention. The stretches here have been modified for you, and the only equipment you'll need is an 8ft/2.4m length of stretch rope and ankle weights. Remember to exhale as you stretch and inhale as you relax.

1

NOTE: DO NOT ATTEMPT THIS EXERCISE IF YOU ARE IN YOUR SECOND OR THIRD TRIMESTER.

Mum's Double-leg Pelvic Tilts

Active Muscles You Contract: Abdominals and muscles from the fronts of your hips down the fronts of your thighs

Isolated Muscles You Stretch: Lower back and buttocks   **Equipment:** Rolled towel

Hold Each Stretch: 2 seconds   **Reps:** 8–10

1 Lie down on your back on a comfortable surface. Pause, take a deep breath and make sure that your baby is not compressing your back. If you don't feel comfortable, skip this stretch. Bend your knees until your feet are flat on the surface. Place your hands behind your knees or thighs to provide a little assistance towards the end of the free movement.

2 Using your abdominals and quadriceps, lift both legs towards your chest, aiming your knees towards the outside of your shoulders. If you feel discomfort in the front of your hips, spread the knees wider. Assist the stretch with your hands, but do not pull. Hold for two seconds, then return to the resting position.

2

Mum's Bent-leg Hamstrings

Active Muscles You Contract: Muscles in the fronts of your thighs

Isolated Muscles You Stretch: Large muscles in the backs of your thighs

Equipment: Rolled towel, exercise strap or rope   **Hold Each Stretch:** 2 seconds

Reps: 10 on the right, 10 on the left

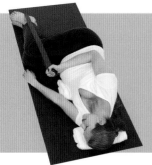

1 Lie down on your side. Tuck a rolled towel under your neck. Bend both knees. Slip the loop of your strap around the foot of your exercising leg, under the arch. Hold the ends and eliminate any slack.

2 Keeping your knee bent, bring the top leg up until your thigh is nearly at right angles to your trunk. Hold the ends of the strap in one hand, keeping it taut to stop it from slipping away from the bottom of your foot.

3 Straighten your leg by contracting your quadriceps until your knee is locked. At the end of your stretch, gently pull on the strap with both hands to add the slightest pressure and extend the range of the stretch just a little more. Hold for two seconds.

3

Mum's Straight-leg Hamstrings

Active Muscles You Contract: Muscles from the fronts of your hips down the fronts of your thighs

Isolated Muscles You Stretch: Large muscles in the backs of your thighs

Equipment: Rolled towel, exercise strap or rope

Hold Each Stretch: 2 seconds **Reps:** 10 on the right, 10 on the left

1 Lie down on your side. Tuck a rolled towel under your neck and head. Your exercising leg (on top) should be straight. The other leg should be bent at the knee to stop you rolling. Loop the strap and slip it over the foot of your exercising leg, under the arch. Straighten the strap to remove slack. Lock your knee.

2 From your hip and using your quadriceps, bring your leg straight out in an arc towards your face. Keeping the strap taut, 'climb' up it, hand over hand, as your leg arcs towards your head. At the end of the stretch, extend the range just a little more, gently assisting with your rope. Don't force it. Hold for two seconds and then relax.

4

Mum's Internal Rotators

Active Muscles You Contract: Deep muscles in the buttocks that externally rotate your hips

Isolated Muscles You Stretch: Deep muscles in the buttocks that rotate your hips; muscles that span the hip sockets to the top of your pelvis, and the muscles that reach from the bottom front of your pelvis to the inside leg halfway down the thigh

Equipment: Rolled towel, exercise strap or rope **Hold Each Stretch:** 2 seconds **Reps:** 10 on the right, 10 on the left

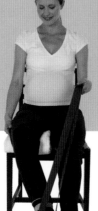

1 Hold the strap taut. Using the hand above your exercising leg, hold the thigh at the knee and grasp the muscle with your thumb on the outside to stabilise the leg.

2 Rotate your lower exercising leg towards the midline of your body. Move from your hip. Gently assist by pulling upwards on the strap to extend the range of motion. Hold for two seconds. Relax the tension on the rope, return to the starting position.

5

Mum's Medial Hip Rotators

Active Muscles You Contract: Muscles in the middle and deep within your buttocks

Isolated Muscles You Stretch: Outer hip and inner thigh **Equipment:** Rolled towel

Hold Each Stretch: 2 seconds **Reps:** 8–10 on the right, 8–10 on the left

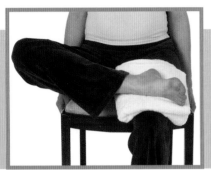

1 Sit on a chair with a small rolled towel between your lower back and the chair back. Place the foot of your exercising leg on the thigh of the opposite leg, with your ankle just above the knee. Use a folded towel on the top of your thigh as a cushion.

2 Contract the muscles in your hip and outer thigh, and press your knee down. Using your other leg as support, gently press your knee down with your hand, using your other hand to hold your ankle steady. Work one side at a time. Be gentle but firm. Return to the resting position.

6

Mum's Seated Trunk Extensors

Active Muscles You Contract: Abdominals

Isolated Muscles You Stretch: Muscles that run up the spine, and the lower-back muscles below your belt line

Hold Each Stretch: 2 seconds **Reps:** 8–10

1 Perch on the edge of your chair with your back straight and relaxed. Place your feet flat on the floor in front of you, shoulder-width apart.

2 Tuck your chin down, as shown, and contract your abdominal muscles to roll your torso forwards.

7 Mum's Seated Thoracic-lumbar Rotators

Active Muscles You Contract: Abdominals, the muscles on the sides of your chest, and the thoracic-lumbar rotators

Isolated Muscles You Stretch: Muscles up the spine; stabilising, rotating and balancing muscles in the back and sides; lower-back muscles

Hold Each Stretch: 2 seconds **Reps:** 10 on the right, 10 on the left

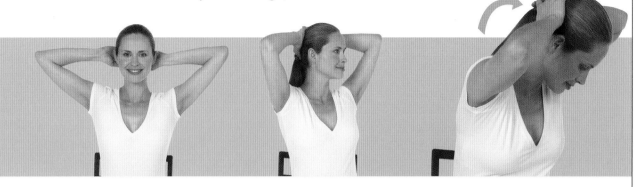

1 Perch on the edge of a chair with your back straight and relaxed. Place your feet flat on the floor in front of you, shoulder-width apart for stability. Lock your hands behind your head with your elbows out.

2 Contract your entire abdomen, including the muscles in your side, and twist your upper body in one direction as far as you can go. Repeat this warm-up four or five times in one direction until you feel loosened up.

3 Rotate again and hold, then flex your trunk forward, leading down between your knees towards the ground with your elbow. Return to an upright position. Work one side at a time, completing all reps, then change sides.

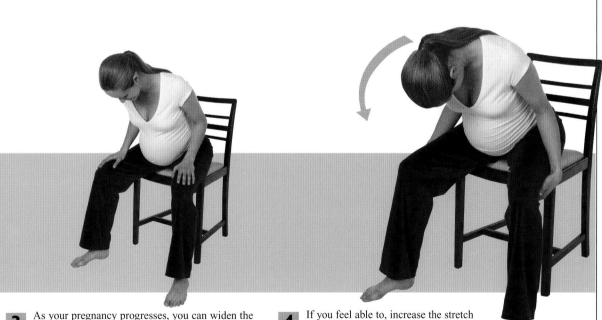

3 As your pregnancy progresses, you can widen the distance between your feet. Put your hands on your knees to steady yourself. Pull forwards gently. Don't bounce. Hold each stretch for two seconds.

4 If you feel able to, increase the stretch slightly. Gently roll your torso forward until your head is as near your knees as you can get. Hold the stretch for two seconds and then return to the resting position.

8

Mum's Trunk Lateral Flexors

Active Muscles You Contract: Abdominals; muscles on the sides of your chest; the thoracic-lumbar rotators on the non-exercising side

Isolated Muscles You Stretch: Muscles along your spine and the muscles in the sides of your trunk opposite the exercising side

Hold Each Stretch: 2 seconds   **Reps:** 8–10 on the left, 8–10 on the right

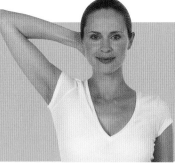

1 Perch on the edge of a chair with your back straight and relaxed. Place your feet flat on the floor, shoulder-width apart. Raise one arm, placing your hand behind your head with the elbow pointed away from your body.

2 Bend at the waist so that the hand of your straightened arm is lowered towards the floor. You'll feel a gentle stretch on the opposite side of your trunk. Hold for two seconds then return to the resting position. Work one side at a time.

9

Mum's Neck Routine

Active Muscles You Contract: Muscles in the front and back of your neck and the top of your back between your shoulders

Isolated Muscles You Stretch: Muscles in the front and back of your neck and the top of your back between your shoulders

Hold Each Stretch: 2 seconds   **Reps:** 8–10

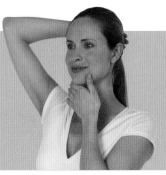

1 Perch on the edge of a chair with your back straight and relaxed. Place your feet flat on the floor, shoulder-width apart for stability. Place one hand on the back of your head and one hand on your chin to assist the stretch.

2 Tuck your chin down and roll your head forwards until your chin meets your chest, as shown. Gently assist the end of the stretch by pressing lightly at the back of your head. Return to neutral position.

10

Mum's Rotator Cuffs 1 (Rhomboids)

Active Muscles You Contract: Muscles in your shoulders

Isolated Muscles You Stretch: External shoulder rotators, commonly called the rotator cuff, and the upper back

Hold Each Stretch: 2 seconds **Reps:** 8–10

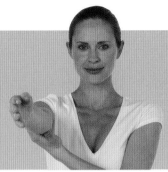

1 Perch on the edge of a chair with your back straight and relaxed. Cross your legs at the ankles or place your feet flat on the floor, shoulder-width apart for stability. Lift one arm and hold it straight out. Lock your elbow.

2 Keeping your elbow locked, move the arm straight across your chest towards the opposite shoulder. Don't rotate your torso and keep the shoulders down. Use the other hand to give assistance at the end of the movement.

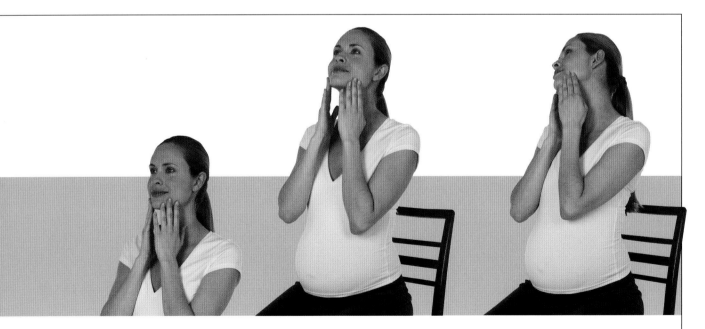

3 Now move your hands to your chin and spread your fingertips along your jawbone.

4 Then roll your head straight back over your body – chin straight up. Again, you can gently assist the stretch by pressing with your fingers. Return to the neutral position again.

5 Rotate your neck and head slightly to one side, then roll it down towards your chest. You can assist the end of the movement with your hands at the back of your head. Return to the neutral position. Keep your shoulders down and relaxed.

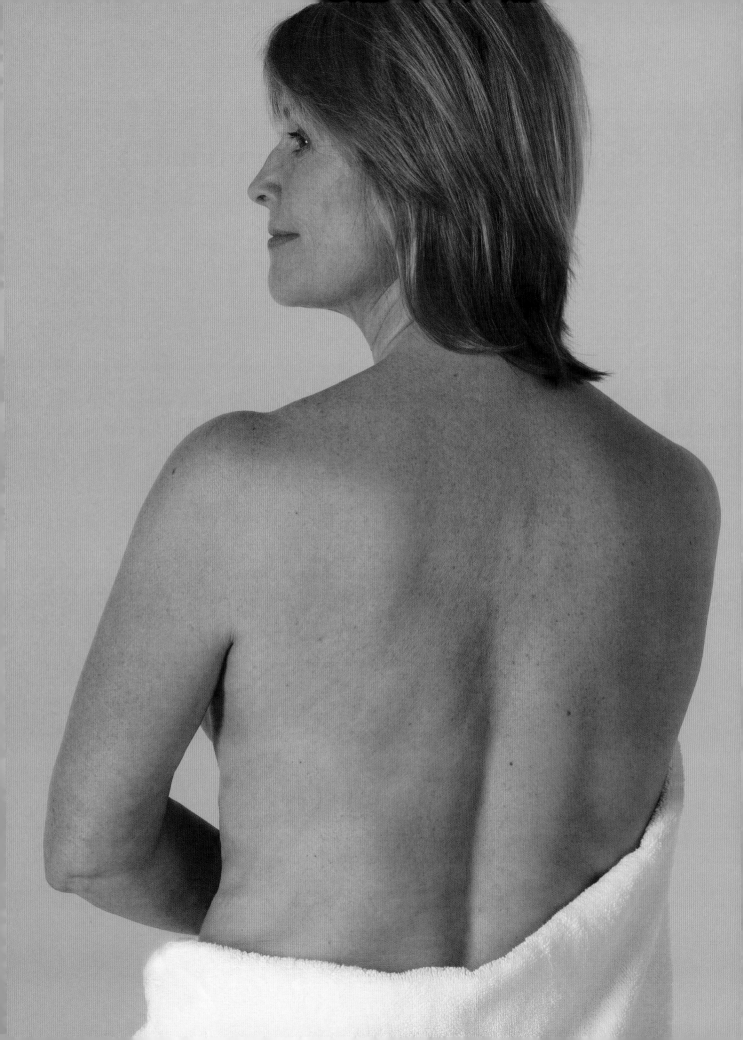

CHAPTER 10

STANDING TALL AGAINST OSTEOPOROSIS

Osteoporosis used to be called the silent killer, *but there's nothing silent about osteoporosis any more. The press and the medical profession are succeeding in getting the word out about this disease (it literally means 'porous bones'), and on account of effective prevention, earlier detection and advances in medication, it's less a killer than it once was. But it's still dangerous.*

The treachery of osteoporosis lies in decreasing bone mass, which increases the risk of fractures, especially in the hip, spine and wrist. When left unchecked, osteoporosis quietly and insidiously steals bone mass until a person is so fragile that a deadly fracture can occur just by moving the wrong way. One in three women over the age of 50 will suffer a fracture of the hip, wrist or spine as a result of osteoporosis. Fifty per cent of those who suffer a fractured hip lose the ability to live independently, and around 20 per cent die within a year.

Yet the disease is largely preventable, chiefly through regular exercise (such as the Active-Isolated Stretching, Strengthening and cardio programme) and a diet rich in calcium and vitamin D. Doctors are also optimistic that medicine will improve in the future and that detection methods will become less expensive and more widely available than they are currently.

And for those who have osteoporosis already, its destruction can be certainly be slowed or halted. We help many of our patients arrest osteoporosis with Active-Isolated Stretching and Strengthening, so that they can reclaim their independence and enjoy life again. A little education can help you halt osteoporosis in its tracks. First, let's look at where it comes from.

ARE YOU AT RISK?

Although one in 12 men suffer from osteoporosis, women with low levels of oestrogen face the greatest risk for osteoporosis. That includes not only women who have reached menopause naturally or surgically but also women who earlier in life had delayed or irregular menstruation. Other risk factors include the following:

A family history of osteoporosis. If your grandmother and mother had osteoporosis, chances are that you will, too. Heredity is responsible for 70 per cent of peak bone mass; the remaining 30 per cent is up to you.

Chronic disease. Some chronic diseases that alter hormone levels and affect the kidneys, lungs, stomach and intestines – such as end-stage renal disease – increase bone loss.

Age. As a natural part of the life cycle, bone loss increases with age, with fractures more common after the age of 50. Breaks that aren't the result of hard falls or blows may be the first signal that bone health is in decline. It's better to be evaluated before you have a fracture, but every fracture – especially if there was no obvious cause – should certainly be a warning.

Insufficient calcium. The UK Food Standards Agency recommends that the Adequate Intake (replacing the old Recommended Daily Allowance) is 1,000mg a day for adults aged 19 to 50, and 1,200mg for the prevention of osteoporosis and those over 50. For those already suffering from osteoporosis, 500–800mg twice a day is recommended.

As few as three alcoholic drinks per day fill you up with empty calories and impair your ability to make good choices regarding food, which can contribute to poor general nutrition, including low intake of calcium and vitamin D. Alcohol also inhibits the liver's ability to absorb calcium and to activate vitamin D. Without access to these vital nutrients, osteoporosis sets in.

Inadequate exercise. One study reported that women who were less active had a 0.25 to 2 per cent increase in bone mass, compared with a 6 to 8 per cent increase in more active women.

Overexercising. Exercise – especially load-bearing exercise – is important, but overdoing it can impair bone building. Studies show that some female athletes with low body fat are unable to store sufficient oestrogen and can even stop menstruating. Once oestrogen levels drop, women are at risk of osteoporosis. You want to keep your body fat higher than about 16 per cent – although most of us won't have any trouble with that, as the average fit woman's body fat percentage is between 20 and 25 per cent.

Smoking. This nasty habit changes the liver's metabolism of oestrogen, making it less biologically active. Women who smoke actually enter menopause a year or two earlier than non-smokers. Also, there is conclusive evidence that cigarette smoking inhibits bone cell formation.

Body build and race. Women who are thin, small-framed, Caucasian or Asian are statistically at greater risk.

Prolonged use of certain medications. The aluminium in some antacids can bind to phosphorus and lower its levels, which would cause your body to excrete more calcium. Other medications having this effect include thyroid hormones, anticonvulsants, steroids used for asthma or arthritis, certain diuretics, tetracycline and long-term use of the anti-tuberculosis drug isoniazid. Your doctor will help you determine which medications put you at risk.

PREVENTING BONE LOSS THROUGHOUT YOUR LIFE

For the past few decades, the best lifelong prevention for women has been a three-way approach: oestrogen, a good diet and plenty of exercise – especially load-bearing exercise. However, recent research about supplemental hormones indicates that oestrogens need to be approached with caution.

In younger women, hormones – including oestrogens – should be in perfect balance. As a woman ages, however, oestrogen levels drop, signalling the end of menstruation and childbirth years. Unfortunately, the drop in oestrogens also reduces the body's ability to remodel bones. For postmenopausal women, oestrogen, in the form of HRT, is one of the treatments given for the prevention of osteoporosis. Essentially, oestrogen slows bone loss by acting directly on the bones. It blocks bone-dissolving hormones and helps activate vitamin D, which in turn enhances calcium absorption. Oestrogen increases collagen

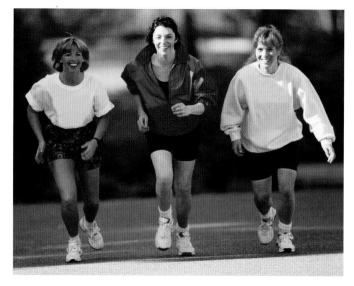

▲ Prevention through exercise
Osteoporosis, like many other conditions, is largely prevented by aerobic and weight-bearing exercise, along with a healthy diet.

as well, a substance that helps form new bone tissue. The 'bone mineral age' of a woman who takes oestrogens is on average 10 to 12 years younger than her biological age.

But there's a problem. A big one. A major study of the effects HRT on women aged 50 to 70, run under the auspices of the US National Heart, Lung and Blood Institute of the National Institutes of Health (NIH), was halted three years early when preliminary results demonstrated that the risks for the study group on combined HRT (a combination of both oestrogen and progesterone) outweighed the benefits.

The main goal of this trial had been to see if HRT would help prevent heart disease and hip fractures, and to examine the effect of HRT on breast cancer. Researchers discovered small but significantly increased risks of breast cancer, coronary heart disease, stroke and blood clots for the group of women on HRT. While the benefits of HRT did include a decrease in vertebral and other osteoporotic fractures, NIH officials concluded that the risks were significantly high enough to justify stopping the study for public health reasons and for the sake of the women who participated. If you are taking HRT solely for the prevention of osteoporosis, you and your doctor might consider stopping it, because other medications exist that can help prevent osteoporosis and fractures and that appear to carry fewer risks for breast cancer. (See 'Damage Control' on page 191.)

Although oestrogens might not be right for you, there is still a good choice of other things to try for healthy bones.

A good diet. A diet rich in calcium is a valuable weapon against osteoporosis. Calcium keeps the bone replacement process in balance so that your body stores more than it

Choosing the Right Calcium Supplement

When you first step up to the shelf in your local pharmacy to choose a calcium supplement, you'll be dazzled by the selections. . . and confused. It's important that you select the calcium that's right for you. Not all supplements contain the same amount of elemental, or pure, calcium. Some forms of calcium are more bioavailable than others – meaning that they are quickly dissolved so that your body can easily use them.

If you want to conduct a comparison test of the calcium you're considering so you'll know how easily the mineral will dissolve, simply drop one tablet into room-temperature vinegar and stir every five minutes. The US Pharmacopeia (USP), a non-profit organisation that sets standards for medications, reports that at least 75 per cent of the calcium should dissolve within 30 minutes. If it doesn't, the tablet contains little bioavailable calcium and is probably not of much use to you. If you don't have the time, here's our handy list of calcium supplements, listed in order of percentage of elemental calcium.

- **Calcium carbonate.** With 40 per cent elemental calcium, this is the least expensive, dissolves quickly, and is the most concentrated tablet. It is absorbed best with food.
- **Calcium phosphate.** Although it has 31 per cent elemental calcium, this is one of the least soluble and least bioavailable.
- **Calcium citrate.** With 21 per cent elemental calcium, this dissolves the fastest and is best absorbed on an empty stomach.
- **Calcium lactate.** Though this dissolves more reliably than calcium carbonate, with 13 per cent elemental calcium, it will require taking more tablets to get a good result. It's not advised for women who are lactose intolerant.
- **Calcium gluconate.** With 9 per cent elemental calcium,

this dissolves more reliably than calcium carbonate, but because it contains less elemental calcium, getting the best result will require taking more tablets.
- **Bone meal, dolomite, oyster shell.** Avoid these unless your doctor directs you to take them. They are high in calcium but potentially contaminated with toxic metals and generally not recommended.

Calcium absorption is improved by vitamin D, so your supplement should contain some of this important nutrient. Calcium is also hard for your body to absorb, so rather than take all your calcium in one go, you'll increase absorption if you take 750mg twice a day with food. And if you suspect that calcium is causing digestive upset – constipation, bloating or wind – be sure to wash it down with lots of water.

loses in waste. Low-fat dairy products, such as skimmed milk and low-fat yoghurt, are good sources of calcium, as are leafy green vegetables (except spinach), nuts, tofu and fish. But if none of those sounds appetising, many fortified foods will do, including some orange juices, breads, dairy and soya milks.

Calcium (and vitamin D) supplements. As we stated before, you'll want to aim for 1200mg if you're over the age of 50. Because the body can absorb only about 600mg at once, doctors recommend dividing the doses: 600mg in the morning and 600mg in the evening. There are many different types of calcium available on the market and it is important to buy the right one for you. Please refer to 'Choosing the Right Calcium Supplement' on page 189 for more information.

Calcium, no matter how you get it, is boosted by vitamin D, which is activated by the liver and kidneys. Your body manufactures vitamin D naturally, with the assistance of ultraviolet sunlight. Getting your daily requirement takes only 10 minutes of exposure a day, but it's very easy for your levels of vitamin D to get too low, especially if you can't get outside very often during daylight hours. Some studies also suggest that the older we are, the more difficult it is for the body to translate sunshine into activated vitamin D. So why take the chance of becoming low in D?

For those without any special needs, it is considered that enough vitamin D can be obtained from food and the sun. For older people or pregnant women, the UK Adequate Intake (AI) requirement of vitamin D is 10 micrograms (or 0.01mg). However, a daily supplement of up to 25 micrograms (0.025mg) is considered to be safe.

Exercise. If you already have osteoporosis, there's no question that you're more fragile than you used to be, but you can still work out. Just go easy, and talk to your doctor about any necessary precautions.

Exercise is crucial for keeping muscles toned so that a fall is less likely or at least less severe. Some research suggests that load-bearing exercise such as walking or weight-lifting stimulates bone formation by triggering the same kind of remodelling that would occur with stress and rest.

Load-bearing exercise places the resistance of weight on bones. But as the body adjusts to load, the exercise that was once beneficial to your bones can suddenly becomes less so. Take walking, for example. At first, your bones – from your feet to your back – work against gravity and the weight of your own body, and all your bones benefit and

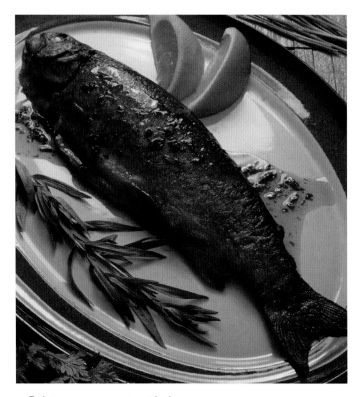

▲ Fighting osteoporosis with diet
Fish, especially those with edible bones, offer an excellent source of calcium. Fish oil capsules improve the body's absorption of calcium.

remodel. But as you grow fitter, the bones become used to this load. Gravity and the weight of your own body will no longer challenge them. It's your responsibility to keep your routines challenging to your bones by mixing up your activities or by progressively increasing the work your body has to do. The key is to continuously create resistance, enough to make your bones – and the rest of you! – feel challenged.

If you don't have osteoporosis, load-bearing exercise is a great way to ensure that you'll never have it. Experts agree that, no matter what activity you select, it should be fun so that you'll be more likely to stick with it.

In many cases, women who have begun experiencing some of the more unpleasant symptoms of osteoporosis – such as a dowager's hump – will stop doing exercise because of pain or discomfort. If this is your situation and you want to begin slowly, we recommend the four exercises on the opposite page to start you off. Do these for two weeks, and you're certain to feel your back and hips loosening up. Once you feel better, you can start the full Active-Isolated programme.

If you have begun to experience symptoms of osteoporosis, try these stretches on a regular basis.

FOUR EXERCISES FOR OSTEOPOROSIS

1. Single-leg Pelvic Tilts

See complete instructions for this two-step exercise on page 50.

2. Double-leg Pelvic Tilts

See complete instructions for this two-step exercise on page 50.

3. Pectoralis Majors

See complete instructions for this two-step exercise on page 60.

4. Anterior Deltoids

See complete instructions for this two-step exercise on page 61.

DAMAGE CONTROL

Our prevention recommendations will go a long way, but if bone demineralisation has begun, medications other than oestrogen are available to slow down or even halt the loss.

We include this information here as an overview of your pharmaceutical options. Of course, the best place to find out which drug (if any) is right for you is your doctor's office.

Alendronate (Fosamax). A member of the bisphosphonate family, this drug is used to treat both women and men. Bisphosphonates stop or slow bone breakdown of osteoporosis but don't slow the build-up of new tissue, so they allow the bone to 'catch up' with the natural remodelling cycle. These medications are probably more effective than oestrogen in slowing and preventing bone loss, especially if your risk factors are unusually high. In research trials, alendronate not only reduced bone loss but also increased bone mass in the spine and hip. Taking 10mg daily of this medication reduces fractures by 50 per cent.

One problem is that alendronate is absorbed through the intestine and can be irritating. You must therefore take it with 6–8fl oz (180–240ml) of water first thing in the morning on an empty stomach, and you must stay upright for at least 30 minutes to keep it from irritating the oesophagus. Other side-effects might include musculo-skeletal pain, nausea, heartburn and abdominal irritation. The other reservation about alendronate is that, once taken, it sticks to the bone – probably for life. Although researchers think that it is unlikely to be harmful, no one knows for sure.

Alendronate is approved for treatment or prevention of osteoporosis caused by prolonged use of steroids and glucocorticoid medications in both men and women. A once-a-week form is now available, and it might be just as effective as the daily dose but with fewer side-effects.

Risedronate. Taken at a prescribed dose of 5mg a day, this drug, also a bisphosphonate medication, slows bone loss, increases density and reduces the risk of fractures. Like alendronate, it has to be taken with plenty of water first thing in the morning, and you may not eat, drink or take any other medications for an hour. Some side-effects include upset stomach, nausea, vomiting, diarrhoea and headache. Like alendronate, it is approved for use by men and women for the treatment or prevention of osteoporosis caused by prolonged use of steroids and glucocorticoid medications.

Raloxifene (Evista). One of the new designer oestrogens known as selective oestrogen receptor modulators (SERMs), raloxifene is taken as a pill once a day to prevent bone loss and increase bone mass throughout the body.

Raloxifene, along with calcium and vitamin D, appears to reduce the risk of first spinal fractures by about 55 per cent within three years. Women who have already suffered one spinal fracture appear to reduce their risk of subsequent fractures by 30 per cent, although there's no proof yet that hips are as well-fortified.

Like oestrogens, raloxifene appears to reduce blood lipids, thereby reducing risk of cardiovascular disease. But unlike oestrogens, it does not appear to increase risk of breast and uterine cancers. In fact, researchers are suggesting that raloxifene reduces the risk of breast cancer by 76 per cent among postmenopausal women who use it.

Raloxifene doesn't reduce the incidence of hot flushes – and might make them worse. Side-effects appear to be few, although SERMs have been associated with some deep vein thrombosis. Because SERMs are relatively new on the scene, long-term effects of raloxifene are not yet known. Speak to your doctor for more information.

Calcitonin. This naturally occurring protein hormone is best taken as a nasal spray. It regulates how much calcium is in the body and how bone metabolises it. If you are a woman more than five years beyond menopause, taking calcitonin may inhibit the breakdown of your bone and increase your spinal density, but it may be of little benefit to other bones. Women who use it, however, report that it also reduces pain associated with fractures.

Unfortunately, while none of the delivery methods is that pleasant, the nasal spray may win out. It might cause a runny nose, but the injections might trigger an allergic reaction, flushing of the face and hands, rash, nausea and the need to urinate frequently.

Parathyroid hormone. This hormone, taken in a daily injection, stimulates bone growth by building new bone faster than old bone is broken down. In a recent 21-month study involving 1,637 women, those who received the injections had up to 13 per cent more bone in their spines than those taking a placebo. They also reduced their risk of new spinal fractures by up to 69 per cent.

MAN-TO-MAN TALK: OSTEOPOROSIS IN MEN

While osteoporosis is considered to be a woman's health hazard, the truth is that it affects up to one in 12 men at

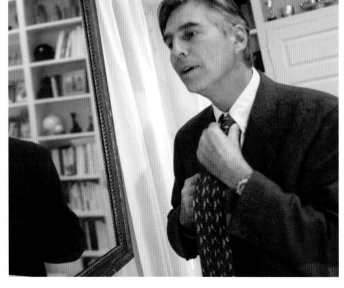

▲ Osteoporosis affects men too
Although less common than in women, osteoporosis affects one in 12 men. Caucasian men are at the greatest risk.

some stage of their life. Twenty per cent of all vertebral (spine) fractures and 30 per cent of all hip fractures are endured by men, and, of these cases, a third will not survive more than a year. Clearly, this disease is a killer, yet a diagnosis of osteoporosis remains commonly overlooked among men. Part of the problem is that men have larger, stronger bones than women. When evaluating simple fractures in men, or even while doing annual physical examinations, doctors traditionally have not been quick to consider the possibility that osteoporosis could be setting in. We hope that's changing.

The causes of osteoporosis in men are similar to those in women: a low peak bone mineral density when they were younger and excessive bone loss as they age. Like women, if men don't have a good base before they start to lose mineral density, then the onset of osteoporosis is certain. Diagnosis is also the same: If you notice a little loss in height, a change in your posture – head forwards and a slouch – or sudden back pain with no real explanation, osteoporosis could be the culprit.

Risk factors are also similar to those of women, with a couple of additions: osteoporosis in men can be caused by insufficient levels of the sex hormone testosterone, especially if undiagnosed and never balanced. And Caucasian men are at greatest risk, although all ethnic groups are vulnerable.

In order to protect yourself, there are several things you can do: get treatment for medical conditions that cause bone loss; stop smoking; drink only moderately; get active with load-bearing exercise; take 1,200mg of calcium a day if you are over the age of 50; and make sure that you either have plenty of exposure to the sun or take at least 10 micrograms of vitamin D every day.

At this time, alendronate and risedronate are the two most common drugs used in the treatment of osteoporosis in men, mainly for steroid-induced osteoporosis. But even though there aren't as many medications available for men as for women, you have other options to consider.

Your doctor might suggest testosterone replacement therapy. Both genders have the hormone oestrogen, and it's thought that testosterone contributes to the circulating levels of oestrogen in men. As a man ages, and testosterone decreases, so does the oestrogen. By increasing the naturally diminishing levels of testosterone, it might be possible to increase the levels of circulating oestrogen and slow bone loss. A simple blood test can determine testosterone levels and tell you for sure if you're a little low.

Another medication your doctor might suggest is calcitonin, which has been used for a long time in women to slow or stop bone loss. It may relieve some pain of fractures, if they've already occurred. Your doctor might administer it as an injection or send you home with a nasal spray.

Besides adjustment in medication, osteoporosis is treated exactly the same in men as women. Because many men have grown up in a tradition of sports and physical prowess, it's hard for a guy to think in terms of his body being fragile, but it is… for now. You have to take it easy, and tuck your ego in. If you're gung ho, back off the heaviest weights and the impact of exercise, and add duration instead. It's possible for you to enjoy building strong, flexible and balanced muscles, knowing that stronger bones will follow. When we work with osteoporotic men, we subscribe to the 'less is more' school of thought. Stick to the programmes in this book and avoid injury so that you can stay in the game every day, and you'll be surprised.

OSTEOPOROSIS PREVENTION HAS A BRIGHT FUTURE

Doctors expect that within the next decade better medications will be available to prevent and treat osteoporosis. Some of the most promising include bisphosphonates and activated vitamin D, but keep in touch with your doctor to talk about the latest advances.

While you're waiting, ask your doctor to refer you for a bone scan, eat a calcium-rich diet (including supplements), take enough vitamin D or spend 10 minutes in the sun when the weather allows, and enjoy the Active-Isolated Strength programme that will help build bone and prevent falls.

▼ Healthy and restful
Vitamin D is a useful weapon in the fight against osteoporosis. A good source of this is sunshine – on holiday or in the garden!

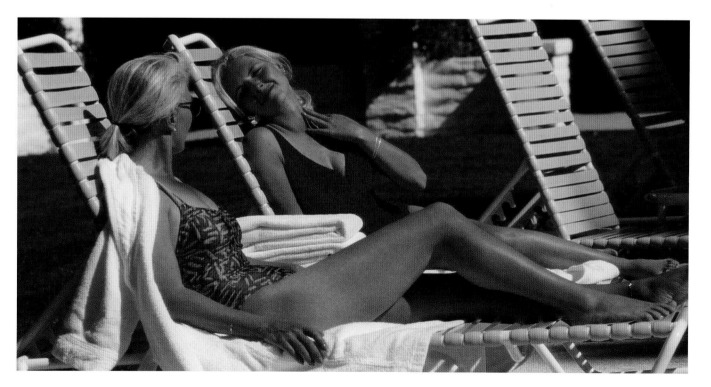

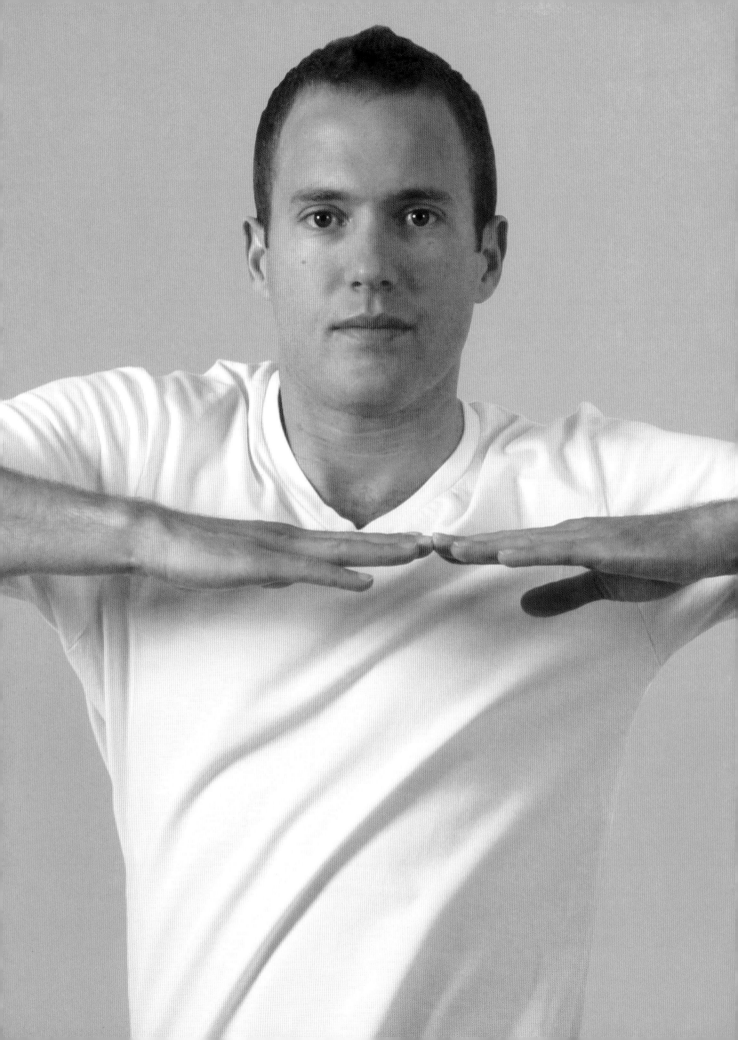

CHAPTER 11

SUPPLE BACK, YOUTHFUL BODY

The limit of our natural life span and how we *can expand it is a hotly debated topic. Many experts believe that the maximum that can be achieved with healthy humans is about 120 years of age. Others believe this upper level can be increased to 150. Regardless of the upper-limits issue, the fact is that it's now very possible to keep older human beings more active and alert in their final years.*

Of particular interest to us in our discussions about the back is that cells shrink as we age. The gelatin-like centres of the discs in your spine condense, and you become a little bit shorter. While your spine shortens – even just a small amount – the ligaments and tendons that surround the bones might not shrink at the same rate. When you're younger, those connective tissues support and hold everything tight, and in alignment. But when the spine shortens and the connective tissue does not, the spinal column literally becomes loose. It becomes easier to throw your back out or suffer other aches and pains. Also, without their plump cushions, your discs are less effective as shock absorbers.

Normal activity brings about an acceleration of wear and tear on the bone, causing jagged edges called bone spurs. As the bone spurs get worse and expand, they can cause a narrowing of the spinal canal and the spaces between the vertebrae. Before you know it, you could be suffering nerve impingement and some loss of function. People who experience this describe it as first an awareness of pressure, then pinching, then pain.

Can this deterioration be avoided? Unfortunately not. It's part of the natural process of ageing. When researchers examine a vertebra from a young person, by all accounts, the interior of the disc is firm and whole. When they examine a vertebra from an older person, the interior of the disc, as one researcher described it, is like 'sawdust and crabmeat'.

Before you slam this book shut and run for cover, believe us when we tell you that there's a lot you can do to make sure you're well and healthy with a strong, flexible, comfortable back throughout your later years.

STAY STRONG, LIVE LONG

As we age, we lose muscle mass – about one per cent per year after age 30. Not only do the sizes of the individual cells decrease, the total number of muscle cells diminishes. This phenomenon is called sarcopenia. Researchers are not certain why it happens, but they suspect the combined effects of several factors. Reduced levels of physical activity, declining testosterone in men, declining oestradiol in women, declining growth hormone in both genders, an ageing central nervous system, a reduction in the synthesis of muscle proteins, and poor diet all contribute to the decline.

But scientists tell us that it's no longer acceptable to blame ageing for a decline in fitness. Rather, it's the other way around: a decline in fitness accelerates ageing and certainly accounts for many of the 'symptoms' we associate with ageing.

It's not uncommon for a sedentary man to go from 18 per cent body fat at age 20 to about 38 per cent by age 65. Women are capable of even worse. They can go from 23 per cent at age 20 to almost 44 per cent by age 65. These increases in body fat alone can put a human being at risk of Type 2 diabetes, high blood pressure, stroke and heart disease.

You may ask yourself, 'Why put in all the effort if ageing is inevitable?' If living a longer, healthier life is not enough of an incentive, remember that good muscle tone, strength and flexibility are critical to maintaining independence. It's a matter of 'Use it or lose it.' So, let's use it!

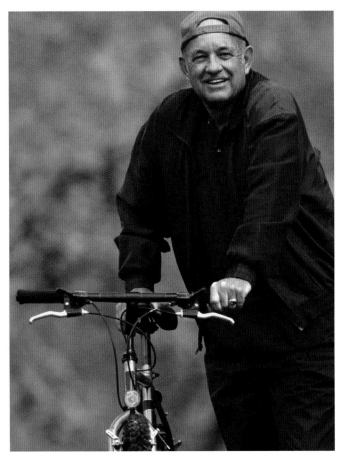

▲ Use it or lose it!
Although ageing inevitably slows us down, keeping fit will give us a longer, healthier life with more independence.

MAINTAINING THAT CRITICAL MUSCLE MASS

Fitness can be defined as a combination of good health, flexibility, strength, endurance and cardiovascular vitality. To be honest, no single component is more important than any other, but strength training is the only way to build muscle mass. In fact, studies of master athletes over 60 who regularly engage in aerobic exercise and have done so for a long time tell us that although these masters are leaner and healthier than their sedentary counterparts, they have the same amount of muscle mass and strength. The only way to build muscle mass is to lift weights, no matter what your age.

Studies have found that the density of the lower spine and thigh bone in postmenopausal women who strength train is much higher than in their sedentary counterparts. While other methods of preventing bone loss, such as medications and calcium, are effective, none has the additional benefits of strength training. The fit women not only improved bone mass but also added muscle mass, strength, balance and an overall sense of well-being that goes with being active and confident. And exactly the same holds true of men. The good news is that it is never too late to begin a fitness programme, especially one that involves strength training.

FLEXIBILITY: THE FOUNDATION OF SENIOR FITNESS

At any age, but particularly as we get older, flexibility is the key that unlocks all the other components of fitness. If you can get your body to move, you can put in place the other workout pieces – strengthening and cardio work – providing that you are medically able to participate. The Chinese say, 'You are as young as your spine is flexible'. We would add, 'and strong'.

The Active-Isolated Stretching routines you'll find in our exercise section (see pages 48 to 65) are the perfect way to begin. Most of the stretch routines can be accomplished from sitting or reclining positions, so the programme may be started slowly and gently if you're not used to working out or if you have physical limitations.

Stretching requires no special equipment except your stretch rope or strap. You don't need special clothing and you can do it almost anywhere. The benefits of the Active-Isolated method are many.

- To elongate a muscle (the antagonist), you must fire the opposing muscle (the agonist). The effect is a relaxed, lengthened muscle and a slightly strengthened opposing muscle.

STARTING SLOWLY

1. Single-leg Pelvic Tilts

See complete instructions for this two-step exercise on page 50.

2. Double-leg Pelvic Tilts

See complete instructions for this two-step exercise on page 50.

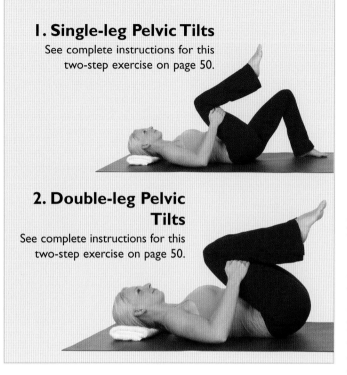

- The rhythmic action of your routine pumps blood throughout the area you are stretching.
- Your heart works a little harder, and you breathe a little more deeply – exhaling on the extension phase and inhaling as you relax the position.

The more you do, the more you are able to do. Add the strength component of the programme when you feel ready, and then eventually start the cardio training as well. Before you know it, you'll feel better than you thought possible.

MAKE IT SAFE

If you've been sedentary for a while, you should start physical activity slowly. Exercise at short intervals (5 to 10 minutes) and gradually build up to your desired level. Work out gently, with no straining. Remember that *some* exercise – even if it's a brief session with small movements – is better than none at all. You'll soon be up to speed.

Clear it with your doctor. Take this book to your doctor and talk to him or her about your plans. If you are on any medication that might affect your blood pressure or heart rate, make sure your doctor explains what will happen when you start working out, so you'll know what to expect. Discuss risk factors, illnesses and injuries that might make it necessary for you to start slowly or modify or skip an exercise.

Take your time. A few small movements will get you there, especially if you've been inactive for a while. If you push a workout, you risk getting injured or so seriously fatigued that you'll have trouble showing up for tomorrow's session. Just as getting out of shape took some time, getting back into shape will not happen overnight. Be patient.

Don't ever hold your breath. This concern is particularly important if you're straining during the strength exercises, which causes a sharp rise in blood pressure that could be problematic for you. Keep breathing: exhale as you bring the weight up, inhale as you let the weight down.

Be sure to drink plenty of water. If you wait to drink until you feel thirsty, it's too late. Thirst is a symptom of dehydration, not some early-warning system to let you know that it's time to drink. Staying hydrated is especially important as we grow older; research indicates that our ability to discern thirst is compromised as we age. Remember to drink at least eight glasses of water per day – about 1.2 litres (40fl oz).

Follow instructions specifically. They're designed to keep the strain off your back. We've spent our entire careers studying athletes and clients with varying degrees of ability and disability. Your workouts are engineered to work muscles – one or a few at a time – in small movements organised in very specific sequences that activate muscles and unlock joints when they're ready. Don't rush in feet first.

Most important: don't skip around. Do everything in order. Little by little, you'll see real results.

Avoid painkillers before exercise. Pain is a useful tool for evaluating your body. Masking it can give you false information, which could lead you to bad decisions. While using painkillers can make you more comfortable so that you can keep moving, using them to mask a profound pain and let you 'push through' can lead to injury. We had a client who regularly took ibuprofen before exercising to mask the pain of a stress fracture in her pelvis and allow her continue to train for and run marathons – with disastrous and long-term consequences. Her career ended because of this bad judgement.

MAKE IT REALISTIC

The biggest downfall we see among people starting to exercise, or getting back to it after a long hiatus, is to have grand illusions that can be dashed immediately. Know that this is a journey that will yield rewards at every stage, as long as you're patient and pragmatic about your expectations.

Make your goals attainable. That way, every workout will be a success and make you feel great. If it's been a while since you worked out, just focus on showing up every day and 'stepping up to the line'. Look at every workout as a step ahead of where you were. It's taken a lifetime to lose the high level of fitness you once had. You're working now to regain the integrity of your body, to learn how to use it again, and to teach it that you're going to put it back to work. Everything else will fall back into place in its time.

If you experience pain in a move, you've gone too far, and you're damaging something. A measure of caution is not only prudent, but also necessary. So go slowly and gently. But go.

Don't forget to rest. When you feel exhausted, drop back the routines or just skip a day. Rest will allow your body to rejuvenate, refresh and rebound. You'll be able to get right back to the workout when you're ready.

Rest is valuable for athletes of all ages, but especially true for the older athlete. Because recovery is a little slower, you'll need to give yourself extra time. We tell our older athletes that their bodies respond to training progressively, not aggressively. You have to give the neural pathways a chance to 'remember' how to move, and you have to give your muscles a chance to work up to the demands you're now making. It takes time. If you overdo it, you risk injury, which could sideline you even longer. We would rather have you in the game. Just make sure that you come back to working out.

EATING FOR ENERGY AND LONGEVITY

A balanced diet is just as important for you as for any of our athletes. The trick is to make sure you get everything you need, because as we age, we tend to have a problem opposite to one in our younger years: we tend to eat *less*. Sometimes this happens because we gradually lose some of our sense of taste and smell.

Eating just isn't as much fun, so meals tend to be smaller and less frequent. Consequently, it's increasingly difficult to get all the nutrients that a healthy body needs. Studies of ageing are particularly focused on a decrease in protein intake because one of the effects of inadequate protein is an accelerated loss of muscle, where protein is stored.

When you are stressed, have an infection, or are consuming too little protein, the body draws on stored protein in muscles to keep organs functioning. Although it's not clearly understood why, when you strength train, your body is able to store more protein, even if you aren't eating enough. The more protein you have on reserve, the better able you are to maintain muscle mass. The more muscle

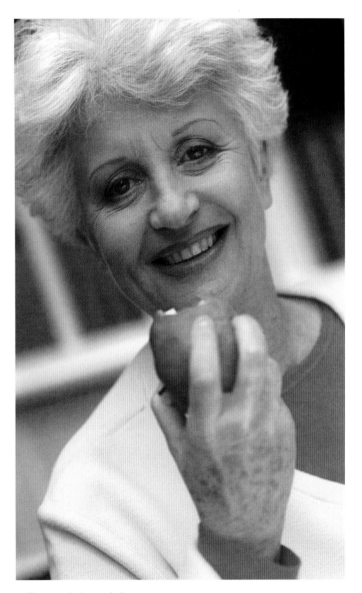

▲ Eating a balanced diet
Older people tend to eat less as they age, making it more difficult to get all the nutrients necessary for good health. Plenty of fruit and vegetables, along with more protein, will help keep you strong.

Fight Free Radicals with Antioxidants

You've heard a lot about free radicals. Free radicals are molecules in the body, usually of oxygen, that have lost an electron. Whereas most molecules have their electrons in pairs and are balanced, the free radical has only one and is unstable. Because the natural order of the universe is for electrons to be in pairs, the free radical goes in search of electrons to steal. They are like evil little bandits that career through the body, looking to raid the other molecules. When they find one, they attack and snatch an electron. The hapless molecule that has been raided is crippled and can no longer function properly. It can even die. If this sounds terrifying, realise that free radicals are unavoidable. If you want to see them in action, cut open an apple, let it stand, and watch it turn brown.

Free radicals in the human body form in the lungs and enter the bloodstream through metabolism. By damaging cells in the lungs and oxidising cholesterol to form plaque in the arteries, free radicals are thought to contribute much to the process of ageing in individual cells and, consequently, the entire human mechanism.

If free radicals are indeed a factor in the ageing of cells, then it is possible that antioxidants might help mitigate that damage. They are your body's warriors and protectors. Antioxidants combine with free radicals to neutralise them and convert them into harmless waste products. Some antioxidants actually repair damaged cells. The key antioxidant vitamins are C and E, and beta-carotene. Beta-carotene is converted by the body into vitamin A. Antioxidants are naturally abundant in vegetables, fruits and nuts. A good rule of thumb is that the deeper the colour of the plant, the more likely it is to be rich in antioxidants. (Additionally, green tea is a great source.)

Copy the list below and take it along to the supermarket to stock up on the richest sources for these important antioxidants. Please note that although it is always preferable to get all your nutrients from food, a simple, inexpensive supplement might put you on the winning side.

■ Vitamin C
Asparagus
Broccoli
Brussels sprouts
Cantaloupe melon
Commercial vegetable juices
Cranberries
Kiwi fruit
Oranges
Papaya
Potatoes
Red peppers

Spinach
Strawberries

■ Vitamin E
Almonds
Cereals fortified with vitamin E
Hazelnuts
Spinach
Sunflower seeds
Sweet potato
Vegetable oils
Wheat germ

■ Beta-carotene
Cantaloupe melon
Carrots
Commercial vegetable juices
Kale
Mangoes
Peas
Pumpkin and squash
Spinach
Sweet potato

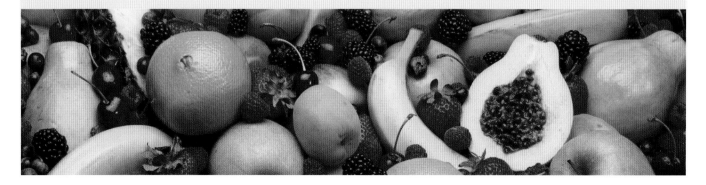

mass you maintain, the stronger you are, the more protected you are from osteoporosis and the more calories you burn. The more calories you burn, the more food – of all types – you can eat. What a wonderful cycle! Ask your doctor or better still, a nutritionist to recommend an appropriate number of protein servings per day, based on your age, gender, weight and any persistent health conditions you may have.

In order to stem the tide of muscle loss, in addition to getting an adequate amount of protein, be sure to take a multivitamin formulated for mature adults every day. Good-quality, inexpensive vitamin and mineral supplements abound. And, frankly, some vitamins are more difficult for the body to absorb from food after the age of 50. Taking supplements greatly increases your chance of benefit.

Experts suggest that taking a single multivitamin/mineral supplement is a good idea because vitamins and minerals work together in very specific proportions. If you aren't sure about what you need or how much to take, it is best to seek the advice of an expert and let them arrange the combinations for you.

FOR GOODNESS SAKE, STOP SMOKING

We know that smokers are tired of hearing about lung cancer and heart disease, but there's yet another insidious side-effect of smoking. For reasons not yet fully understood, smoking deteriorates the spine.

Researchers from Johns Hopkins University in Baltimore discovered that a history of smoking, high blood pressure and coronary artery disease are risk factors for atherosclerosis, or clogging and narrowing of the arteries.

Quit the habit for the sake of your back. Doctors are now certain that there is a link between smoking and spinal health. Along with the other risk factors associated with smoking, you should stop immediately.

What About Joint Health Supplements?

You may have heard about joint health supplements that contain glucosamine hydrochloride, glucosamine sulphate or a combination of glucosamine sulphate and chondroitin sulphate. If the claims are true, backs could theoretically be made more stable and, therefore, more comfortable. This promise is particularly attractive to people who have osteoarthritis and other degenerative disc diseases that cause pain and dysfunction. Let's take a closer look.

These supplements are available in capsules and pills and do not require a prescription. They have been in use in Europe since the 1960s and appear to live up to their claims, although no long-term studies have been done.

A word of caution: if you choose to take these supplements, make sure your doctor knows and has given you the green light. Glucosamine may cause upset stomach, heartburn or diarrhoea. Glucosamine sulphate also appears to increase insulin resistance, so people with diabetes, beware. And people on blood thinners need to avoid chondroitin sulphate.

- **Glucosamine sulphate.** Found naturally in the connective tissues of the body, glucosamine sulphate is responsible in large part for cartilage's ability to provide buffering and gliding of bone against bone without friction. When taken orally, it is absorbed easily and moves straight to the cartilage within a few hours. It boasts unique anti-inflammatory properties, and research suggests that when taken orally, it may stop the erosion of cartilage, soothe the inflammation, and promote regeneration of cartilage.

- **Glucosamine hydrochloride.** This supplement has been studied less than glucosamine sulphate, but it appears to be as effective. It has the advantage of more rapid absorption.
- **Chondroitin sulphate.** Although it has been less studied than glucosamine sulphate, chondroitin appears to have all the same properties: it may stop the erosion of cartilage, soothe the inflammation and promote regeneration of cartilage. It is also found naturally in cartilage.

No big secret here, right? The shocker is that these same risk factors are also significantly associated with the onset of lower-back pain and degenerative disorders of the discs between the vertebrae. Additionally, researchers have linked high cholesterol to the development of lumbar spondylosis, or degenerative osteoarthritis in the lower spine.

While studies continue, indisputable evidence suggests that injury and degeneration of the lower back are caused by damage to the vascular structures of the discs and joints – and that damage is caused by atherosclerosis and smoking. Although the exact mechanisms of the links between back pain and smoking are still unclear, every doctor we've spoken to regarding spinal health has emphatically stated that any person with a back problem has to stop smoking.

STAYING SAFE ON YOUR OWN

Studies tell us that falling poses a serious health problem for adults over 65 years old and is a leading cause of accidental death in adults over 75. One out of three will take a tumble. Even if there's no injury, once having fallen, an older person is statistically more likely to fall again.

Without having to resort to packing yourself in cotton wool, you can do plenty to avoid falls. In fact, people of all ages can benefit from a few tips for preventing a stumble and tumble.

Stay fit and healthy. Keep bones healthy with calcium and vitamin D. Keep your weight under control. Exercise regularly. It's never too late to start, but it's always too early to give it up.

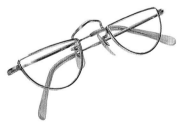

See your optician regularly. He can make sure your glasses are the correct prescription. And be sure that both your regular glasses and your sunglasses are the same prescription.

Be a good housekeeper. Keep your house clutter-free, and make sure the areas where you walk are wide and clear. Immediately wipe up spills on the floor. Keep your bed linen simple so that you won't get tangled up in it as you try to get out of bed.

Slip-proof your home. Make sure your carpets, rugs and bath mats are skid-proof and flat on the floor. Make sure

towel racks are secured tightly to the bathroom wall, so that if you need to hold onto one, it will support your weight.

You want to look slick, but your clothes shouldn't be. Select clothing and footwear that is easy to put on and take off without having to be a gymnast, and make sure that wearing it allows you free and easy movement and doesn't get in your way.

Let there be light. Make sure your environment is well-lit and that you have easy access to plenty of light switches. Install night-lights everywhere you might wander in your home after bedtime.

Hang on tight. If you stand on a chair to reach something, make sure it's stable and not wobbly. If you climb a ladder, make sure it's firmly and securely stabilised at both ends. If you're unsteady at heights, invest in an extension 'grabber' for reaching and gripping small items above your head.

Prepare for winter. If it snows, keep snow and ice off your porch, steps, walks, drive and pavements – anywhere that you will walk. If you must navigate alone, try to choose a route that is bordered by stable things onto which you can lean or cling.

Keep alcohol under control. Avoid drinking alcohol to the point that you're tipsy. Not only will you be off balance, your judgement will be impaired.

Stay in communication. As we grow older, we tend to be alone more than when we were younger. Establish regular contact at least once a day with someone who will check on you.

Stay in the game. Action breeds action. Sure, things may take a little bit longer. They may even be a bit more difficult. But in the end, your life is worth it. Stay active.

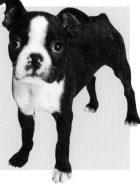

Encourage your furry friend to refrain from jumping on you unexpectedly or getting under your feet as you move. You may well have to be very firm, but with training your dog or cat will gradually learn that these potentially dangerous actions are not allowed any more.

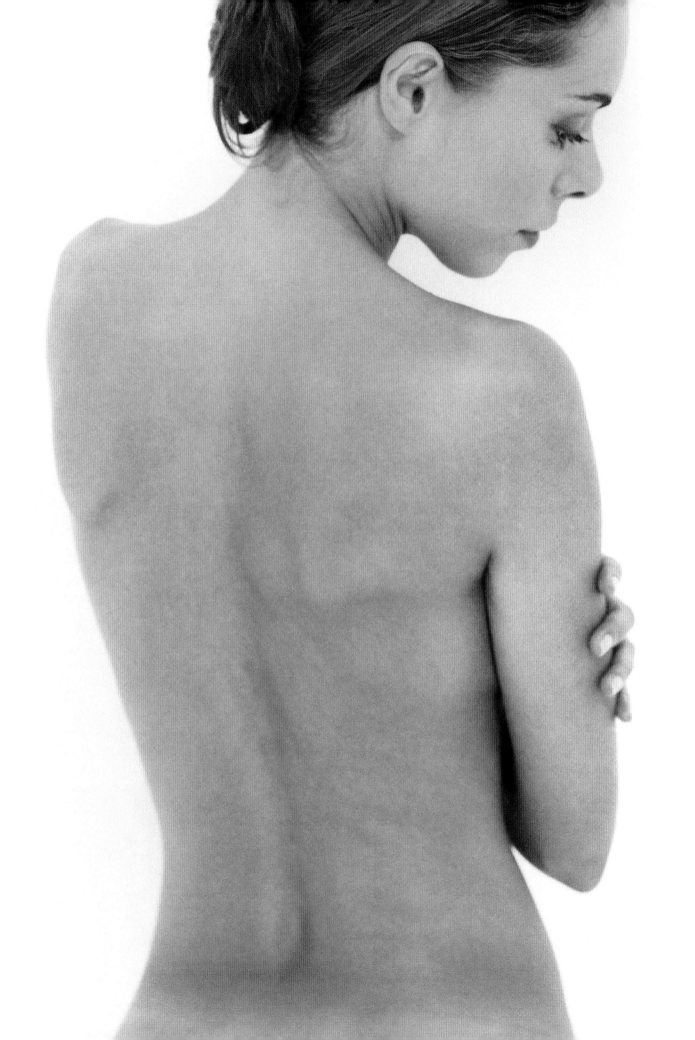

5

STRESS AND SLUMBER

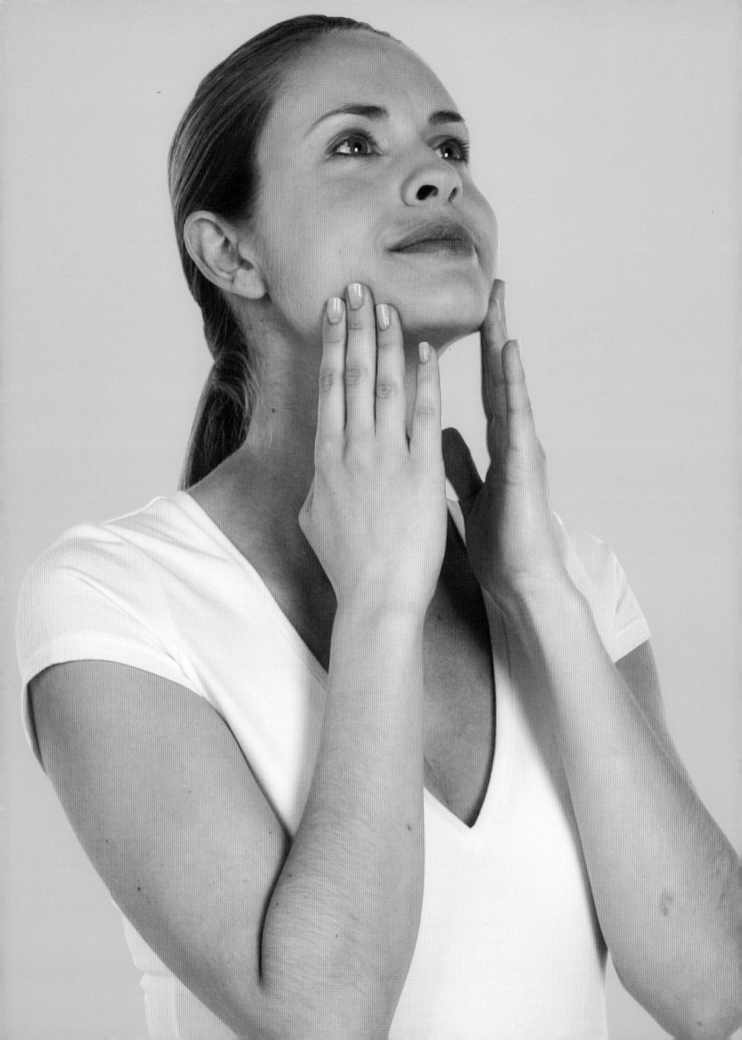

CHAPTER 12

PUTTING TENSION BEHIND YOU

In the dark days that followed 9/11 and the attack on *the World Trade Center, we, like all New Yorkers, struggled to find a way to help our city stand up and fight back, to heal a gaping wound that was kept raw by fear and exhaustion. As did most New York City businesses, ours fell silent, so we had time to join the massive volunteer effort. Our offering was therapy for weary workers.*

We could do nothing at Ground Zero, but we could do a little for the men who struggled to deal with it every day – the firefighters who were grieving for their dead while searching for survivors in the twisted, smouldering rubble of the World Trade Center.

Rarely did any of our team have the luxury of an uninterrupted hour of treatment with a firefighter, but between alarms that signalled scrambles to the truck and polite apologies, we helped them to relax their bodies with the same techniques we use to get elite athletes on to Olympic tracks.

Keeping the body operating at peak efficiency through stress features two components: first, physically preparing for the immediate demands, and second, overcoming the fear and tension that can take an insidious toll on the body, especially the back.

WHY DOES TENSION ATTACK THE BACK?

If you ask most people what happens when they tense up, they'll tell you what you already know: we carry our tension in a small zone of pain right between our shoulder blades up to the base of our necks. But why does tension take up residence in this very specific place? There are many theories.

Tension can be emotional. Tension in the back is directly related to state of mind. Instinctively, when we're upset, we curl up. This posture takes a lot of effort, straining and fatiguing the muscles in your upper back and neck. The longer you despair, the more strained and tired those muscles get. And worse, the muscles in the front of your chest will begin to shorten, pulling you even lower. It's no accident of language that we refer to an unhappy person as being 'down'.

We're going to tell you something shocking: unhappy people are prone to injury and illness. Nearly 80 per cent of all the physical problems we treat are related, directly or indirectly, to tension and pressure. When we treat a client who falls into this category, we make friends, because we know we're likely to see them again. No matter what we do to unlock the body or how successful we are in restoring function, sooner or later, this client is going to come back unless he gets a handle on life. We aren't saying that getting happy will guarantee you a lifetime of health and injury-free fitness, but it helps. Big time.

Tension can be physical. The emotional aspect of carrying tension between the shoulder blades is not the only culprit. Fitness, or lack thereof, plays an even bigger part.

When your back is in pain, your abdominal muscles are the suspected cause. Weak abs cause your pelvis to be unstable, so your back – all the way from your sacrum to your skull – has to compensate to keep your body balanced and erect in posture, sort of like a gyroscope. But without the assistance of supporting abdominal muscles, your struggling back becomes a very unstable gyroscope.

While the problem originates at your pelvis, it qualifies as a full-blown disaster by the time it reaches your head. Weighing in at 8–12lb (3.6–5.4kg), the head is heavy. When your abdominals are weak and your back is struggling to compensate, that heavy head pulls your spine forwards.

Shoulders follow suit as the front of your shoulders foreshorten and collapse. This sag may be subtle at first, but it doesn't take long for your upper back, designed to stabilise, to become fatigued from trying to support weight. It will short out. A strong, fit body ensures that all your muscles are doing their jobs and that they are sparing your back from having to compensate.

Tension can be postural. People can even make tension between shoulders worse by postural mistakes. When you sleep on your side with a pillow that fails to support your head and neck, you collapse your lower shoulder, folding it towards your chest and straining the muscles in your back for hours. When you work at a desk, you sit and put all action in front of you, so that you reach out and down towards the desk – and your upper back is stressed. When you drive, you reach forwards and up to steer – and your upper back is stressed. When you eat, your plate is on the table in front of you, so you reach down and towards it – your upper back is stressed.

Case Study: **Harry Stetz**

Back and shoulder problems aren't always the result of a postural imbalance or an incorrectly performed exercise; sometimes the root cause can be a lot deeper.

Harry Stetz is a successful mortgage broker. He came to us with a frozen shoulder and mid-thoracic spine pain after a bus door accidentally closed on him. We were able to use Active-Isolated Stretching to unlock his cervical spine, and then we started working lower. But we could sense a terrible fear.

As we touched him, Harry would recoil. It's not uncommon in deep-muscle massage to press our hands into someone and cause an explosive emotional release, or trigger the recollection of a long-forgotten memory of pain, sorrow or fear. It's one of the mystical links – between

mind and body – that we cannot prove. We just know it's there.

Our work on Harry's back released memories of being trapped and severely beaten as a fearful child. He had been storing pain, injury and fear that were locking up his back and probably had little to do with the injury.

Although the pain was in his upper back, Harry's shoulder was locked and his neck was very painful. We started unlocking his neck through stretching very gently and slowly. When his neck eventually released through stretching, his shoulder then let go. We were able to begin stretching his shoulder. Again, very

gently and slowly. As we released his muscles, he began to release his hurt.

We don't know why this happens, but we do know that when Harry accepted and healed the hurt of his childhood, his back stopped hurting. And we got his shoulder unlocked.

When Harry was flexible from doing his Active-Isolated Stretching, he was able to add strengthening exercises to his workout. We put a special emphasis on his upper back and shoulders. He felt better immediately, but every day got even better. In three weeks, he got his arm over his head and could put his shirt on without assistance.

In fact, there's a *lot* you do to stress your upper back. If you switch positions frequently and keep your back relaxed and moving, there's usually no problem. Problems can start when you are sedentary and still and you sustain stress for long periods of time. Add personal tension to biomechanical mistakes and long-term fatigue, and you have a knotted, cramped upper back.

YOU CAN'T AFFORD TO IGNORE TENSION-RELATED BACK PAIN

Stopping tension-related pain in its tracks is very important. While many back problems originate in that upper-back zone, they don't necessarily stay there. Back problems beget back problems. Just when you thought you couldn't be more locked up and incapacitated, this pain sneaks down to your lower back to hobble your step, creeps up your neck to inflict a world-class tension headache, or radiates down your arms in an exhausting ache or a shooting pain.

When those muscles between your shoulder blades become fatigued, they begin to shut down in a process that is a little like strangulation. The area becomes *hypoxic*, or deprived of oxygen, as blood flow is slowly squeezed off when tissues constrict. This condition poses a double threat, because not only does blood carry oxygen to the muscles so they can function properly and thrive, it also helps carry away metabolic waste generated when the muscles fire. When metabolic waste, like lactic acid, accumulates, you

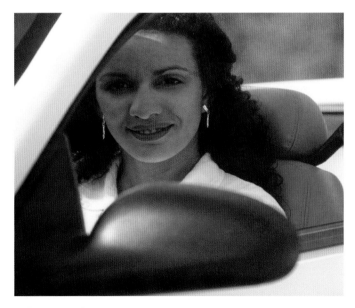

▲ Driven mad
Poor posture when driving is one of the chief culprits behind tension-related back pain.

experience cramping – your body's alarm signal that you have moved beyond fatigue and are approaching full-blown injury. It doesn't take much longer before signals from your brain through nerves to the muscles are cut off and a debilitating, painful loss of function follows.

Up to the point of hypoxia, you might have recruited blood flow to the area by reducing the swelling and getting yourself moving. Now it's too late for an easy way out. Your muscles can't pick up the signals they need to fire. You'll have to get serious now – and that means getting rid of that tension. Luckily, we have the answer.

GET OUT OF PAIN FAST: EIGHT QUICK RELEASES

These quick-release techniques can be done at your desk or even standing right in front of another person, who won't be able to tell that you're stretching.

Quick releases are not exactly exercises. They don't constitute a workout. They're fast, subtle moves, which are powerful and effective. Because they fly below the radar of conventional fitness, we call them 'stealth health'.

This series is *not* a routine. These small moves that release tension can be done individually, in any order. Whenever you feel tension in your back, just move quickly to release it. Just as you scratch an itch, you release a tense muscle.

You'll get the most out of these movements if you remember the basic principle of releasing tension: all muscles work in pairs. When one muscle contracts and shortens, another must relax and lengthen. One muscle is activated; the opposite muscle is relaxed into a stretch, allowing more circulation of blood and oxygen. So when you have a spasm or cramp between your shoulders from tension, it makes good sense to relax it by activating opposite muscles.

For example, when the muscles on the left side and back of your neck are in spasm (which they always are when your upper back is locked), you'll want to fire the opposite muscle group on the right side and front of your neck. By repeatedly activating the opposite muscle group in a sort of pumping action, the muscles in spasm are isolated and soothed. In addition, they are gently stretched, which begins the all-important restoration of circulation.

Continuing further down in a tension lock are the upper back extensors. To isolate and relax them, we have to activate the opposite muscles on the front side of the body, which are the pectoralis majors in the chest. Again, the key here is movement.

If you're looking for a rhythm to which you can pace these movements, the mantra is 'Let it go, feel the flow'. Recite it a few times, and you'll understand the rhythm.

Roll Your Shoulders

Active Muscles You Contract: Inner muscle group that steadies and controls your upper back and your shoulder

Isolated Muscles You Stretch: Outer muscle group that steadies and controls your upper back, your chest and your shoulder

Hold Each Stretch: 2 seconds **Reps:** 10 forwards, 10 backwards

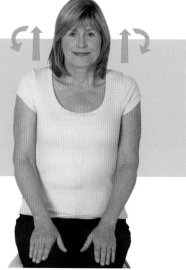

1 Sit on a chair with your back straight. Relax and dangle your arms straight down. If the arm of the chair is in the way, move forwards. It's better to sit back, however, so that your tailbone is directly underneath you.

2 Roll the shoulders forwards, up, around and back. Breathe in on the up, then out as you roll back. Lead with the hands and don't hunch your shoulders. Keep your head up and aligned with your spine. Relax your neck, then repeat.

Roll Your Neck

Active Muscles You Contract: Nothing specific. This is a warm-up

Isolated Muscles You Stretch: Nothing specific. This is a warm-up

Hold Each Stretch: 2 seconds **Reps:** Roll from right to left and then back to the right 10 times

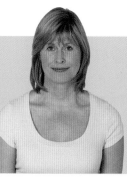

1 Sit on a chair with your back straight. Relax your shoulders. Tuck your chin in. Roll your head towards your shoulder – around and up. Inhale on the upward roll. Hold for two seconds.

2 Roll towards the other shoulder. Exhale in the middle of the roll. Stop when your chin is parallel to the floor above your shoulder. Don't tilt your head back and stop if there is discomfort. Roll your head back and forth.

TIP: When you roll your neck, you might hear grinding noises or a tendon or ligament flipping. Don't panic. Your skull magnifies all sound and your ear picks this up from the inside. As you continue, this will lessen.

3

Reset the Back of Your Neck

Active Muscles You Contract: Muscles in the back of your neck

Isolated Muscles You Stretch: You're resetting your upper cervical vertebrae

Hold Each Stretch: 2 seconds **Reps:** 10

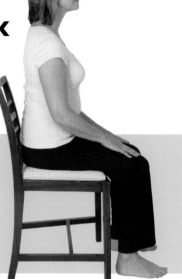

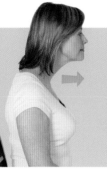

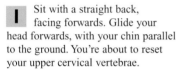

1 Sit with a straight back, facing forwards. Glide your head forwards, with your chin parallel to the ground. You're about to reset your upper cervical vertebrae.

2 When you can go no further, lead with your chin and gently roll your head back until your nose is in the air. Elongate the front of your throat. Hold for a moment.

3 Return to the neutral position. Glide your head back until it's in alignment with your spine. Hold, and then glide back out again to repeat the lifting and lengthening.

4

Relax the Sides of Your Neck

Active Muscles You Contract: Muscles in the side of your neck (flexors)

Isolated Muscles You Stretch: Muscles in the opposite side of your neck (flexors)

Hold Each Stretch: 2 seconds **Reps:** 10 to the right, 10 to the left

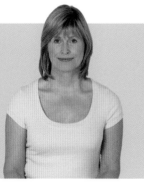

1 Sit on a chair with your back straight. Your head and neck should be in alignment with your spine.

2 Lower your ear to your shoulder as you exhale. Inhale as you slowly bring your head up. Do the full reps on that side, then swap. Finally, quickly shrug the shoulders up to the ears, then drop and relax them. Do this three times in rapid succession.

5

Promote Neck Rotation

Active Muscles You Contract: Muscles in the side of your neck (rotators)

Isolated Muscles You Stretch: Muscles in the opposite side of your neck (rotators)

Hold Each Stretch: 2 seconds **Reps:** 10 to the right, 10 to the left

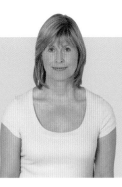
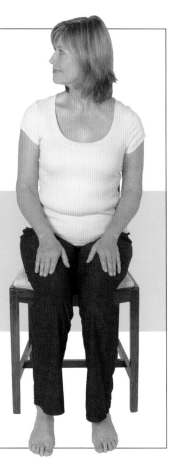

1 Sit on a chair with your back straight. Align your head and neck with your spine. Elongate the neck and bring your head up, as though your crown were attached to a helium balloon. Keep your chin parallel to the ground.

2 Keep your shoulders forward. Turn your head straight to the side until your chin is over your shoulder, while exhaling. Lead with your eyes. Hold for two seconds. Inhale as you return to neutral and then repeat. Do the full reps on that side, then swap. Stop if there is discomfort.

6

Release the Back and Side of Your Neck

Active Muscles You Contract: Muscles in the front of your neck

Isolated Muscles You Stretch: Muscles in your upper shoulders at the base of your neck, including trapezius muscles

Hold Each Stretch: 2 seconds **Reps:** 10 to the right, 10 to the left

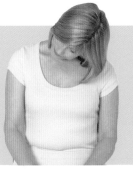

1 Sit in a chair with your back straight and your head aligned with your spine. Turn your head 45 degrees, then drop it forward, with your ear close to your chest.

2 Put your hand on your head and press. Hold for two seconds. Do 10 reps on one side, keeping your head in rotation as you return to the neutral position, then swap. Please note that momentum will take your trunk down with your head, so you'll have to concentrate to isolate the head and neck movement from the torso.

7

Stretch the Back of Your Shoulder

Active Muscles You Contract: Muscles in the front of your shoulder

Isolated Muscles You Stretch: External shoulder rotators

Hold Each Stretch: 2 seconds **Reps:** 10 to the right, 10 to the left

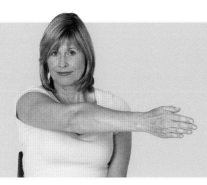

1 You can do this one from either a seated or standing position. (This one isn't too subtle, but its benefit is worth the potential embarrassment if someone catches you doing it.) Simply lift one arm, with the elbow locked, and raise it straight across your chest towards the opposite shoulder.

2 Use the other hand to gently assist and get the most out of the stretch. Hold for two seconds and relax. Return your arm all the way to the starting position. Relax a moment. Do all 10 on one arm before moving on to the other arm.

8

Stretch Your Whole Back

Active Muscles You Contract: Abdominals, muscles on the sides of your chest, and the thoracic-lumbar rotators

Isolated Muscles You Stretch: Muscles that run from your pelvis to the base of your skull along the spine, and the muscles throughout your back and sides that stabilise your torso

Hold Each Stretch: 2 seconds **Reps:** 10 to the right, 10 to the left

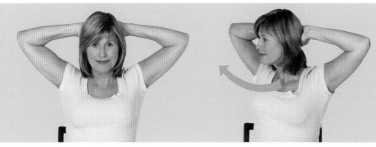
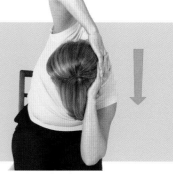

1 Sit in a chair with your back straight. Your head and neck should be in alignment with your spine. Lock your hands behind your head, with your elbows pointed straight out. Tuck your chin down very gently.

2 Rotate your upper body to the side as far as you can twist. Do this three times, trying to go a little further each time, until you're warmed up.

3 Then rotate, hold, and flex your trunk forward towards the floor, moving your elbow between your knees. Hold, then unwind the rotation until facing forwards again. Repeat this rotation and dip 10 times, then swap sides.

OTHER FAST TENSION RELEASERS

Quick releases are great, but they may not work for everyone, every time. Here are some other quick fixes that can help to quickly lessen the tension in your back.

Ice it. When your shoulders are locked up, people usually head for the hot-water bottle or heating pad. It's easy to get fooled into thinking that because heat feels good and relaxes you, it's doing the job. Besides, ice is initially uncomfortable. We'll even admit that the first few seconds can take your breath away. We advise our clients to persevere, however.

When you're battling a cramp between your shoulders, ice helps to reduce swelling and promotes circulation. The body is designed to run extra blood to areas that are cold.

(This is why your nose turns pink when it's cold.) You need that blood flow to remove metabolic waste and reoxygenate your muscles. Additionally, ice numbs the skin and reduces pain so that you'll feel less guarded about moving your back. The more you move, the better off you'll be.

Ice can be applied directly to a painful site for up to 10 minutes, which is sufficient time to numb the skin and recruit healing blood flow, without causing damage to your skin. If you're still in pain after the first application, try icing the site every hour on the hour. Three times should yield good results, but use your own judgement. (For a professional athlete with a serious injury, we've maintained a 24-hour schedule, but this is rarely necessary.)

If you don't have a conventional ice pack, take a paper cup and fill it with water. Freeze it, and peel away about

How Tight Are You?

Most of us do not know what 'normal' flexibility is. Only by knowing where you start will you have any sense of progression towards your goal, once you undertake a simple exercise programme. Instead of the standard sit-and-reach test, which is not an accurate measure, we suggest three other ways to evaluate your flexibility.

■ **Let's check your back.** Sit on the floor with your feet flat and your knees flexed. Contract your abdominals, bend at the hips, and draw your torso slowly down, pointing your head towards the floor between your feet. Don't bounce to get there. It doesn't matter how long you can hold it.

If you can roll your back forwards and get your head past your knees, your back is fairly flexible. If you can get your head past your midshin, your back is very flexible. If you can't get your head down to your knees, you have work to do. Here's another hint that your back is tight: if you can't sit upright in this position without putting your hands back on the floor behind you, you have a *lot* of work to do.

■ **Now, let's check your calves.** Stay seated on the floor. Put your legs straight out in front of you. Bend one knee and draw your foot towards your buttocks with the bottom of your foot flat on the floor. Bending at the hips, lean forwards over the straight leg. Reach down and take the ball of your foot in your hands. Keep your heel on the floor and pull the ball of your foot towards your torso. You want to get a 15-degree range of motion on the ankle by drawing your toes to your nose.

If you can't reach your foot, the calf is too tight. A tight calf means a tight hamstring, which means that your hip rotators and glutes are having to overcompensate and are shortened. Remember, no back is an island. It's all connected. If your calf is tight, your back will follow. You have some work to do.

■ **Finally, let's check the flexor muscles.** In order to check their flexibility, and also that of the muscles in the sides of your trunk, stand with your feet slightly apart and your knees slightly bent and relaxed. With both arms at your side, contract your trunk at the waist and slide the palm of one hand down your thigh, bending sideways from the waist without shifting your pelvis. Stand back up, then slide that palm down the front and the back of your thigh. You should be able to get your fingertips just below your knee from all three angles. The less able you are to hit that target, the less flexible your lateral trunk flexors are. You have work to do.

Case Study: **Sam Zomber**

Knee surgery would not seem a likely culprit when treating searing back pain. But one leg may compensate for the weakness of the other until, eventually, the back locks up.

Sam Zomber is a businessman who spends most of his time hunched over a desk. When we met him, he had undergone two knee operations that had made walking difficult and painful. As his mobility decreased, Sam gained weight. His biggest complaint was that his back hurt. It was constantly fatigued and was occasionally seized by a screaming spasm.

Sam's knee injury was wreaking havoc. We immediately identified the weakened knee as the culprit. When the knee is weak, the thigh is strained and the hip flexors have to compensate. When the hip flexors compensate, the pelvis is thrown out of alignment and strains the lower back. A knee injury usually moves right up the chain of mystical links, but Sam's also moved *down* the chain to his ankle. Remember, when one part of the body falters or fails it sets off a chain reaction of compensations and imbalances. And although we can usually identify the obvious injury as the lowest and weakest link on that chain, sometimes the injury works its mischief all the way down the line. In Sam's case, his left ankle was frozen in a muscular fusion from misuse, disuse and compensation.

Before we could strengthen Sam, we had to unlock him, so we started with some stretching exercises. When we had restored range of motion to the joints of his body, we added strengthening exercises to his workout. Although we helped Sam learn to stretch and strengthen a back in spasm, we made sure that he was diligent about everything below the belt from his hips all the way down to his ankles. We also worked to strengthen his abdominals, so they could once more support his back. The net effect was that when we balanced his gait and tightened his midsection, his back stopped hurting. He walks now with only a slight limp and carries an exercise strap for stretching.

1in (2.5cm) of the cup's top to expose the ice. As the ice melts, keep peeling. Hold the ice by whatever is left of the cup to keep your fingers comfortable, and massage your back with the exposed end. If you can't reach your back and have no one to help you, place ice in a plastic bag, put it on the floor, and lie down on it.

Alternatively, you might try taking a sealed bag of frozen peas and draping it against your back. The pack remains neat and tidy because it is sealed up and conforms to the contours of your body. You can, of course, reuse your bag of frozen peas – just put it back in the freezer.

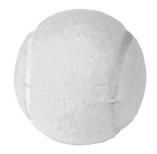

Try 'floor tennis'. You can sometimes work out tension between your shoulders by lying on a tennis ball. Place a tennis ball on the floor, then lie on it, positioning the ball just outside the point of tension, not on the spine, but in the depression on either side of your spine, between your vertebrae and your shoulder blade. Relax your weight down on the ball very slowly. Keep your knees bent so that you can lift your pelvis off the floor and glide back and forth with the weight of your upper back on the ball. It's a sort of self-massage done upside down.

This massage feels great as long as you don't roll the ball directly under your spine. You'll be putting painful pressure on the vertebrae, where there's no muscle to benefit from massage. Roll as long as you enjoy it or until the tension releases. If you can't get the tension to release within 10 minutes, move immediately into a full Active-Isolated Stretching routine, and see if the combination of floor tennis and a stretch rope or strap does the trick. Our bet is that you'll be all right before you know it.

Shrug it off. One interesting theory holds that muscles have cellular memory. They 'know' where they're supposed to be and how they're supposed to feel. Assuming this is true, it's possible to lead a muscle quickly into pain and tension in order for it to access its cellular memory to recoil and rebound back into comfort, back into its perfect state of being. In other words, you are using your body's memory to quickly, dramatically demonstrate to it that pain is very wrong and then, following that moment, letting your body show you what will make it right.

The action is painful, yet simple: tense and release. Hunch your shoulders up as high and as tightly as you can lift them. Exhale as you bring your shoulders up. Hold for a few seconds. Let it hurt, hurt, hurt! Then inhale completely as you quickly drop your shoulders down. Breathing deeply is very important because you need oxygen in your blood to help your muscles fire properly and to help carry away the metabolic waste from a fatigued muscle that has been in a full clinch. The body uses the 'sigh' to release tension naturally. If you don't feel like engineering a few deep breaths, just sigh the same way you always do. Repeat until you feel the tension relax.

Breathe deeply into relaxation. Our friend Dr Andrew Weil believes that tension is the culprit in many cases of illness and injury. As the director of the programme in integrative medicine at the University of Arizona College of Medicine in Tucson, Dr Weil devotes a great deal of time to training his patients to relax, body and soul. We share techniques.

As we've told you, when you're tense and upset, you jack your shoulders up and carry that resulting tension in your body. When you're relaxed and serene, you don't do that. Thus, it stands to reason that personal serenity would do much to prevent or mitigate tension in one's body and, more specifically, in the area of the upper back between the shoulders.

Achieving a peaceful state of mind might be as easy as practising Dr Weil's Yoga Breath. Get comfortable and close your eyes. Breathe through your nose, one nostril at a time. Start with the left nostril by blocking the right. Inhale to a slow count of four. Hold to a slow count of seven. Exhale to a slow count of eight. Switch sides. Block the left, breathe with the right. Switch sides again.

Do this four times per side. Imagine with each breath that you are filled with energy and that your muscles are relaxing, lengthening, strengthening and getting organised – fibre by fibre.

Treat it with over-the-counter analgesics. Sometimes the fastest remedy is the tried-and-true pill. A number of over-the-counter analgesics or painkillers can help take the pain out of a tension backache.

Drink more water. The body is largely made up of water. When you are dehydrated, healthy cells that are normally plump and juicy dry out and shrivel up. Their composition and function are disrupted. They don't slide as easily against each other, and, in fact, they actually shred. If your upper back is tight because you're tense, and you're also dehydrated, you'll exacerbate the damaging effects of the tension on your muscles. Make sure that you drink plenty of water. As an added benefit, you'll feel better in general if you keep yourself hydrated.

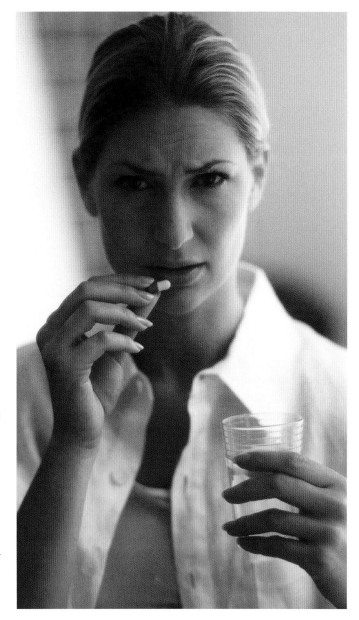

▲ No-pain gain
If you're suffering from back tension, don't be proud – take over-the-counter painkillers. These can be effective in quelling the pain.

Not only should you drink throughout the day, you should plan to hydrate before, during and after every workout. Plain water is good, but some athletes prefer sports drinks that hydrate as well as replace electrolytes lost in sweating and carbohydrates such as glucose, sucrose, fructose and glucose polymers. These drinks can help boost energy immediately. Some experts believe it is best to drink water before your workout to hydrate you, and the sports drinks later, during your workout, when your body needs the carbohydrates and is prepared to handle and use the sugars you're taking in.

There are plenty of good sports drinks on the market. Because results and reactions vary with individuals, test them during training. By the way, studies indicate that no matter what you drink, it will absorb more quickly from your stomach and into your cells if you drink it cold.

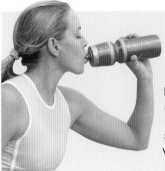

Sports drinks are widely used by athletes and casual exercise enthusiasts alike. They help to rehydrate the body, as well as replace electrolytes lost through sweating. Try out a few and see which brand works best for you.

Be sure to rest. When you're tired, you droop and keep the muscles in your shoulders and upper back in tension. The more tense and in pain you are, the less likely you are to get good rest. The less rested you are… well, you get the picture. This cycle of pain and exhaustion is a catch-22. An exhausted person can't hold posture properly. Muscles don't fire properly. Fatigue erodes everything in your body, mind and spirit.

Rest. You'll be amazed at how breaking the cycle can help ease the tension from your shoulders.

Sleep in the right position. When you sleep on your side without proper support for your head and neck, your head drops down. With your head dropped, the shoulder on which you're resting will collapse forwards towards your chest, compressed under the weight of your body, and blood flow to your shoulder becomes constricted.

This position throws your body into automatic contraction, with the centre of gravity balanced on your hip and folded shoulder, which strains your upper back. If you hold this position all night, the constriction and tension will take its

toll. Either get a pillow that supports your head and neck, keeping them in alignment, or sleep on your back.

We also recommend that you avoid sleeping all night on your abdomen, with your head turned to one side, propped up on a pillow. This position hyperextends the neck and causes fatigue. (See page 223 for our recommended sleep positions.)

A FRIEND IN KNEAD

At one time or another, nearly every human has been recruited as a massage therapist. We have all grabbed a friend behind the neck and kneaded those upper-back muscles with our thumbs to relieve a searing spasm or, even more commonly, a knot in the back. But what exactly is a 'knot' and how exactly should you massage someone who has got one?

Knots feel like small, firm lumps within soft, smooth muscle fibres. For the person that's suffering with them, they feel like ignited charcoal embedded under your skin. Acutely painful to the touch, knots are adhesions – sort of like scar tissue – that are caused when the muscle is microscopically torn. Muscles are fibrous, like bundles of rubber bands. When a few of these fibres are injured and tear, they recoil into snarled disruptions. As they try to heal, they reconfigure out of their smooth pattern. The torn ends of the individual fibres stick together (adhere) in a disorganised knot, like a scar. You don't have to suffer trauma for it to happen; fatigue or overuse can cause a little tear in muscle fibres. In fact, it's pretty common. In areas that are used heavily or have generous blood flow, a microtear is no big deal. But in an area like the upper back, where blood flow is less generous than other areas of the body and easily impeded, microtears cannot heal quickly and easily. They develop into adhesions, or the knots we all know so well.

To break up these adhesions and restimulate blood flow, you need to gently and firmly massage the knot. The muscle fibres will eventually relax and smooth out; the adhesion will loosen and let go. Eventually, the knot will disappear along with the acute pain.

The fitter you are, the less tension you'll carry in your body. The less tension you carry, the easier and faster fitness will come to you. Letting go of a lot of unnecessary strain will allow muscles to respond to training and restore your vital energy. Let us show you how to do it right with our three tried and tested massage routines. Not only will you help your friends, you'll be the most popular person around.

Massage 1

1

Muscles You Relax: Upper trapezius and rhomboids

Duration of Massage: 10 minutes or until tension eases

Equipment: None

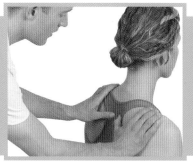 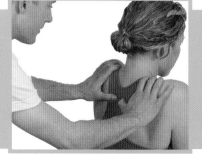 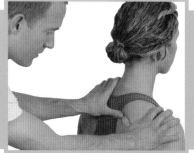

1 Stand behind your seated friend. Place your palms on top of her shoulders resting your fingers over the shoulder and your thumbs on the muscles between the shoulder blades.

2 Squeeze, pressing the shoulders with your thumbs, while your friend contracts her shoulders, like a shrug. Hold for three seconds. Let go as your friend relaxes. Repeat. You want her to feel the squeeze, but no pain.

TIP: After the first two steps, if there is a specific point of pain, keep your fingers high on the shoulders, but slide your thumbs down over the 'knot'. Press firmly and gently for a few seconds. Release. Repeat until the tension eases.

Massage 3

3

Muscles You Relax: Upper trapezius, rhomboids, neck

Duration of Massage: 10 minutes or until tension eases

Equipment: None

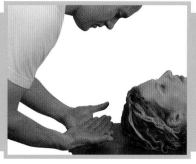 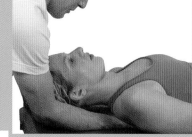 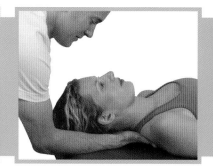

1 Remove all jewellery and make sure your nails are trimmed. Get your friend to lie flat on her back. Position yourself above the top of her head. Cup your palms together with the palm of your dominant hand on top, facing up.

2 Get your friend to lift slightly so that you can slide your cupped palms under her back before she relaxes her weight down on to your hands. Rest your friend's head on the upturned insides of your forearms.

3 Contract your fingers until they're over the muscles to one side of the spine. Draw your hands back, pressing your fingers into the muscles. Run your hands from the shoulder blade to the top of the shoulders three times. Change sides. Repeat.

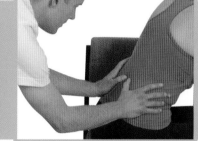

Massage 2

Muscles You Relax: Erector spinae

Duration of Massage: 10 minutes or until tension eases

Equipment: None

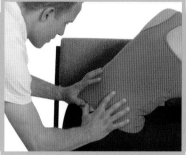

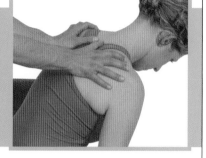

1 Stand behind your seated friend. Get her to roll forwards and down from her hips, aiming her forehead to her knees. When she's fully curled down, put your thumbs on either side of her lower spine.

2 As your friend rolls her back up slowly, slide your thumbs firmly up her back. Make sure she is okay with the pressure. Advance your thumbs up only 6–8in (15–20cm) by the time your friend is fully upright.

3 Get your friend to curl down again and then roll back up as you advance your thumbs up another 6–8in (15–20cm). Continue this progression until you've reached the base of her skull.

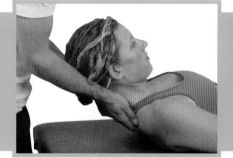

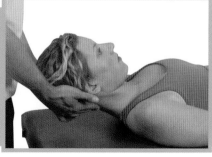

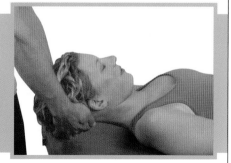

4 On the third pass, uncup your hands and put one hand on each side of the spine. Slide your fingers continuously from the back up the neck as your friend tucks her chin and lifts her head.

5 Then, using gravity and the weight of your friend's head in your palms, knead the base of her skull with the tips of your fingers in short, firm, gentle strokes.

6 Finally, lock your fingertips under the base of her skull and gently, firmly pull towards you as she exhales. Do this to the count: 'Pull, two, three, four. Release, two, three, four.' Beginners need to be careful. Nothing should ever hurt.

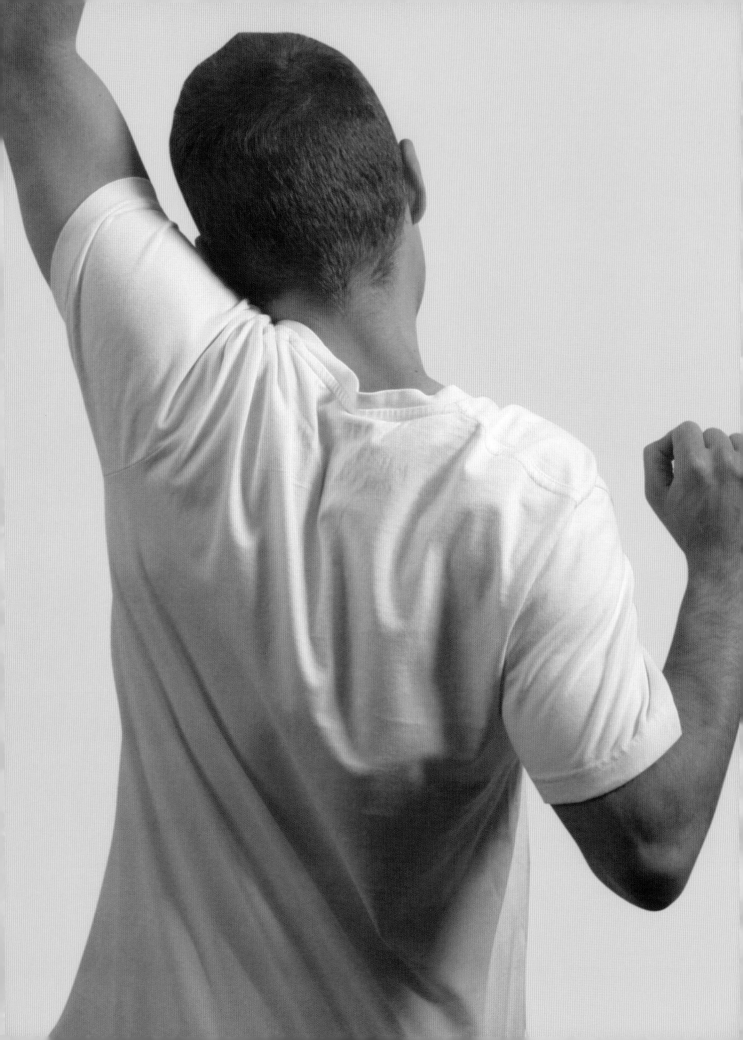

CHAPTER 13

NOW I LAY ME DOWN TO SLEEP

Sleep is the way the human body heals and restores.
If you can't sleep because your back is bothering you, you're not alone. One in five of us suffer sleep problems, and 15 per cent of doctor visits are due to sleep problems. For most patients, back pain is the number one culprit, followed by headaches and muscle pain. To make matters worse, some medications used to ease an aching back also disrupt sleep.

If **your back is bothering you,** it's likely that you will not sleep well. Researchers who study pain management tell us that falling asleep is the toughest part. You would think that clearing that hurdle and finally drifting off would assure a restful night. But even if you manage to get to sleep, one toss or turn the wrong way can cause pain that awakens you as suddenly and surely as the rude jolt of an alarm clock. If you can't get comfortable enough to drop back to sleep, or if it happens more than once a night, the net effect is a brutal, restless sleep. In the morning, you emerge from between the tangle of sheets, exhausted and angry – so not only is your back aching, but you spend the day emotionally drained, mentally dulled and cranky. Being tired will heighten your perception of pain, making it noticeably less manageable, and lessen the energy with which you usually carry your body, further aggravating your back. But there's more.

Under normal circumstances, your body uses the time you've spent horizontal to enjoy a reprieve from the effects of vertical gravity on your back – and the time you've spent asleep to refresh and rejuvenate on a cellular level while your metabolism is slowed. Deprived of those opportunities, your body's ability to heal is diminished. It takes only a few nights of disturbed sleep, or no sleep at all, for some serious erosion in body, mind and spirit to set in.

We have studied sleep and integrated it in a very deliberate way into every training and rehabilitation programme we supervise. We've learned that if you are going to take successful control of healing, you have to take control of sleeping. This begins with understanding why sleep is beneficial and how you can become good at getting a good night's sleep. Then, because we live in a 24-hour-a-day society that values constant activity into the wee hours and regards resting as slacking, we have to teach you to be unapologetic about going to bed.

SETTING THE STAGE FOR SLUMBER

In times gone by, people would go to sleep when the day was literally done: when the sun had gone down and the fire faded into glowing embers in the dark. The temperature of the room would drop, cooling the air. Bodies, physically tired from a day of hard work and full from an evening's meal, would slow metabolically. People would curl up into their blankets to sleep. Hours later, at sunrise, light and warmth would gently, naturally raise metabolism and stir people to get up, rested to face another day, and hungry.

Today, in sharp contrast, we have pushed back the darkness to create a 24-hour society without such clear distinction between day and night. At night, we create day. We flip on a light, turn up the thermostat, order a pizza, and continue to work and play in darkness. And we can turn day into night – we turn off lights, block out the sun with shades, make the room colder with a simple command, and drop into soft, fragrant sheets to sleep at high noon. No problem.

But all this efficiency, flexibility, ingenuity and joy come with a price, for although times have changed, human need for sleep has not. Most of us are so out of touch with the natural rhythms of the universe and our own bodies that we are sleep-deprived to some degree.

People today get an average of 20 per cent less sleep per night than 100 years ago. We've also added a month per year to the time we spend working and commuting. So here are ways you can counteract these changes to get more sleep.

Turn your bedroom into a sacred space. The room should have only two purposes: sleeping and making love. If you are using your bedroom for any other activities, put an end to them now. No television. No computer. No bill paying. No library filled with adventure novels. No football table. Nothing that excites the imagination or provides a distraction. The space should be serene and well-ordered.

Create a tranquil environment. Your bedroom should be peaceful. If you are disturbed by outside noises – like the sounds of the street right outside your window – consider investing in an electric fan or some CDs that produce relaxing sounds such as ocean waves, rainforest, whale song, babbling brooks and so on. It doesn't matter what you listen to as long as it drones softly and lulls you to sleep.

Adjust your thermostat. Although scientists suggest that you'll do better if your bedroom is a little cool, it's entirely up to you. We're not trying to influence you, but the golden numbers are 60°–65°F (16°–18°C).

The trick is to find a temperature you like and stick with it. A very warm room will signal your body metabolically that it's time to get up. A very cold one will cause you to tighten up muscles. You might sleep, but you'll awaken exhausted and sore. Find the middle ground.

▼ Bedroom space should be well-ordered
A tidy, peaceful bedroom is more conducive to relaxation and a restful night's sleep. Keep electronic equipment to a minimum.

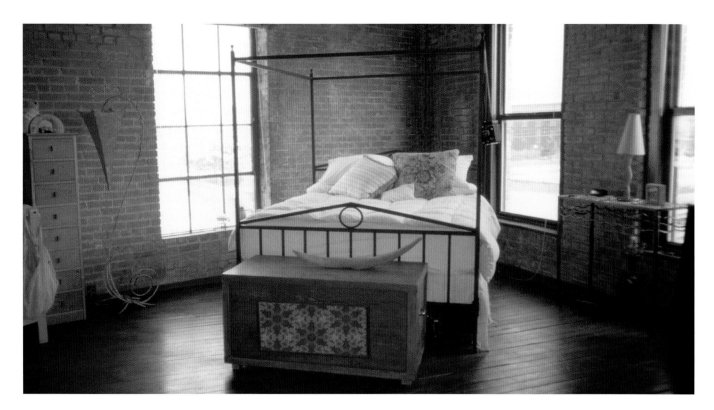

Do You Need More Sleep?

You might think that you're getting enough sleep, even when you're not. (Remember, when you have a sleep debt, your judgement might be impaired.) Here's a short self-test suggested by Peter B. McCullagh, director of the North Florida Regional Medical Center Sleep Disorders Center in Florida, USA. If three or more of these statements describe you, you might need more quality and consistency in your sleep hours. If your sleep problem is extreme, seek professional advice.

- I don't feel refreshed after a night's rest.
- I frequently feel tired.
- I forget things.
- People remark that I look tired.
- I am cranky, irritable and short-fused.
- I have trouble concentrating, especially on quiet projects.
- I sit through meetings, lectures and sermons, but I can't tell you what was said.
- I am completely reliant upon my alarm clock to get up in the morning. I hit the snooze button more than once.
- I feel lethargic until I've had more than one cup of coffee in the morning.
- I have trouble calculating numbers.
- I snore so loudly that I disturb my bed-partner… or the neighbours.
- I keep the volume on my car radio so loud that it startles me when I first turn it on.
- I fall asleep when I'm bored or relaxed.
- I sometimes awaken myself with a single loud snore.
- I have to keep my room or office cool to stay alert.
- I often wake up in the morning with a headache.
- I am sometimes inexplicably weepy.
- I sometimes have difficulty getting my thoughts organised.
- I fall asleep in under five minutes after I go to bed.
- It takes me longer than 15 minutes to fall asleep after I go to bed.
- When I'm driving, I sometimes realise that I've covered miles without being aware.
- On my days off, I sleep longer than I do when I am on a work schedule.
- I sometimes need to nap to get through the day.
- Naps don't really refresh me.

Keep your bedroom as dark as possible while still feeling safe. Don't apologise if you need a little light. If the room is too dark for your personal sense of safety and causes you to feel insecure, you'll be on guard all night and will not sleep well. The room doesn't have to be pitch black, just darkened to the point where your human instinct to sleep when it's dark is triggered.

Sleep in a comfortable bed. We're not just talking about clean sheets and a firm mattress. We also expect you to control every variable of the environment. We once had an athlete with continuing sleep difficulty even after several meetings, so we went through a step-by-step review of his plan. He was doing everything right, he insisted. In fact, even his dogs were sleeping better! His four golden retrievers were really enjoying the new bedtime programme and were less restless all night than usual – on *his* bed!

Go to bed within one hour of the same time every night. This includes the weekends. If you stay awake too long, you'll find yourself, ironically, frustratingly, too tired to fall asleep. If you go to bed too early, you'll not be sleepy. You'll lie awake and toss and turn.

Gradually decrease your exposure to bright light. Throughout the course of the evening, in the hours leading up to bedtime, gradually dim the lights. When we are around low light, our natural instinct is to wind down and move towards rest. Bright light is neurologically stimulating and signals that it's time to get up.

Cool off. Wear lightweight clothing, if anything at all. Even if you've taken a warm bath to relax, take a few extra minutes to dry off, allowing the water to evaporate, which will drop your skin temperature a little.

Cut off your caffeine in the very early evening. If you still have trouble falling asleep after doing so, back up the cut-off to late afternoon. If you still can't sleep, back it up to the middle of the afternoon. Shortly, you'll find the magic cut-off time. Remember, caffeine is not only in coffee and tea but also hidden in chocolate and some medications. Be aware.

Cut off or limit alcohol consumption in the evening. Some people think that a glass of wine will relax them and help them sleep. It may, but it also interferes in their ability to get into and stay in deep sleep, where the benefits of rest are the greatest.

Avoid nicotine. This stimulant delays sleep. Of course, we have other issues with it, but that's another book. Please don't smoke. Not before bed. Not ever.

Avoid napping if you're not used to it. A quick snooze might seem like a good idea at the time, but it will certainly interfere with your ability to fall asleep later and stay that way. Unlike eating, sleeping is not as effective if it's parcelled out over the course of 24 hours. For most of us, it's best done all at one time. There are people who are great at napping and enjoy tremendous benefits, but you would have to try it and decide for yourself.

Go to bed tired. This one is tricky because there are several kinds of fatigue: mental, emotional and physical. Any one of the three is sufficient to trigger your need for sleep, but you will sleep better if you are *physically* tired.

In the grand design, humans were built to toil all day and sleep all night. In today's culture, we work, but we don't expend a great deal of physical energy. You might feel wasted by bedtime, but your body – tethered to a desk all day and driven home in a car and then plopped in front of a television set all evening – simply isn't tired out. You need to get some heart-pumping, butter-burning, blood-rushing, sweat-inducing exercise some time during the day on a regular basis in order to command good sleep. You'll be stunned by the difference it makes.

Be aware of your exercise schedule. Pay attention to the timing of exercise in relation to your ability to sleep, and adjust your workout schedule if it interferes with your ability to settle down. Most scientists recommend that you exercise early in the day, suggesting that rigorous activity in the late evening stimulates you too much to allow sleep. But, frankly, this has not been our experience. Often, the only time *we* have to exercise is late at night, after our last client has left the clinic. We've found that a hard workout dissolves away the tensions of the day, tires us out physically, and allows a better night's sleep. We would say that you have to do what works for you. Simple experimentation will quickly yield an answer.

Have a bedtime snack high in carbohydrate. Hunger pangs and a growling stomach will keep you awake. We suggest carbohydrates because they trigger the production of serotonin, the neurotransmitters in your brain that cause sleepiness. Keep the snack light – a few crackers, a rice cake. Speaking of cake, avoid chocolate when searching for bedtime snacks. Hidden caffeine will defeat the purpose.

Finish your mental tasks. Do all you can do to wind up your day so that you can go to bed with a clear conscience. Fretting is useless. Sleeping isn't walking away from your battles. Sleeping is preparation. If you are wrestling with a challenging problem that is affecting your ability to sleep, decide to deal with it in the morning, when you are rested and prepared to do battle again. Give yourself permission to sleep so that you'll be better able to think creatively and energetically in the morning.

Get some sun today. Studies suggest that exposure to natural light during the day contributes to the body's ability to make the most of sleep. In fact, it's thought that the benefits of exercise in the broad light of day are greater than exercise in an enclosed gym. We aren't saying that you have to buy a deckchair and move your computer to the roof of your building, but we are suggesting that you poke your nose out the window once in a while.

Wind down. It's a rare person who can step away from engaging activity and flop into bed to fall asleep immediately. Many of us need to wind down at the end of the day, when activity requires no 'output' from us, no participation required of us except presence. Try reading, watching a little television or listening to music.

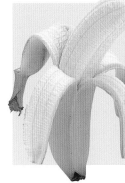

Bananas are an ideal snack to have before bed. They are high in carbohydrates, which raise the levels of trytophan, an amino acid that helps the body to produce serotonin, a natural sleep inducer and relaxer. Bananas are also easily digestible. Avoid milk drinks as they inhibit the uptake of trytophan.

Do some stretches before bed. Once you've set the stage for slumber, doing some gentle, rhythmic stretching releases tension and puts you on track for a good night's sleep. If you're having trouble sleeping, try the four stretches at the top of the opposite page that we use to help relax us before bedtime.

SLEEP POSITIONS THAT TAKE THE STRESS OFF YOUR BACK

Although we have had clients who have slept in chairs while their backs were healing, for the purposes of this

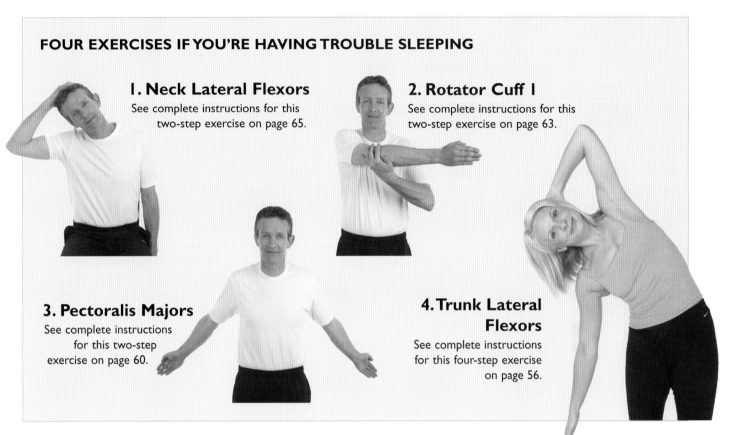

FOUR EXERCISES IF YOU'RE HAVING TROUBLE SLEEPING

1. Neck Lateral Flexors
See complete instructions for this two-step exercise on page 65.

2. Rotator Cuff 1
See complete instructions for this two-step exercise on page 63.

3. Pectoralis Majors
See complete instructions for this two-step exercise on page 60.

4. Trunk Lateral Flexors
See complete instructions for this four-step exercise on page 56.

discussion we're going to assume that you'll be sleeping in your bed. Unless your doctor suggests otherwise, you need to experiment until you find a position that feels good. Here are a few tips.

Consider a firm mattress. 'Firm' does not mean 'concrete slab', but the mattress should support your body comfortably. Old, soft mattresses might have sentimental value but lumpy feathers and foam will cause you to tense and 'guard' a tender back out of alignment. If you simply cannot give up an old favourite, consider sliding a full sheet of plywood between the mattress and box spring.

Sleep on your back or your side. You might be more comfortable when your spine is aligned as closely as possible to its natural curves. We urge you to try to stay off your stomach, not just because it puts your spine into a sort of concave arch, but because you have to spend the night with your neck rotated, face to the side, to keep you from suffocating. This puts added strain on your neck.

If you sleep flat on your back, you might consider putting pillows under your knees and neck to take some of the tension off your lumbar spine. If you sleep on your side, we

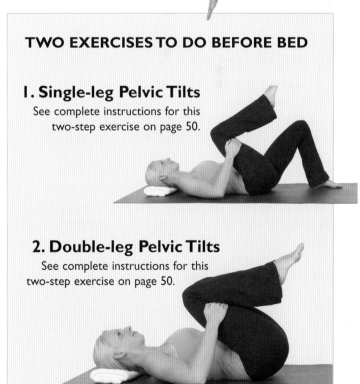

TWO EXERCISES TO DO BEFORE BED

1. Single-leg Pelvic Tilts
See complete instructions for this two-step exercise on page 50.

2. Double-leg Pelvic Tilts
See complete instructions for this two-step exercise on page 50.

suggest you put pillows between your knees and under your neck to keep the tension off your lower back and pelvis.

Many people use body pillows, which are the length of your torso. Not only are body pillows very comforting, they take the tension off your lower back and pelvis. Additionally, they give you something against which to 'lean' so that you can find the right position, lock it in with your body pillow, and relax.

Consider a pillow that supports your neck. Traditional pillows, although wonderfully fluffy and soft, do very little for vertebral alignment. They either lift your head, arching your cervical spine to the ceiling; fail to support your head at all, arching your cervical spine to the floor; or get it just right for most of the night. You have a one-in-three chance of sleeping without strain.

You and your doctor might determine that you would benefit from a firm cervical pillow that is sculpted of a single piece of foam and shaped like a roller-coaster as opposed to the traditional pillow that is pliable, stuffed with fluff, and shaped like a muffin (most of the night). A cervical pillow rises to conform to your neck and then forms a trough to cradle your head. If you were to take an X-ray of your spine while you were using this pillow, you would notice that the vertebrae are in straight alignment. Some people do very well with them.

Home Remedies for a Sleepless Night

We know that when your back hurts and you're ragged from tossing and turning, desperate measures can seem tempting. Good judgement can get clouded. But if you're having trouble sleeping and decide to do something about it, slow down and use your head. When you're suffering from back pain and you're under the care of a doctor, it's likely that he has already prescribed painkillers. They'll help you relax to fall asleep and stay that way. If you are still having trouble sleeping, do *not* self-medicate on top of prescription medications. See your doctor and have a heart-to-heart chat.

Try relaxation techniques. Get comfortable and close your eyes. Breathe through your nose, one nostril at a time. Start with the left nostril by blocking the right. Inhale to a slow count of four. Hold to a slow count of seven. Exhale to a slow count of eight. Switch sides. Block the left, breathe with the right. Switch sides again. Do this four times per side. Imagine with each breath that you are filled with energy and that your muscles are relaxing, lengthening, strengthening and getting organised – fibre by fibre.

Another favourite of ours is to imagine yourself in a hammock between two trees. Peaceful. Swaying back and forth. Back and forth. Deeply relaxed. More relaxed with every sway. Now eliminate the trees. You're still in the hammock, swaying back and forth. Back and forth. Even more deeply relaxed. Now eliminate the hammock. You're still swaying back and forth. Back and forth. Profoundly, deeply relaxed. Before long, you'll be lulled into sleep.

Take aspirin or NSAIDs. Aspirin and non-steroidal anti-inflammatory drugs (NSAIDs), such as ibuprofen, can reduce pain and inflammation by blocking the production of prostaglandins (chemicals that cause inflammation and trigger transmission of the pain signal to the brain). Of course, when you feel comfortable, you'll sleep better.

A few words of caution: pain is your body's way of communicating clear messages to you about the status of an injury. Don't use over-the-counter painkillers to mask pain that you and your doctor need to be evaluating and using for information. NSAIDs have possible side-effects of which you need to be aware: nausea, indigestion, diarrhoea and peptic ulcers. Aspirin can cause clotting disorders, prolonged bleeding, colitis, gastrointestinal disorders, ringing in the ears, and aggravation of asthma, hives and gout. Both interact with other medications. Be careful.

Look into over-the-counter sleeping aids. If you read the packet carefully, you might notice that over-the-counter sleeping pills are largely a combination of aspirin and antihistamine – not a bad combination for a sleepy person with an aching back. Generally, they have been found to be safe for healthy people, but their effectiveness may vary. Avoid them completely if you plan to end your evening with a glass of wine or any other drug. Follow packet instructions very carefully.

Apply a heating pad. Usually, we recommend ice for treating injury by reducing swelling, slightly numbing and promoting blood flow, but an aching back at bedtime presents an unusual challenge. Low in subcutaneous fat and rich with nerves, the back muscles sometimes tense up when they're iced – especially if you're trying to do it yourself. The better solution might be to warm the back and relax it by applying the heating pad.

Consider antihistamines. Antihistamines, usually used to combat allergy symptoms, are sometimes used for relaxation as they cause drowsiness. A low dose will do the trick. The quality of sleep is pretty fair. Read the packet instructions and make sure you follow them to the letter. Also, be sure that you time the dose carefully. Once you've taken it, your day is done. No more operating heavy machinery for you.

Take a hot bath. If you don't have a heating pad, you might achieve the same relaxation with a hot, but not scorching, bath. Do make sure you are careful getting in and out of the tub – one slip will jar a back that's already in trouble. For added comfort, why not roll a towel and tuck it under your neck. If you plan to spend a long time in the tub, keep a plastic bottle of cold water within easy reach and keep drinking from it. Heat causes you to sweat. And, of course, sweating causes you to dehydrate, but you might not notice if you're already wet.

Look into botanical supplements. Several nutritional supplements are thought to calm the nervous system and support sleep. Among them are camomile, valerian, passion-flower and skullcap. Just as with herbal teas, we urge you to do as much research as you can before taking an unregulated botanical, which may have potential drug interactions. Over the years, we have

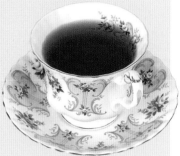

There is a huge selection of herbal teas now available in health food shops and supermarkets, especially those aimed at sleep and relaxation. Try to find one that contains camomile, a substance well known for its calming qualities.

encountered enthusiasts who swear by them, but sadly clinical research is still lacking. Without it, we can't endorse or recommend these supplements.

Sample some herbal teas. Some herbal teas may promote sleep and relaxation. We can see no real harm in drinking these teas, and they are certainly very popular now, but be aware that their production isn't regulated. If you trust the company, drink the tea in moderation.

▼ **Relaxing in the tub**
A hot soak will soothe and relax the back. For added comfort, roll a towel and tuck it under your neck.

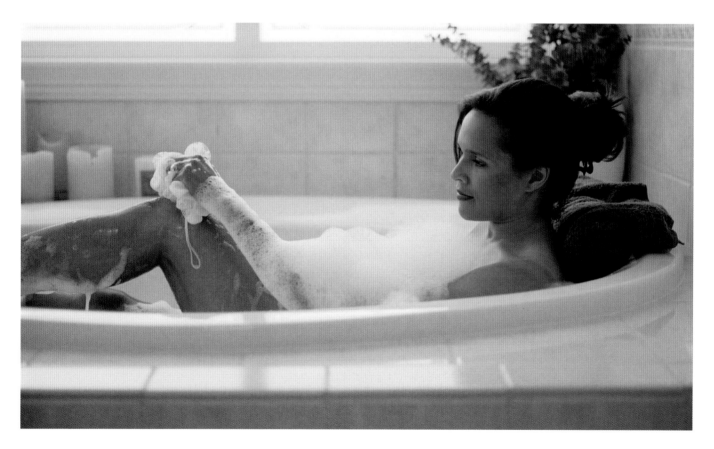

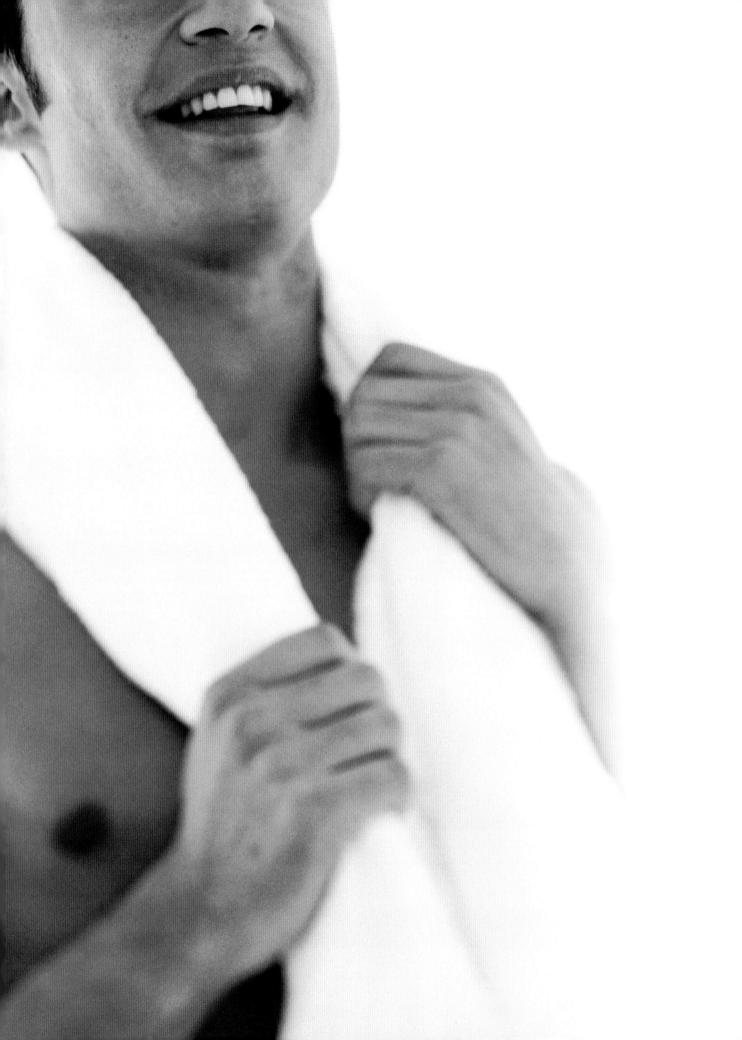

6

EVERYDAY LIFE – WITHOUT PAIN

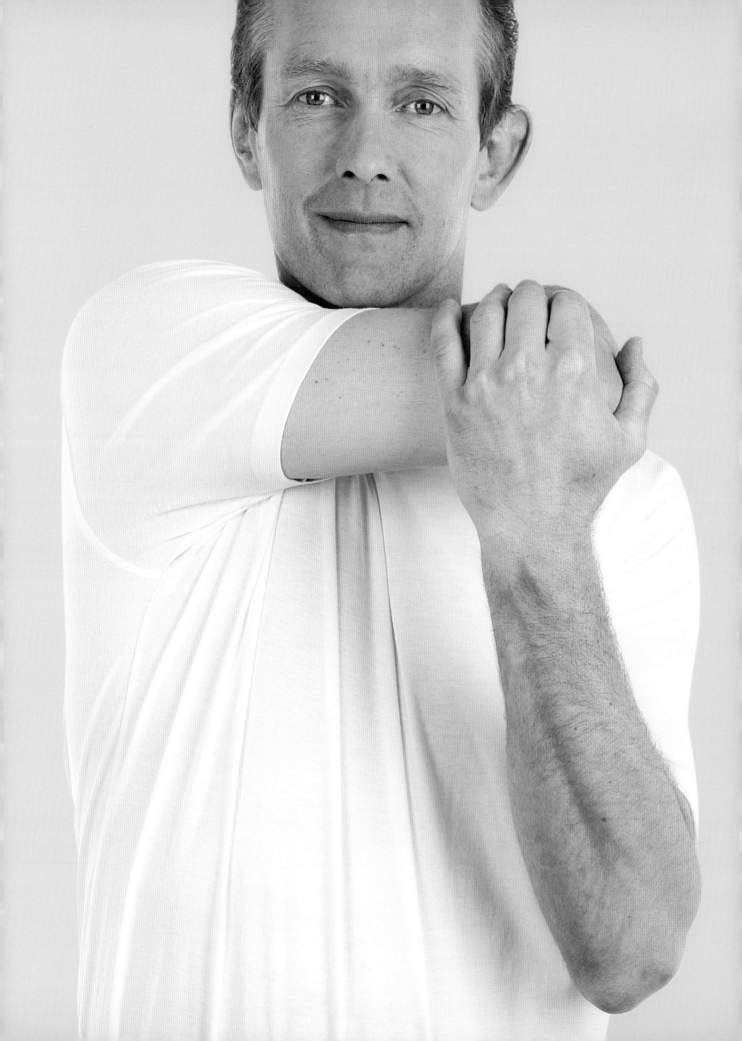

CHAPTER 14

PROTECTING YOUR BACK AT WORK AND HOME

Sitting is a way of life for many people. While many *activities could just as easily be accomplished while standing, we choose to sit. We could stand at the counter to eat, but we sit at the table. We could stand while we watch television, but we sit on the sofa. We could raise our desks and stand while we work, but we sit in chairs. We don't stand, we sit. And sit. And sit...*

Whether you are in a sedentary job that demands you sit at a computer all day, or whether you are based at home doing a variety of tasks, you need to respect the job you are doing – it is a way of life for you. If you are sitting incorrectly at work or constantly tripping or falling over clutter at home, you are putting unnecessary strain on your back on a regular basis. The good news is that there are many easy ways to prevent this.

YOUR HEALTHY BACK AT WORK

Sitting at a desk all day can take a terrible toll on an unprepared body, putting more stress on your lower spine than standing. And, no matter how ergonomically designed and seemingly comfortable your chair is, your back, hips, legs and buttocks are going to suffer fatigue and tighten up if you don't give them a break.

The other problem with sitting is that all your work is contained within a small, specific space – usually right in front and just below your face on a desk. Your arms and hands are usually up on the desk, and your neck is flexed downwards towards your work. This bad situation is made even worse by your locking into this position and moving very little and very infrequently. Your shoulders and the area between your shoulder blades suffer fatigue and strain as you maintain and sustain this torturous posture.

As long as we sit so much, we might as well be good at it. So let's take a look at ergonomics, the science of applying engineering principles to environments, tools, furniture and equipment so that people are safe and productive at work and at home. It's a booming industry. In America, Occupational Safety and Health reports that 1.8 million workers suffer from injuries that result from mistakes in ergonomics – a seemingly harmless desk too high, a chair too low, a mouse the wrong size.

As workers become more efficient at simplifying and streamlining operations, requiring less physical effort to get a job done, they're hurting themselves more. For example, 20 years ago a secretary had to type on a manual typewriter, run back and forth to the filing cabinet, carry an office diary into the boss's office to review appointments, and dash to the bank to transfer money. On her way home, she stopped by the office supply shop to order stationery. Today, all that can be accomplished with one computer in minutes.

There's no question that we're getting more done, but there's a heavy price to pay for all this efficiency. That price is paid in human suffering. Experts in ergonomics have identified the problems that occur from sitting at desks which affect circulation, muscles, bones, connective tissues, eyes, ears and nerves.

Most of the problems are caused by cumulative stress and fatigue. The most common are neck and shoulder pain, back pain, eyestrain and repetitive stress injuries such as carpal tunnel syndrome. (See 'Protecting Your Back When You Use a Computer All Day' on page 236.)

Working at your desk all day means that you are not getting enough exercise, so put together an after-work programme that combines strength, flexibility and cardio work. To get the kinks out of your back after sitting, try the exercise opposite.

AN EXERCISE TO DO AFTER SITTING

1. Trunk Extensors
See complete instructions for this two-step exercise on page 55.

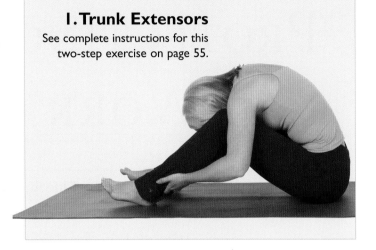

Protecting Your Back While at a Desk

Some simple changes to your work environment will make a big difference. These ergonomic guidelines will help you maintain good posture and keep your back safe.

- **Use a towel or pillow to create the right angle.** To support and balance your lower back, place a pillow or rolled-up towel at the back of your chair to lean against. Also, set the angle of your seat so that your knees are slightly lower than your hips and your feet are flat on the floor. This forward angle tips your pelvis forwards and takes a lot of strain off your lower back.

- **Choose your chair well.** The best chairs have seats that don't tip when you recline the back, so you won't have pressure on the backs of your knees and thighs. If your chair has arms, make sure they are adjusted to the proper height so that when you rest your arms on them, your shoulders are relaxed and comfortable with no pressure on your upper back. Try to avoid crossing your legs. Pull your chair in very close to your desk, so that you don't have to lean forwards to reach your work.

- **Position your computer and other tools appropriately.** Make sure your computer screen is level with your face so you don't have to extend or flex your neck to get a good look at it. Place your keyboard at a height that allows your elbows to be flexed at 90-degree angles. Don't wedge the phone between your shoulder and your ear.

- **Keep moving.** Equally important as designing the perfect workspace is moving around whenever possible. Use every excuse you can find to stand up and walk around. File things. Stroll down the hall to ask a question rather than use the phone. If it is inappropriate for you to stand, wiggle and flex while seated. Roll your shoulders. Lift your arms over your head. Extend your legs, rotate your ankles and feet, crunch your toes up and then relax them… do anything that gets blood flowing. Use your breaks and lunchtime to walk and relax your shoulders and back. Take a few deep breaths.

- **Use the quick releases.** If you want real tension busters that take only a few minutes, require minimal space and draw only a little attention, go to page 207 in chapter 12. These moves will work the kinks out and get your blood circulating.

- **Treat your back gently.** A word of caution: ergonomic experts who specialise in preventing back injuries warn us that back fatigue is tricky. It can sneak up on you when you least expect it, so always try to avoid sudden, jerking movements after you've been sitting for a while. To pick up objects from the floor, gently slide to the edge of your chair and place a hand on your knee or your desk to support your back. Keep one foot in front of the other for additional support.

Case Study: **John Tierney**

John is a newspaper columnist. His back was killing him from years of sitting at his desk and using a keyboard. He was gravely worried about an upcoming assignment.

John was to accompany an expedition to the North Pole and cover the story. The trip would require a lot of cross-country skiing, and, because he was out of shape, John was concerned that his back would never withstand the exertion.

Sitting seems like a relaxing posture, but it's a killer on the body, especially when it's done at great length by professional 'sitters'. John's glutes, hip rotators and hamstrings were in constant compression and he had only 25 degrees range of motion. He also had nerve pain down his leg from pressure, and his abdominals were weak. The problems originated in the zone from his knees to his pelvis, but his back was where he felt the pain. There was really nothing wrong with his back that a little balancing act couldn't correct.

John's biggest relief came from increased flexibility. We started to work with stretch ropes, training him to increase his range of motion, joint by joint. We focused on his hamstrings, glutes and hip extensors. He was out of pain nearly immediately.

When John was flexible enough, we added strengthening. Initially, he was unable to do one abdominal curl, so we had to modify the move. This was particularly important because the abdominals support the back. We needed all his muscles back on duty, but especially his lower abdominals. Even with the modified exercises, he progressed very quickly – little efforts add up fast.

John is an athlete at heart and he felt better after being stretched out. He improved quickly. Four weeks later, all of the back pain was gone, and in just a few more weeks, he was in shape and ready for the expedition.

John's trip was a success. He sent us a photo of the campsite with a dogsled and exercise strap. Apparently, the expedition team members had been queuing up to use the strap!

PROTECTING YOUR BACK WHEN YOU STAND ALL DAY

We once attended a naval training ceremony in a large, stiflingly hot auditorium. Young men and women stood to attention for over an hour through speeches and presentations. They started to drop like flies. If it hadn't been so disturbing, we could have started taking bets about which sailor would hit the deck next.

While you might not have to stand rigidly to attention without moving a muscle, we are going to assume that you are upright and on your feet throughout a work shift of some duration. So what happens now?

Your foot is literally a shock absorber, designed to take the vertical forces of your weight and gravity and translate them into horizontal force. When you walk, the arch of your foot sort of flattens out and then springs back up to give you a little lift with each step you take. It's a physical dynamic that is really quite remarkable. But when you stand all day and never lift those vertical forces off your feet, the arch flattens under your weight but never springs back into shape. As you move around, it might spring a little, but never fully. The arch and all the muscles that surround it become strained and exhausted.

Any imbalance in your foot, such as a slight roll of your ankle inwards caused by a weak or flattened arch (inversion) or a slight roll outwards (eversion), will be aggravated by standing for long periods of time. Those imbalances will travel up your ankle to your knee, which will eventually strain to try to keep you in balance. The strain in your knee will travel to your hip, and your hip could then throw your back out. This chain of unfortunate compensations sends the pain and strain straight up.

Your circulation is also affected. The heart does a remarkable job of pumping blood down the body and usually does a remarkable job of pumping it back up, but gravity is a formidable foe. Being on your feet all day can make circulation sluggish. Metabolic waste from firing muscles in your legs and feet may not be flushed sufficiently. Fluids may pool in muscles and around joints, and you may find yourself swollen from the knees down, a condition called oedema. When leg and feet tissues swell, nerves are compressed, and you may experience aching.

Additionally, the fainting sailors remind us that when blood and fluids are accumulating in your lower half, they're not supplying your upper half. When blood can't make its way back to your brain in sufficient amounts, you faint. Getting your heart pumping and your blood circulating is a matter of moving once in a while. But if you wait too long and feel as if you're about to keel over, sit down and put your head between your knees or lie down and elevate your feet. Gravity will do the rest. As soon as blood gets back to your brain, you'll feel better. Don't allow pride to keep you from preventing a fall. When you faint, you have no control over how or where you will fall. It's better to have hurt pride than to have a hurt back

To get the kinks out of your back after standing, try the exercise opposite.

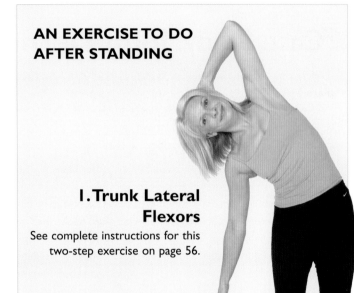

AN EXERCISE TO DO AFTER STANDING

1. Trunk Lateral Flexors

See complete instructions for this two-step exercise on page 56.

Case Study: **Ed Matthews**

Ed is a massage therapist and a musculoskeletal therapist. When he came to us for treatment of a painful back, he thought he had already determined the cause.

Ed attributed his lower-back pain to constant flexion and exhaustion. He thought his upper back kept going into spasm from years of massage that tired his shoulders and arms. Ed was right about the stresses of massage. But we suspected that the real culprit was that he stood on hard surfaces every day.

The foot is far from the heart, so gravity and distance had caused some circulation problems as well as tired feet. As a successful skilled therapist, he had worked hard, and the result was a punished body. However, Ed told us that he had dislocated his ankle several years earlier. The injury had been severe and had left him with a fallen arch in his foot that rotated his ankle towards the midpoint of his body. We smiled at each other — Ed was about to learn something.

When the ankle is unstable and the arch falls and rolls the foot in, the knee gets strained. When the knee is strained, the hip compensates. When the hip compensates, the lower back is strained and weakened. And that will shoot right up to the neck.

In addition, when the arch isn't stable, it's not able to do its job at first point of impact in a foot strike. It's the shock absorber for the body. It's supposed to take the weight, dissipate the shock and then spring back into shape to give lift to the step. Ed's couldn't do it. All that shock was travelling straight up the leg. The body finds the weakest link, and Ed's was in his shoe.

Instead of throwing Ed on the table and working on his back, we used Active-Isolated Stretching to unlock his body. We needed to restore range of motion to his joints and get circulation going again. Then we taught him a couple of exercises specifically to strengthen the foot and lower leg.

Once we had Ed feeling better, we added the full strength routine with emphasis on glutes, adductors, abductors and hamstrings. His back stopped hurting very quickly, but full recovery took six weeks because Ed had so many levels of dysfunction from years of being hard on his body.

We're proud to say that Ed made our systems his own. In fact, he now works in our New York City clinic.

Keeping Your Back Healthy at Work

Combating back problems is a matter of proper planning. Here are a few tips for a safe back.

- **Wear suitable shoes.** Good footwear that balances support with comfort will go a long way in preventing problems. Whether you are wearing shoes or boots, you need to make certain that they fit properly and provide support and cushioning appropriate to your job and the surface on which you must function.
- **Investigate insoles.** Beyond the shoes themselves, you can buy gel insoles and slip them into your shoes to help take some of the strain off your feet. Make sure they fit the shoes you'll be wearing and feel comfortable.
- **Cushion your standing area.** Try a padded mat on the floor where you stand. Mats made of a soft gel diffuse vertical force and feel cushioned beneath your feet. Available from commercial suppliers, these mats are slip-proof. They will not correct imbalances in your feet and ankles, but they can make you more comfortable, since your feet are protected from the hard floor.
- **Put your feet up – but not for long.** By the end of the day, you'll be tired of standing and want to get your feet and legs up. Not a bad idea, as long as you don't stay there too long. Being tired is one of the most common excuses for skipping a workout. We urge you to push through fatigue if you can. Don't be tempted to cut the below-waist exercises, thinking that you've had enough for one day. Becoming stronger, more flexible and more balanced will help you withstand the rigours of standing all day.

PROTECTING YOUR BACK WHEN YOU LIFT AND HAUL ALL DAY

Recently, we had the opportunity to work with a highly trained dancer from a Broadway show. In each performance, one of his most spectacular moves was to catch a leaping female dancer and lift her over his head before she slid down from his upreached arms and into his embrace for a showstopping moment of romance. He did it eight times a week. But one night came when the tiny, leaping female dancer leaped, he caught her in mid-air, but he couldn't lift her. She slid down his face, and he slid down right next to her for a showstopping moment of disaster.

His lower back had simply shut down in a painful spasm, and he could no longer support her weight. How could a strong, experienced professional dancer suddenly become so weak? Easy.

Like most of us, he lifted all his weights in front of his body… including his partner. His back side, imbalanced and weaker than his front side, struggled to participate in the lifting. He had become so weak that to lift her, he had to arch his back to create a sort of fulcrum with his body to balance her weight. His lower back, buttocks and hamstrings stayed continually contracted, impinging nerves and shorting out, getting weaker and even more imbalanced with every lift, until things started shutting down.

When the muscles in his lower back could no longer handle the load of the lifts or support the forces of impact and lift, muscles in the front had to work harder. But they weren't strong enough to carry the whole load by themselves. Plus, he started having difficulties with muscles in his arms and shoulders, and then his lower back was in real pain as he arched and absorbed the forces of lifting another dancer. From that point forwards, his lifting days were numbered. This was a man in need of balance.

We can't assume that a person who lifts and hauls for a living is totally fit, despite having a highly physically demanding job. Frequently, the opposite is true. Fitness is defined as health, strength, cardiovascular fitness (endurance) and flexibility. A person who lifts and hauls for a living could well have only one of the components – strength. Someone might look great and still fall far short of being fit. If you want to do well in your profession and work injury-free, you must make sure that you have all the fitness pieces in place.

In lifting and hauling, there are two types of injuries: acute (like sprains) and overuse (like tendinitis). Most common are sprains, strains and soft-tissue injuries of the lower back, shoulders, biceps, deltoids, elbows, forearms, wrists, hands, groin, thighs and hamstrings. If it looks as if we just listed every body part as being in serious jeopardy, don't panic. Notice that we did not mention knees, ankles and feet. This is because it is harder to get hurt in your lower extremities. Still, it's important to remember that although lower extremities are not the targets of injury, they can be the causes. Remember that imbalances in your lower extremities can translate right up through your hips and back as your muscles try to compensate and soft and connective tissues are strained.

Be advised that lifting and hauling can also cause one-sided muscle hypertrophy. This means that the muscle is highly developed in the lift (concentric contraction), but not nearly so developed in the opposite direction – say, when you lower whatever you've lifted (eccentric contraction). Because this muscle develops only half of its functional strength, it isn't flexible. And because it's inflexible and firing on only half of its pistons, other muscles are continually recruited to assist whatever task is at hand. Imbalances are common. A truly strong muscle can shorten to lift a weight and then lengthen to lower that same weight with the same speed and control as the lift, with both phases of movement through the full range of motion. All the way up, all the way down. Nice and easy.

Using common sense should help you avoid many of the injuries associated with lifting and hauling, but here are several useful tips to keep in mind.

Stay well. Don't lift and haul if you are injured or feeling under the weather. When you're not well, your body diverts energy into healing. In this weakened state, you're out of balance and your muscles might not be able to fire at full capacity.

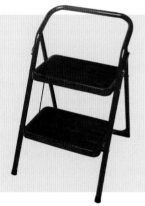

If you have to lift something from a level higher than your shoulders or place something higher than your shoulders, stand on something stable, like a stepladder, which will support your weight and get you where you need to be. Stay balanced and in control. No 'heave-ho'!

Don't rely on a back belt to give you support. These belts keep your waist and lower back warm, but they don't live up to their promises. They give the illusion of support, so that you might feel invulnerable and try something that ultimately will hurt your back. Also, they restrict range of motion and cause muscles to get lazy and atrophy from disuse. Make no mistake: you *are* muscularly developed enough, especially your abdominal muscles, to support the weight you are lifting or hauling. The only back belts we endorse are those worn by competition weight lifters. These are specifically designed for well-trained athletes who use them for one purpose: to protect the lower back in a lift.

Know your limits. If something is simply too heavy to lift, use your brain, not your brawn. Either figure out another way to move it (like with a pulley) or ask for help.

Put your body against the object you're lifting. This tightens your centre of gravity and removes some of the load from your lower back. Never stand away and reach out for something heavy. Instead, pull the object close to you, bend your knees and lift with your legs. Focus your energy. Don't hold your breath. Lift slowly and smoothly.

Use your feet. If you're carrying something and you have to change directions, don't twist or turn your torso. Keep the load of this weight distributed right where it is – directly in front of you and close to your body. Change directions with your feet.

Lower with your back straight. When you're ready to put the weight down, keep your back straight, hold the object as close to your torso as possible, bend your knees and lower slowly and smoothly. (It's okay to make the 'ughhh' sound!)

Don't forget your stretching. No matter how much you lift and haul during the day, you need *total* stretch work for balance, so include an Active-Isolated Stretching workout in your training. A tight muscle, especially one with one-sided hypertrophy, takes more effort to move and can't move as fast.

Also, don't forget: no matter how hard you work or how you huff and puff, lifting and hauling are not a form of aerobic exercise. You need to do cardio training for that.

To get the kinks out of your upper back after lifting and hauling all day, try the stretch below.

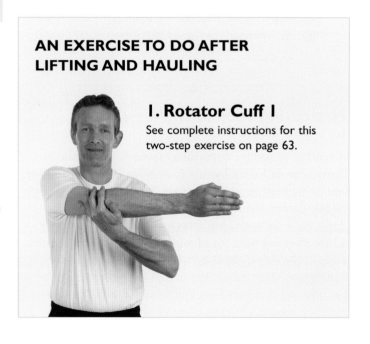

AN EXERCISE TO DO AFTER LIFTING AND HAULING

1. Rotator Cuff 1
See complete instructions for this two-step exercise on page 63.

PROTECTING YOUR BACK WHEN YOU DRIVE ALL DAY

To those who are stuck in an office job, driving for a living can seem like the ideal lifestyle. You just cruise around, listening to the radio and watching the miles whizz by, right?

Wrong. The truth is that driving is one of the most mentally and physically demanding of all professions. You sit belted into one position for hours with your arms extended in front of you, your hands gripped on the wheel and your eyes glued hypnotically to the road ahead. All the controls for the equipment are within inches of your hands or feet so you don't have to reach for them. Commercial vehicles, especially lorries, seem to be designed so that you *never* have to get out. The only problem is that efficiency and convenience leads to a very sedentary driver whose only exercise is to walk to the toilet and back to the cab.

From the standpoint of physiology, driving makes several specific athletic demands upon the driver. Pressing on the clutch puts your left leg and foot to work, using ankle flexors (gastrocs in your calves) and knee extensors (quads in the fronts of your thighs). Braking engages hip rotators and adductors. Changing gear also engages your arm: wrist flexors, arm extensors, triceps and upper rear shoulder. Steering requires development in your chest (pectoralis) and shoulders (deltoids and rotator cuffs).

With arms out in front of you as your hands grip the steering wheel, you tend to relax arm muscles and rely on your grip to support their weight. Try this posture for a moment, and you'll notice a slight pull in your back between your shoulders. If you hold this posture for long periods of time, this slight pull becomes a big problem. Tension will set in. As the muscles in your upper back tense, blood supply is restricted. The muscle fatigues and starts shutting down, and metabolic waste from the effort is not easily flushed away, so pain sets in.

Your neck may be holding steady, rotating and extending as necessary, but it's never enough. It will short out, for sure. The problem with neck fatigue while driving is that you cannot relieve it by rolling your head or rotating it to get the kinks out. Doing this will not only take your eyes off the road (never a great idea), it will also upset your equilibrium to the extent that you'll be a road hazard all on your own.

The sitting position puts more stress on your lower spine than standing. And, no matter how ergonomically designed and seemingly comfortable your seat is, your back, hips, legs and buttocks will fatigue and tighten up if you don't give them breaks regularly to stimulate circulation. Worse than that, with more work to do, one foot is dominant over

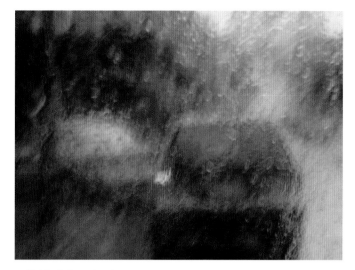

▲ Behind the wheel
If you drive for a living, it is important to be aware of the many demands being placed on all parts of your body.

the other, so you'll sit at an angle on one hip to get that foot ready to move. You'll stay that way throughout the drive – vigilant and prepared to move fast. With one hip hiked up, you've put your back into slight rotation. It fatigues from tension, even if the drive is under an hour. You've created a serious imbalance because the side opposite the dominant side is suffering fatigue while trying to hold you there.

When tension and fatigue set in, the piriformis muscle, which runs from your sacrum to your femur bone in your thigh, constricts in a spasm and clamps down on the sciatic nerve, which runs from your buttocks down the back of your leg. In piriformis syndrome, as it's called, your back aches, your bottom and the back of your thigh hurt, and you'll start to notice that you're losing function. This can cause a potentially dangerous lag between the moment when your brain tells you to move your foot and when that leg can transmit that urgent signal through a nerve that's no longer communicating well. It disrupts the message between the back and the foot; somewhere in there, the message gets retranslated to 'This hurts so badly, I think I'm going to be sick!' Hitting the brake or clutch becomes difficult.

Piriformis syndrome doesn't automatically go away when you leave the vehicle and straighten up. You'll need to work a little to relieve it, which is your body's way of telling you that it needs flexibility, balance, strength and a break once in a while. Luckily, prevention is simple.

Don't forget to *move*. Whether you drive a police car, fire engine, taxi cab, utility van or an 18-wheel rig, remember to move occasionally. From time to time, shift and wiggle in your seat. Turn up your music and do a little seated dance. Rock your weight from one side of your bottom to the other and back again several times. Roll your pelvis forwards until your back actually arches, hold for a second, and then roll it back as far as you can until it draws your chest slightly down. Clench and release the cheeks of your buttocks several times. This pumping action looks odd, but it recruits blood flow to the area. And get out of the vehicle a *minimum* of every two hours or so and walk around.

Smooth out the transitions. Many professional drivers also load and unload cargo. We can't overemphasise how important it is to make those transitions intelligently from sitting to standing to walking to lifting. Think of yourself as a triathlete who has several physical activities to master; each activity is different, and the transitions between them make the difference between success and failure. In fact, triathletes train for transitions as thoroughly as for their individual sports. You'll have to do the same.

Remember how fatigued your back can get from sitting. You may have weaknesses and imbalances that will make it difficult for you to make sudden demands on your back and upper body. When you get out, use the walk back past the trailer to sneak in a stretch. At the very least, 'shake it out' to remove tension from your back and get blood flowing to your arms and legs. Remember, when you lift, keep your back straight, keep your abdominals tight, and lift from your knees to keep as much pressure as possible off your back.

To get the kinks out of your back after driving all day, try the stretch below.

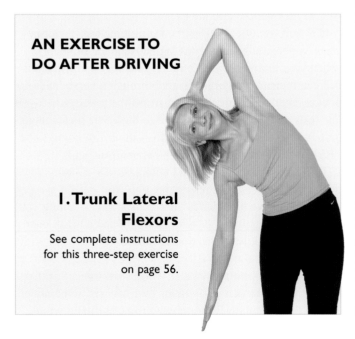

AN EXERCISE TO DO AFTER DRIVING

1. Trunk Lateral Flexors

See complete instructions for this three-step exercise on page 56.

PROTECTING YOUR BACK WHEN YOU USE A COMPUTER ALL DAY

Using a computer, or doing other kinds of keyboarding, can pose a dual risk. Not only will you be sitting at a desk with all the perils that we listed for driving all day, you also add that notorious weapon – the keyboard.

Oh, sure, keyboards look innocent enough. Some even have designations like 'featherlight touch' and 'ergonomically friendly'. But they can wreak insidious damage, better known as carpal tunnel syndrome.

Carpal tunnel syndrome is one of a group of injuries called repetitive strain injuries (RSI). The syndrome develops as fingers repeatedly strike keys over a long period of time. The hands and wrists fatigue; tendons, ligaments and soft tissues swell. Just as stepping on a garden hose slows the flow of water, so the swelling compresses the median nerve fibres and slows down the transmission of nerve signals through the carpal tunnel – the passageway that runs from the forearm through the wrist. The result is excruciating pain and paralysing numbness in the wrist, hand and fingers.

Why are we including RSI in our discussion of backs? Because an alarming number of cases of RSI are directly related to the back. Either the pain of carpal tunnel syndrome sets off a series of compensations that travel directly up the arm to the shoulder to the back, or the back shorts out and sets off a series of fatigued muscles throughout the shoulder and down the arm to the wrist and hand.

We know that the body is an integrated system, with each part linked to every other part. When a wrist isn't operating properly, the lower arm kicks in to move the hands. But the lower arm fatigues. When the muscles start to fail, the arm above the elbow moves in to take up the slack. But that's not what the upper arm is for. It shorts out. When it falters, the shoulder kicks in. But the shoulder isn't good at managing movement in the wrist and hand, so it eventually strains. When the shoulder is strained, the back tightens. See how it works?

These links also work the other way. When the back spasms between the shoulder blades, the body strains to hold the torso up against gravity, particularly in the posture that we assume when typing at a keyboard. As the upper back locks up, the shoulders lose range of motion. When they suffer fatigue, the upper arms work overtime to move the lower arms. When the upper arms tire out, the wrists and hands are strained. Spasm and swelling of tissue impinge the nerves in the wrist. Bingo: carpal tunnel syndrome. Cause and effect, directly linked both to and from the back.

While keyboards have been around for a long time, carpal tunnel syndrome has been epidemic for a mere 15 years. But the reason isn't a mystery. The old-style typewriter keys were harder to strike, so the hands got a better workout. And the carriage return made it necessary for the typist to reach up and whack it at the end of every sentence. In contrast, the computer keyboard has a soft, light touch, so the hands must work more subtly. Without a carriage return, there's no reason to move a muscle.

Computer keyboards are common at work and at home. Many people go from being mesmerised by one computer screen to another with only dinner in between. We can sit for hours without noticing that we're numb from the waist down, so we don't realise that our hands and backs are fatigued until it's way too late.

From your perspective as an athlete, you must view carpal tunnel syndrome as a classic overuse injury. 'Overuse' means just that – used too much, overdone. But the good news is that we can prevent it or, if it's already setting in, we can turn it around.

Don't ignore the signals. People aren't suddenly struck down in the prime of their typing without warning. Indeed, carpal tunnel syndrome develops over a long period of time, settling in while a person ignores clear signals that something's not right.

The first signal is fatigue in hands and arms. You could feel it as 'slowing down' or a slight lack of coordination. Eventually, fatigue will feel like a small ache. The solution is simple: take a short break every hour to get things moving and keep them moving to improve circulation and restore range of motion.

Don't forget your programme. Prevention is a matter of training. Like any athlete, a keyboarder must be physically fit with specific training to withstand the demands of the job. Keyboarding requires strong arms, shoulders and back and flexible wrists, hands and fingers.

Keep your eye on the bigger picture. As we've mentioned, carpal tunnel syndrome isn't the only danger of keyboarding. Sitting at a keyboard all day can take a terrible toll on an imbalanced, untrained, unprepared body, putting more stress on your lower spine than standing. And, no matter how ergonomically designed and comfortable your chair is, your back, hips, legs and buttocks will suffer fatigue and tighten up if you don't give them a break periodically. Your neck, shoulders and the area between your shoulder blades suffer

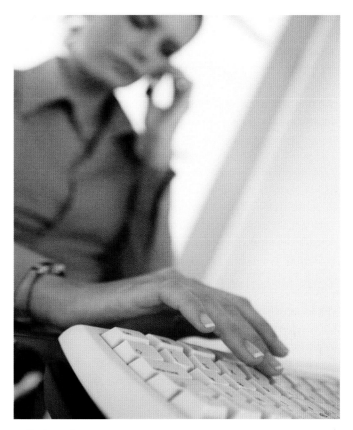

▲ **Keyboards**
Although keyboards look harmless, with constant use they can cause the painful injury known as RSI (repetitive strain injury).

Watch Your Form

Besides frequent breaks, you can also prevent carpal tunnel syndrome by taking a few simple precautions.

- **Keep your mouse** as close to the keyboard as possible and at the same level so that you don't have to reach and strain your back.
- **When you are not using the mouse,** take your hand off it. Move your fingers around to relax them. Don't rest the hand on the mouse or wrist pad if you are not using the computer.
- **Keep your monitor screen** at eye level and straight in front of you.
- **Keep your document holder** as close to the monitor screen as possible. Switch sides occasionally.
- **Keep your wrists straight** so that your hands will relax.

fatigue, and strain as you maintain and sustain an upright posture with your arms in front of you and your hands on the keyboard. You *must* move.

Find and use every excuse you can to stand up and move around. Set a timer if necessary. Never type for more than two hours at a stretch without a 5- or 10-minute break during which you should work out the kinks. Take a look at the tension relievers in chapter 12, starting on page 207.

If you work at a keyboard and are sitting all day, we guarantee that you are not getting enough exercise, so you will want to engage in a fitness programme that combines strength, flexibility and cardio work.

To get the kinks out of your back after keyboarding all day, try the stretch below.

YOUR HEALTHY BACK AT HOME

While most people will tell you that they feel safest at home, every year more than 4,000 people die in accidents in the home in the UK, and nearly three million seek hospital treatment. After road accidents, the home is the second most common place for fatal injuries. Yikes!

Fatalities aside, the most common injury is a back injury caused by a fall, but almost all home injuries are preventable. So why are they so common?

Researchers tell us that most people do not see the hidden dangers within their homes. They may not be in denial, but, on average, people really can't imagine how they could get hurt in their homes, where they feel most safe and secure.

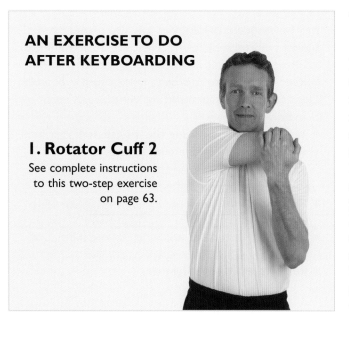

AN EXERCISE TO DO AFTER KEYBOARDING

I. Rotator Cuff 2
See complete instructions to this two-step exercise on page 63.

DON'T LET YOUR BACK DO THE HEAVY LIFTING

When tackling a big load, you may be tempted just to shift it in a surge of effort. Later, your back pays mightily. Use your brain, instead of your brawn. Once again, protecting your back has everything to do with planning. Before you lift, consider the following.

1. First, the obvious: avoid lifting heavy objects whenever possible. Try to figure out ways to shove, roll, slide or drag it. Recruit a helper if possible – two lifters are always better than one. Think about dividing the load into smaller, more easily managed pieces.

2. If you must lift the object, ask yourself these questions:

- Am I fit enough to lift this particular object?
- Am I warmed up properly?
- Is the object awkwardly shaped?
- Is it sharp or does it have things on it that might harm me?
- Is the weight evenly distributed throughout the object?

3. Give it a shove or tip it to test the weight. If you think you can handle it, plan what you'll do with the object once you've lifted it. Look for the shortest path from here to there and make sure it's clear and safe for you to walk there.

4. Decide where you're going to put the object down and make sure that the receiving end of this project is prepared. You don't want to stagger out to your car with a hefty crate, only to discover that you forgot to open the boot.

How to Lift Something Light

If you think it's ludicrous to be concerned about lifting something light, think again. If you simply bend over from the waist and reach to the floor with your hand, you run the risk of straining your lower back. Sometimes the smallest, most simple movements are the ones that trigger spasm or aggravate an imbalance or injury. To lift something light from the floor, such as a magazine, lean over it, slightly bend one knee, and extend the other leg behind you. You'll look sort of like a sprinter on the starting line. Hold on to something or brace yourself against something as you continue to bend your knee and dip towards the object. Once you have it, simply straighten your knee, bring your back leg up, and stand tall. Lifting in this manner may feel a bit unnatural at first but after a few times it will become a habit.

WORKING AROUND THE HOUSE

Some housework tasks can be real back-breakers, so treat them with respect. Do what you can to make sure you're flexible and strong. Pace yourself so that you don't tire yourself out too much. Remember to drink plenty of water.

Cooking: Preparing meals is generally not hard on the back, but it can be if you stand for too long. Ensure that your work surfaces are the right height for you. If you're going to be standing at the work surface for a long time, put a box about 6in (15cm) high under one foot, or open a cupboard and put the foot up on the bottom shelf. This takes the pressure off your lower back. Don't forget to straighten up and shake out the tension once in a while.

Standing to clean floors: Vacuuming, mopping, polishing and sweeping can put pressure on the lower back because you push and pull from your upper body, bending from the waist. Keep your back straight and bend from the hips as much as possible. Make sure that the handles are long enough to allow you to keep an upright posture with as little flexion from the waist as possible. Give your back frequent breaks by standing fully erect. Do a few of the quick-release tension relievers you'll find on page 207 in chapter 12. To get the kinks out of your back after vacuuming, mopping, polishing or sweeping, try the stretch below.

Kneeling to clean floors: Getting down on your hands and knees to scrub requires that your back curves forwards to allow you to reach the floor. But your back also has to support your weight because your hands are occupied and are not helping to keep you in position. Fatigue sets in very quickly, so be sure to take frequent breaks. Stand up fully to take the pressure off your back. To work the kinks out of your back when you've been scrubbing, try the stretches below.

Making a bed: Try kneeling rather than bending forwards to tuck in a corner of the bed. Don't reach across the bed to smooth covers or tuck in a corner on the opposite side. Take the time to walk around. If the bed is against the wall and you can't get to the other side, consider putting the legs of the bed on casters so that you can roll it away from the wall. To get the kinks out of your back when you've been making a bed, try the stretch overleaf.

AN EXERCISE TO DO AFTER VACUUMING, MOPPING, POLISHING AND SWEEPING

1. Thoracic-lumbar Rotators

See complete instructions for this two-step exercise on page 56.

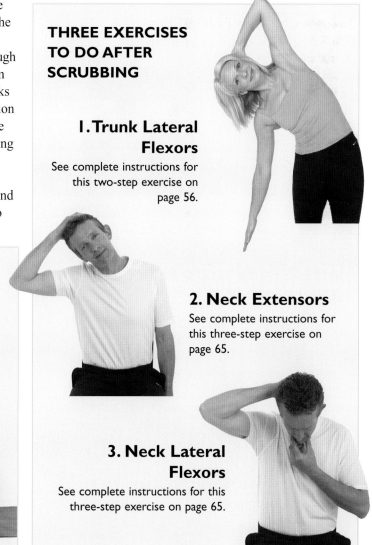

THREE EXERCISES TO DO AFTER SCRUBBING

1. Trunk Lateral Flexors

See complete instructions for this two-step exercise on page 56.

2. Neck Extensors

See complete instructions for this three-step exercise on page 65.

3. Neck Lateral Flexors

See complete instructions for this three-step exercise on page 65.

Doing laundry: Squatting is better for your back than bending over at the waist if you are unloading a front-loading washer or dryer. If your machine is top-loading, try to keep your back as straight as possible, by extending one leg and leaning forwards from the hip on the other one. Keep the toe of your extending foot on the floor as you lean back. Lift it as you lean forwards for counterbalance. These same techniques are good for loading dishwashers. They may feel unnatural at first but will soon become a habit.

To get the kinks out of your back when you've been doing laundry, try the stretch at the bottom of the page.

AN EXERCISE TO DO AFTER MAKING A BED

1. Double-leg Pelvic Tilts

See complete instructions for this two-step exercise on page 50.

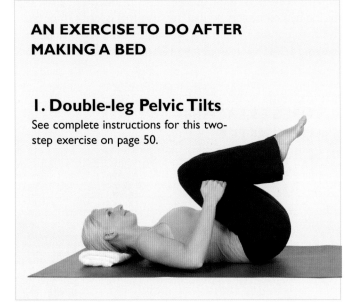

AN EXERCISE TO DO AFTER THE LAUNDRY

1. Rotator Cuff 1

See complete instructions for this two-step exercise on page 63.

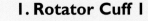

Don't Slip on the Home Front

Homes are private and, therefore, not subject to inspections by experts who could tell us how to make our homes injury-proof. Too bad, because we could all learn a lot from these professionals. Why not act as your own inspector? Try this checklist of common risks found in the home.

- **Are your telephone** and electrical cords tucked out of the way so that no one will trip on them? If you must string out a cord, make sure it's taped securely to the floor, centring wide tape along the entire length of the cord from wall to appliance.
- **Are all your area rugs** and runners secured to the floor with either skid-proof rubber matting or carpet tape? Are all the edges flat to the floor so that no one will trip?
- **Are your walkways free** of clutter? Keep the floor and stairs clear all the time.
- **Are all the legs** of your tables, chairs and stools tightly secured and level?
- **Are you using** maximum-wattage bulbs in all fixtures both inside and outside your home?
- **Is each bath** and shower outfitted with a skid-proof mat or textured strips so that you won't slip?
- **Do you have grab bars** to help you get in and out of the bath or shower? Are they affixed to structural support so that it won't pull out of the wall if you depend on it?
- **Do you have a telephone** next to your bed? If something happens, the ability to call for help is essential.
- **Are the light switches** for your garage located near the entrance? You must not try to feel your way through a darkened garage to get to a switch.
- **Is your garage tidy?** Keep it as neat as your home. Keep all drawers and doors closed. Mop up any oil spillages straight away.
- **Do you have torches** located strategically around your home in case of a power failure?
- **Are the stairs in your home** in good shape? All level? No loose boards? Free from clutter? Repair any problems. Don't put a rug at either the top or the bottom.
- **Are the stairs in your home** well-lit with switches at both the top and the bottom? If not, get an electrician to sort it out. Under no circumstances should you be forced to walk up or down stairs in the dark.

GARDENING

Serious gardeners are athletes, but most don't realise it. Their need for conditioning doesn't become obvious until something goes wrong. The physical problems they present are identical to those of athletes, but that's where the similarities end.

One of the problems is that gardening is seasonal. Spring and summer are more demanding than autumn and winter. Unlike an athlete who spends the off-season training, a gardener might retire to his shed. When it's time to come out of hibernation and get to work, the gardener is deconditioned from months of layoff, yet the work of early spring is especially hard: lifting, hauling, digging, weeding, tilling, planting and pulling out and moving plants. But spring is in the air, so the out-of-shape gardener will leap right back into rigorous labour. Even when the work is not hard, you'll find a gardener kneeling, bending over little plants for hours at a time. Little wonder the back shorts out.

If you want to enjoy gardening and stop referring to it as back-breaking work, you have to train for it during the off-season and then maintain complete fitness when your garden demands your attention. Before your day in the dirt begins, do your workout so that your body is strong, flexible and warmed up, ready for work. If you have time for nothing else, do the Stretch routine. And once you begin, use the right tools for the right jobs. We recommend lightweight equipment.

Different jobs have different remedies. Here are just a few.

Pushing a wheelbarrow: If you're pushing a wheelbarrow, make sure you've balanced the load so that one side isn't heavier than the other. Keep your back straight and let your legs do all the work as you lift the handles and manoeuvre it. To work the kinks out of your back when you've been pushing a wheelbarrow, try the three stretches below.

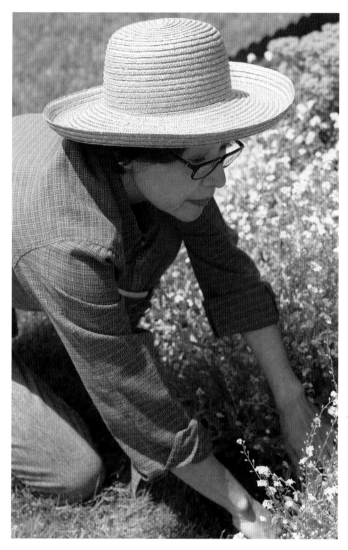

▲ In the garden
The work of a serious gardener involves so much bending that it's very important to warm up beforehand by stretching.

THREE EXERCISES TO DO AFTER PUSHING A WHEELBARROW

1. Trunk Lateral Flexors
See complete instructions for this three-step exercise on page 56.

2. Neck Extensors
See complete instructions for this three-step exercise on page 65.

3. Neck Lateral Flexors
See complete instructions for this three-step exercise on page 65.

Bending over your plants: Weeding and planting involve gipping, pulling and twisting that can irritate muscles and tendons in your lower arms and hands. Work a little while, and then give them a rest. Stretch them a little to get the kinks out. Remember that gripping, pulling and twisting can also irritate the back, so make sure that you're stabilised and that you don't strain. Also be aware of bending over, even at slight angles, for extended periods. Small irritations to the lower back over long periods of time will short it out.

Bending over while kneeling is very hard on your lower back. Take frequent breaks to straighten out your legs and back. If your back is really bothering you, you might be better off using a long-handled tool from a standing position. Or sit on the ground and work. If you're going to be on your knees, put a pad under them to cushion the pressure. (If you are going to be lifting something, please refer to page 238, which describes the proper technique for lifting both heavy and light loads.)

When you're pulling out shrubs, wear gloves. Loosen the soil around the base of the plant. Stand close to the shrub with your feet shoulder-width apart. Keep your back straight and your face forwards. Bend your knees

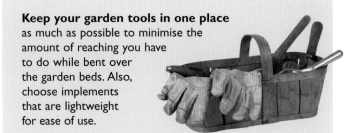

Keep your garden tools in one place as much as possible to minimise the amount of reaching you have to do while bent over the garden beds. Also, choose implements that are lightweight for ease of use.

and lower yourself until you can get a firm grip. Take a firm hold. Straighten your knees and lean back slightly as you rise slowly. Stay alert to that subtle moment right before the shrub lets go, and relax some of your pull. You don't want to keel over backwards with a shrub and a ball of dirt on top of you. When you have successfully pulled the shrub, stand fully upright, relax your back and shoulders, and stretch.

To work the kinks out of your back when you've been bending over your plants, try the stretches below left.

Raking and hoeing: Raking and hoeing are deceptively hard on the back because you reach forwards and pull backwards from a standing position. Additionally, these actions are very rhythmic and repetitive. It's easy to get lulled into underestimating the demands they make on your lower back. Make sure you are sufficiently warmed up, change your position often, and take frequent breaks that involve standing fully upright to take the tension off your lumbar spine.

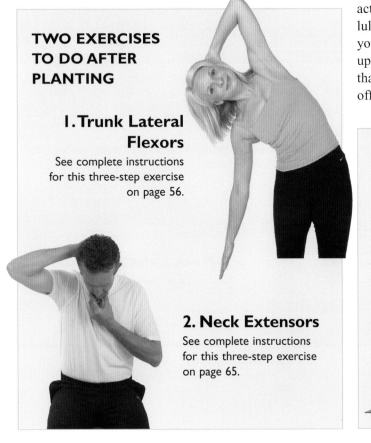

TWO EXERCISES TO DO AFTER PLANTING

1. Trunk Lateral Flexors

See complete instructions for this three-step exercise on page 56.

2. Neck Extensors

See complete instructions for this three-step exercise on page 65.

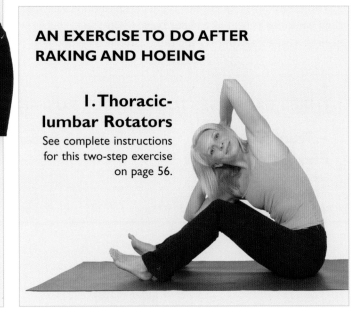

AN EXERCISE TO DO AFTER RAKING AND HOEING

1. Thoracic-lumbar Rotators

See complete instructions for this two-step exercise on page 56.

TWO EXERCISES TO DO AFTER DIGGING AND SHOVELLING

1. Rotator Cuff 1
See complete instructions for this three-step exercise on page 63.

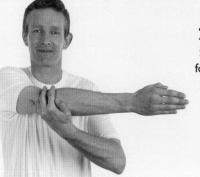

2. Rotator Cuff 2
See complete instructions for this three-step exercise on page 63.

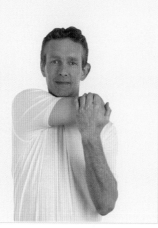

To work the kinks out of your back when you've been raking and hoeing, try the stretch on the opposite page.

Digging and shovelling: Stand with your feet shoulder-width apart when you're digging and shovelling. Be sure to use long-handled tools. Work close to your feet, resisting the urge to bend at the waist and reach out to work. Lift only small amounts of soil with your shovel so that the weight will not strain your back. And always remember to take frequent breaks. To work the kinks out of your back when you've been digging and shovelling, try the stretches above.

Hauling: Hauling is about reaching and lifting, so it's important to protect your lower back from strain. Keep the load close to your body and let your legs do the majority of the work. Keep your spine straight at all times. To work the kinks out of your back when you've been hauling, try the stretch on the right.

AN EXERCISE TO DO AFTER HAULING

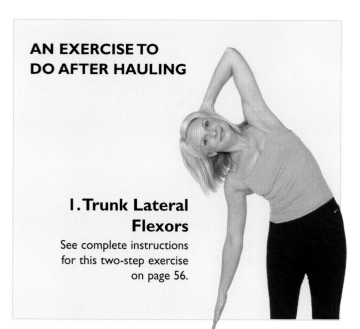

1. Trunk Lateral Flexors
See complete instructions for this two-step exercise on page 56.

A FINAL WORD ABOUT WATER

When you're gardening, it's easy to become so engrossed that you forget to drink. Hydration is as critical for you as it is for your precious plants. If you've waited to drink until you feel thirsty, it's too late. Thirst is a symptom of dehydration, and dehydration decreases plasma volume. With less blood getting to the skin, the systems that control heat dissipation fail. Once this happens, a gardener overheats even more quickly. Work suddenly seems to take superhuman effort.

Symptoms of dehydration include muscle cramping, excessive sweating, dark urine or infrequent urination, weakness, nausea, rapid heart rate, headache, light-headedness, increased body-core temperature, heat exhaustion and heatstroke. If symptoms are too subtle for you, check your urine at the end of the day. If it's darker than the colour of straw, you're not doing a good job of hydrating. Your goal should be urine that is clear or nearly so.

The recommended daily liquid intake is at least eight glasses of water, although you may substitute any other liquid except alcoholic or caffeinated beverages. (These are dehydrating so cannot be included in your eight glasses. If you are going to drink them, do so in moderation.) If you are going to do some gardening or other exercise, you need to drink extra. Plan to hydrate before, during and after your work. Keep a bottle of water next to you. Every time time you water a plant, join in.

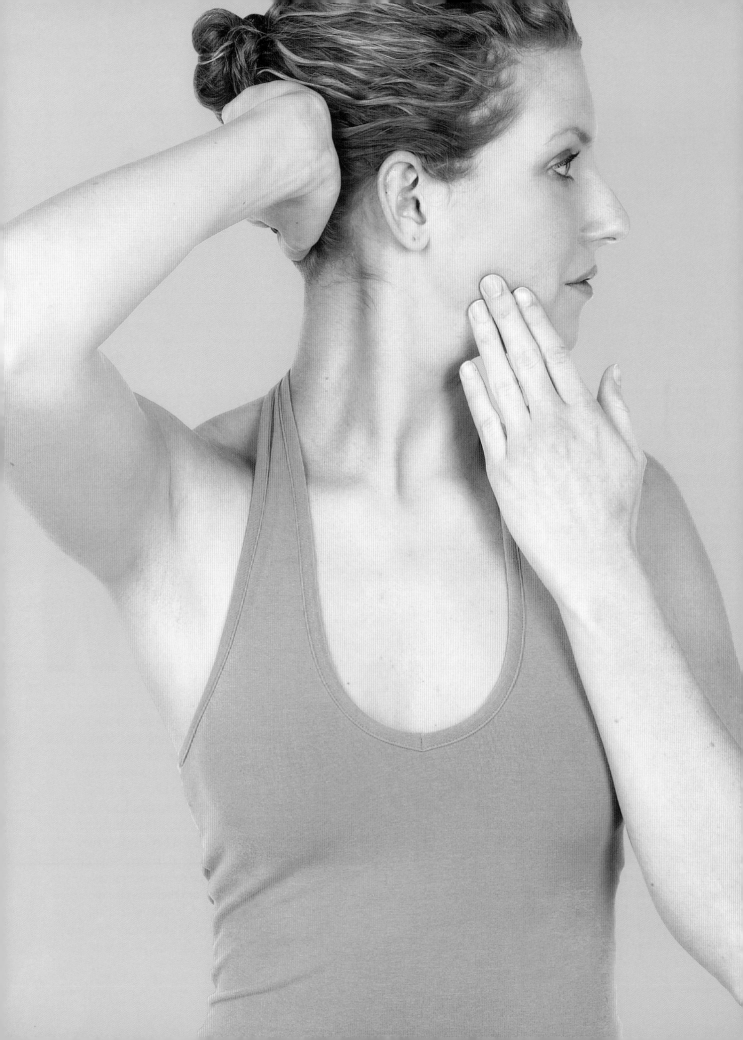

CHAPTER 15

YOUR HEALTHY BACK ON THE ROAD

The travel industry is often called a leisure industry, *but the means of getting to your destination and back home again can be anything but leisurely. Whether it's the cramped indignities of a tiny airline seat or the tense shoulders that come from stressful driving, travel is full of potential pains for the back. The best way to prevent and repair the damage comes down to foresight, planning and some on-the-spot common sense.*

We've culled these strategies from our hundreds of trips around the globe, tending to other peoples' pain while trying to avoid our own, and we're delighted to share them with you. Whether you travel by plane, bus or train, most of these tips will help you keep your back supple, healthy and flexible for the trip and beyond.

GETTING YOUR TRIP OFF TO A GOOD START

Planning is the best thing you can do to make your trip a success. Do your best to plan ahead and get things done in advance so you're not rushing around at the last minute. Tie up loose ends at home and at work so that you are completely relaxed about leaving. Make sure the details of your trip are well-planned and all your reservations and appointments are confirmed.

If you're rushed, you're pushed. We've travelled often enough – and have clients who do as well – to know how rushing to catch a plane or train can really tense up your back. If you think that you can stress out while preparing for your trip until your back is in knots and then relax on the plane, think again. Releasing tension takes some space, which you probably won't have, and movement, which you probably can't have. Strapping into one of those upright seats (with the tray table in its upright position) is practically guaranteed to make everything worse. Upright seat. Upright tray table. Uptight you.

Be on time, if not a little early. Plan not to be panicked, not to rushed off your feet.

Book the bulkhead. When travelling by plane, ask to be placed in the first row, also known as the bulkhead. Because there are no seats directly in front of you, you'll have extra leg room and be more comfortable.

We learned this trick from marathon runners who fly right after they've run 26.2 miles (42.2km), still suffering the effects of the race. With the extra room, they can move and stretch their legs to get the kinks out. You can even lie down on the floor and do a few stretches, provided you are friends with the other passengers sharing your aisle. Caution and courtesy are advised.

PACKING AND HANDLING BAGS TO PROTECT YOUR BACK

The process of moving and hauling your stuff from point A to point B is also rife with threats to your back. Take these steps to protect your back.

Pack as little as you can. If as little as you can is still a lot, at least plan to *carry* as little as possible. If you do have to take a heavy load with you, make sure you use a trolley at the airport to cart your luggage around. Do this, even if it means searching for a trolley.

Roll your suitcases. We don't know how we managed before some brilliant person invented suitcases with wheels and retractable long handles. If you don't have one, buy one. This minor investment will pay off in keeping the strain off your back. When you get to the hotel, tip a baggage handler to help you if there is any lifting involved in getting the bags to your room.

Balance the load you carry. If you're going to carry any bags, always carry two of the same weight so you can balance them. Weight on one shoulder will put tremendous strain on your back and your hip on the opposite side. If you're weighed down evenly, you might huff and puff, but your back will thank you.

Think before you lift. When you reach down to pick up your bags, keep your back straight and bend your knees. If you have two bags, pick them both up at the same time and don't allow anyone who may be helping you to give them to you one at a time. If the bags are heavy, your helper might heave that first one slightly higher than your shoulder and, when it's in position, let go, dropping it on to you. It will hit you quickly and heavily, jarring your back. By the time you receive the second bag, the damage will already be done.

Try to avoid sudden jolts. Even when you put the bags down, be smart: just follow the same advice as picking them up, only in reverse.

Wear your backpack correctly. If you are going to be using a backpack, resist the urge to look very cool with it slung nonchalantly over one shoulder – wear both straps over your shoulders. Carrying all the weight on one shoulder will throw your back off balance and put too much strain on the opposite hip. When you pack the backpack, try

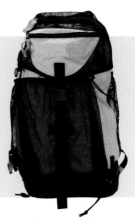

When using a backpack, make sure it is carried on both shoulders to avoid throwing your back off balance. Although it might not look as cool as being slung over one shoulder, it is much better for your neck, shoulders and back. Put any heavy items at the bottom of the bag.

to get the heavier items as low in the pack as possible. This puts the centre of the load near your hips, where it's easier for your body to balance and carry. We encourage the use of bumbags, which always distribute all their weight low on the back.

Send your luggage ahead. If your back is very fragile and any sort of load is problematic, consider shipping your belongings to the hotel by one of the courier services to arrive before you get there. Put your name on the box, the date of your arrival, and the word 'Hold'. Alert the manager that the hotel should expect it and allow plenty of time for the package to get there.

If you want to be really organised, take tape and a mailing label for shipping the package home. Most hotels ship and receive every day and will be glad to help you get this taken care of.

To get the kinks out of your back when your luggage has been too heavy, try the stretch below.

AN EXERCISE TO DO AFTER CARRYING HEAVY LUGGAGE

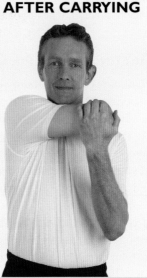

1. Rotator Cuff 2
See complete instructions for this two-step exercise on page 63.

KEEPING FIT AND HEALTHY ON AN AEROPLANE

Here are a few ways to make sure you keep your programme up while you're on the road. (We use the same methods whether we travel by plane, train or bus.)

Use waiting time in the terminal to get some exercise. While you're waiting, walk back and forth in front of your gate. Swing your arms and be sure to stop just short of the place that sells cinnamon buns and chocolate croissants. In fact, you can use that place as a turnaround and quicken your pace as you walk away from it. Get any kinks out of your back by using the stretch below.

Get as much exercise as you can on the plane. We know for sure that plane seats have been ergonomically designed but their one-size-suits-all definitely doesn't fit everyone. How delightful to have to sit with your belt tightened and seat flat, knees jammed, hips thrust forwards and midback arched to the back in a curve that resembles the letter C. Oh, let's not forget that your head is thrust forwards and held there by a pillow that hits you anywhere but where you need it. Nice try, airline industry. Not comfortable or good for your back, especially on long flights.

For this reason, you need to get up and move. Walk up and down the aisle, stand for a while, and do some of the quick releases we showed you on page 207. When we explain to the flight attendants that we're not out of our minds, we're merely suffering athletes, we are always welcomed into the space next to the galley. There's a little more floor space. On

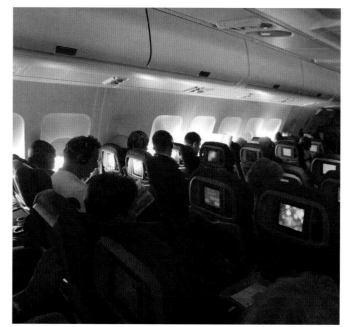

▲ Making the best of aeroplane journeys
Even those travelling in the comparative comfort of first-class need to ensure that they not only get out of their seat to exercise, but drink plenty of water to stay hydrated.

more than one flight, we've been joined by other passengers in the galley to do a small stretch class.

Do everything you can to stay active in flight because, believe it or not, your life might be at stake.

Blood clots can form when blood pools, most often in the legs, during periods of inactivity. Called deep-vein thrombosis, or DVT, these clots can break off and travel throughout the bloodstream to the lungs, brain or heart. Heart attack and stroke can result. Some people have died, although this is rare.

Many DVT victims develop the condition on long flights, considered those over eight hours. But experts have warned that shorter flights do not guarantee safety. If you have poor circulation and sit still for longer than two hours, you, too, are at risk. It's so common, in fact, that it's called economy class syndrome, referring to the cramped seats and minimal leg room.

The key to prevention is to increase circulation by moving around and keeping blood flowing. Additionally, researchers now know that eating and drinking during the flight increases blood volume and helps keep DVT at bay, but eating too much will divert blood from the legs into the digestive system and increase risk. Prevention is simple: don't overeat, drink a lot of water (see overleaf for more on hydration), and move.

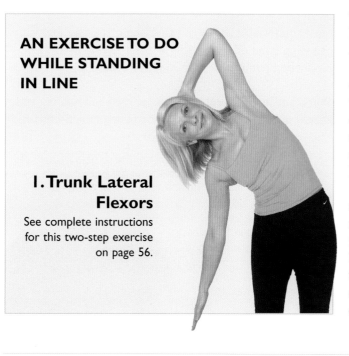

AN EXERCISE TO DO WHILE STANDING IN LINE

1. Trunk Lateral Flexors
See complete instructions for this two-step exercise on page 56.

Drink plenty of fluids. The altitude and dry air in an aeroplane cause dehydration. When you are dehydrated, healthy cells that are usually plump and juicy shrivel up. They don't work as well when their composition and function are disrupted. They don't slide as easily against each other. In fact, they actually shred.

If your back is tight because you're tense, and you're also dehydrated, you'll exacerbate the damaging effects of the tension on your muscles. Avoid this by taking on fluids: ask the flight attendants for water. We carry our own two-litre bottles of water with us. Not only do we stay hydrated even when the flight attendants are busy, we have an excuse to walk to the toilets frequently and get more exercise.

If you are wild for variety, drink decaffeinated beverages and juices. The caffeine found in some carbonated drinks, coffee and tea is a diuretic that will dehydrate you further.

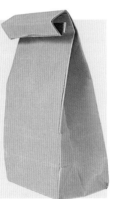

Instead of accepting the peanuts or other salty snacks offered to you on board, why not bring something of your own to enjoy during the flight? Food service has become limited on many flights, so bringing your own bag of snacks might be a great option, as long as you are not breaking any country's restrictions about what you may take on board the plane.

You may think that you need a stiff cup of coffee to keep you going, but please remember to balance it with an equal amount of water.

Alcohol doesn't count at all. Sorry, but it doesn't hydrate you, and it has lots of empty calories. Experts tell us that it's far easier to get drunk at 30,000 feet than at sea level. If you are drunk and fall asleep, you're likely to slump into a posture that strains your back – and stay in that position too long without moving. You'll feel relaxed, but you're doing damage that will affect you once you're on solid ground. It's better if you are sober and conscious just enough to wiggle a little. Save the wine until you're on the ground.

Avoid salty foods the day before your flight and during the flight. Of course, this seems nearly impossible advice, especially considering that a little bag of salted peanuts is traditional, standard fare on an aeroplane. But the sodium makes your tissues retain fluids, which causes swelling of your extremities. You're going to have enough of that to worry about all on your own without the help of salt.

Make sure you're warm enough. If you're cold, you'll shiver and tense up. Before you know it, your shoulders will be up around your ears. Your back between your shoulders will suffer fatigue from tension and eventually begin to short out. When you arrive at your destination, you'll feel tired, but the exhaustion isn't the true exhaustion born of healthy effort – it's from weakness and impeded blood flow to your back.

Once you get to the hotel, you may be tempted to stand under a hot shower or climb into a hot bath – but wait. Stretch first. Then try a little ice to recruit blood to the area and flush out the metabolic wastes that have accumulated while the muscles were constricted. Move a little. Then go ahead with that hot shower or bath.

Take care of your legs and feet en route. Swelling of the lower extremities is caused by sitting still in one position with your feet on the floor. You're sitting so still that your circulation starts to slow. Your heart pumps blood all the way down to your toes, but you don't make it particularly easy to get it back up. If the plane is cold, the situation is even worse – oedema and wretched circulation are the results.

The consequent swelling can be uncomfortable and last more than 24 hours after you get onto the ground. Wear the most comfortable shoes you own and then take them off to wiggle your toes and move your feet around. You want blood flow – as much as you can get. Don't hesitate to lift up your feet and massage them vigorously with your hands.

Dress for success. Always travel in loosely fitting clothes in layers. If it is cold, you can keep all the warm garments on. If you get too hot, you can peel a layer off. Wear the most comfortable shoes you have and make sure that you can wiggle out of them easily without having to make a production out of it in your confined space.

Work out in your seat. To get your blood circulating and keep it going, you need to get moving with the following

Men, take your wallet out of your hip pocket and carry it somewhere else for the duration of your flight. Having a lump on one side of your bottom lifts your pelvis to an angle you'll regret later when your back shorts out. This advice also applies to purses and mobile phones – anything at all bulky will cause your hips to misalign.

four stretches: Rotator Cuff 2 (see page 63), Trunk Extensors (see page 55), Ankle Evertors (see page 250), and Tibialis Anteriors (see page 250). A measure of caution is in order if you're seated next to other passengers who might not appreciate your enthusiastic workout. But if you explain what you're doing, they won't assume you've lost your mind, and might even join you.

Trunk extensors will keep your lower back from fatiguing after being locked in with a seat belt. Be really certain that your tray table is upright for these!

If you must sleep on a plane, support your back and neck. From the perspective of your back and hips, there is no good way to sleep sitting up, but you can help a little. We recommend a cervical pillow that wraps around the back of your neck like a stuffed horseshoe and holds your head in an upright position if you're leaning back slightly. Some are inflatable, so carrying one is easy. And some are stuffed but always light. Additionally, try taking one of the airline's little pillows and placing it at the small of your back for extra support. If you don't have a cervical support or airline pillow, simply reach into your bag and grab a T-shirt or a towel. Fashion anything you need by folding and rolling it until you're comfortable. We do it all the time.

TWO EXERCISES FOR WHEN YOU HAVE BEEN SEATED TOO LONG

1. Rotator Cuff 2
See complete instructions for this two-step exercise on page 63.

2. Trunk Extensors
See complete instructions for this two-step exercise on page 55.

Case Study: **Pat Devaney**

We were impressed with Pat's energy and athleticism, travelling the world non-stop with his footwear business, as well as running marathons. However, it was all taking its toll.

Pat Devaney is a footwear designer for DaDa and Deckers. For years, he has designed the shoes that put the elite-level athletes at the top of their games. He's a high-energy guy who travels the world constantly. We worked with him frequently and were always running into him at trade shows and expos for sports equipment. We started to notice, however, that his back was always in flexion. He was stooped with his shoulders caved in, and he was developing a dowager's hump. What a contradiction – Pat himself is a fine athlete, a competitive marathon runner, in fact.

One day, when he was looking especially tired, we took Pat aside and said, 'Look, you're not supposed to be like this. You don't need to be in this much pain. Let's work on it together.' We examined his lifestyle and discovered that he sat hunched over a drafting board much of the time, but the real culprits were long flights compressing his back, followed by his carrying his own bags – heavy ones loaded with shoes and books. We gave him the Active-Isolated Stretching and Strengthening programme, pointing out that an exercise strap wasn't too heavy to carry. And we advised him to turn *all* his bags over to porters from now on. Pat's taken our advice and he's doing much better now.

Ankle Evertors

Active Muscles You Contract: Insides of your feet and ankles

Isolated Muscles You Stretch: Muscles on the outsides of your feet and lower legs

Hold Each Stretch: 2 seconds   **Reps:** 10 to the right, 10 to the left

1 While sitting in your seat, bring the foot of the exercising leg up and place it on top of the thigh, just above the knee of the non-exercising leg. You may want to use one of the little airline pillows on the top of your thigh, under the ankle of your exercising leg Reach straight down and grasp your forefoot with both hands.

2 From the ankle, rotate your foot inwards, pointing the sole of that foot up. You may use your hands for a gentle assist at the end of your stretch.

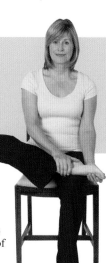

Tibialis Anteriors

Active Muscles You Contract: Muscles in the backs of your lower legs

Isolated Muscles You Stretch: Muscles in the fronts of your lower legs

Hold Each Stretch: 2 seconds   **Reps:** 10 to the right, 10 to the left

1 Bring the foot of the exercising leg up and place it on top of the thigh, just above the knee, of the non-exercising leg. Reach straight down and grasp your forefoot with the hand on the side of the non-exercising leg. Use the other hand to apply gentle pressure on the inside of the knee of the exercising leg to stabilise it.

2 Flex your exercising foot. You may use your hand for a gentle assist at the end of your stretch.

Be aware of the effects of a sleep deficit. Experts tell us that if you arrive at your destination worn out, you will lack concentration and motivation. You'll have trouble following instructions and directions. You won't remember details, you'll be irritable, and your immune system will be compromised by fatigue, leaving you susceptible to illnesses. These misfortunes can't be good for either conducting a business meeting or enjoying a piña colada on the beach.

Crossing time zones is especially problematic. Every human has an inborn personal clock, called a circadian rhythm. That clock is set in your own time zone, so when you pass from one zone to another, your circadian rhythm is disturbed, resulting in what's known as jet lag.

NASA scientists say that you need one day for every time zone you crossed to reset your circadian rhythm and feel normal. If you travel six hours out of sync with your own time zone, you'll need six days to equalise.

Flight attendants advise that if you're travelling east, don't rush to your hotel and go to sleep. Try to 'push through' and stay awake and active. Eat on a local schedule and tuck in for the night fashionably early. If you're travelling west, just go to bed at the time you normally do when you're in your own time zone.

Stick to your normal routine. If you're on holiday, breaking away from your normal routine would seem precisely the point. A break does you a world of good.

But when you eat and sleep on a different schedule, your body will be confused. You'll have to cope with adjustments that might take a few days to work out. We aren't suggesting that you should be rigid in adhering to a disciplined schedule, especially if you've changed time zones. We're suggesting that you try to keep within the broad range of basic functions, or adjust slowly to changes.

Make sure your hotel bed is a good one. Try it out. Like Goldilocks, you'll find some too hard, some too soft, and some just right. If the bed is too hard, call housekeeping and ask the chambermaid to put three or four blankets under the mattress pad for you. If the bed is too soft, pull the mattress on to the floor.

If the bed is just right, check out the pillow. Order extra pillows if you need them or take the cushions off the chairs and couch. Even a rolled-up towel from the bathroom will sometimes give you the support you need.

If you have back problems and always find hotel pillows unacceptable, consider travelling with your own. We have one friend who ships his favourite pillows to the hotel in advance of his arrival. They are too bulky for him to handle in luggage, so he packs them in a box and sends them ahead. He's never had a problem.

▼ Make sure your hotel bed is right for you
Don't be afraid to ask housekeeping for extra blankets or pillows to make your bed more supportive for your back.

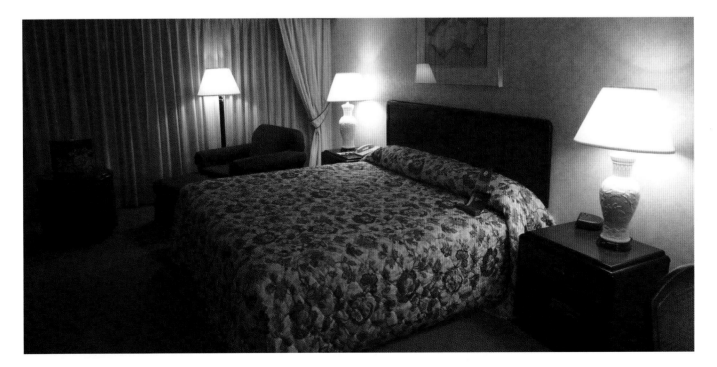

DRIVING WITH A HEALTHY BACK

For people who spend the majority of their work time behind the wheel, the effects of driving on the back are discussed in more detail in the previous chapter, but we thought it would be helpful to give some advice here to those of you who have to do long car journeys on an occasional basis.

Automotive engineers have made sure that you can do everything without moving from a seated position. You can honk your horn, roll down your windows, lock your door, get into gear, put on the headlights, release the hand brake, signal, see behind you, and adjust the speakers on your CD player with the smallest of movements. This efficiency is nothing if not hard on your body.

While driving, you're also susceptible to all the physical difficulties of an aeroplane passenger: dehydration, swelling in your feet and legs, fatigue in your back and shoulders, and deep-vein thrombosis (DVT). But when you drive, you can add a couple more hazards.

You learned in your driving lessons to hold the steering wheel at 10 o'clock and 2 o'clock and to grip it firmly so that you are in full control at all times, especially in case you need to steer quickly. Because your arms are out in front of you as your hands hold the steering wheel, you tend to relax your arm muscles and rely on your grip to support their weight. While this works very well, you'll notice a slight pull in your back between your shoulders. If you hold this posture for long periods of time, this slight pull becomes a big problem. Tension will set in. As the muscles in your upper back tense, blood supply is restricted. The muscle starts shutting down and gets fatigued, and the metabolic waste from the effort is not easily flushed away, so pain sets in.

When you drive, you extend your legs so that your feet can reach the accelerator, clutch, brake and anything else mounted there. Whether your car is manual or automatic, one foot is far more active than the other, so you'll push up on one hip to get that foot ready to do its job. The bad news is that you'll hold that position, with your back in slight rotation and your hip pushed up, for the duration of your drive.

When your back is held in this odd position, even if the drive is under an hour, it fatigues from tension and creates an imbalance. If, like most people, you hike up on the right, the left is working hard to hold you there. Then the piriformis muscle, which runs from your back to your hip and buttocks, constricts and impinges a nerve that runs from your buttocks down the back of your leg. In this painful and debilitating condition called piriformis syndrome, your back aches, your bottom and the back

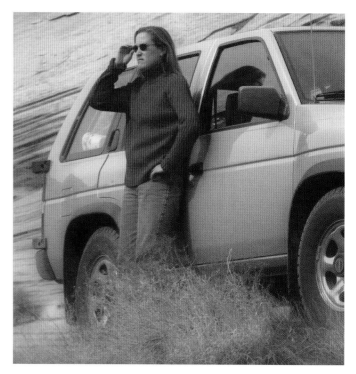

▲ Protecting your back on the road
Long-distance car journeys hold your back in an unhealthy position for too long. Get out and stretch at regular intervals.

of your leg are in pain, and you start to lose function. Suddenly, hitting the brake or clutch with your left foot is difficult. Most disturbingly, there's a lag between the moment your brain tells you to move that foot and when that leg can transmit that urgent signal through a nerve that's no longer communicating well. You won't be paralysed, but you'll be slowed down. Dangerously so.

Prevention is simple. Here are a few suggestions for how to do so without disrupting your trip too much.

Just move. From time to time, shift and wiggle in your seat. Consciously shift your weight from one side of your buttocks to the other and back again several times.

Take a picnic with you.
It's not just the driver whose back suffers from being in the same position on a long trip. A picnic will bring exercise and fresh air that will benefit the whole family, hopefully making for an all-round less tense car journey!

Do a pelvic tilt. Roll your pelvis forwards until your back actually arches, holding for a second, and then rolling it back as far as you can until it draws your chest slightly down. It might also help to clench and release your buttocks several times. (If you do it right, it will actually elevate your body. Don't worry that you'll look like you're bobbing up and down – just focus on the fact that it recruits blood flow to the area.)

Take a pit stop. Get out of the car and walk around at frequent intervals, no longer than two hours in between breaks. It's important to get out of the car because you cannot relax your neck, back and shoulders while driving. Rolling, rotating and nodding your head will throw off your equilibrium – and you'll get pulled over for weaving all over the road.

Stopping for petrol. Always get out and put in your own petrol – in some garages an attendant will still try and do it for you. Walk around and check your tyres. Vigorously wash your windows. Clear the interior of the car of rubbish. And walk into the building to use the toilet. Work hard to be as active as you can while you have the chance.

Remove that wallet. We mentioned this earlier when we talked about planes, but, please, guys, take your wallet (or mobile) out of your back pocket and carry it somewhere else. Having a lump on one side of your behind lifts your pelvis to an angle you'll regret later when your back shorts out. Small things like this can make a real difference.

To get the kinks out of your back when you've been driving for too long, try the stretch below.

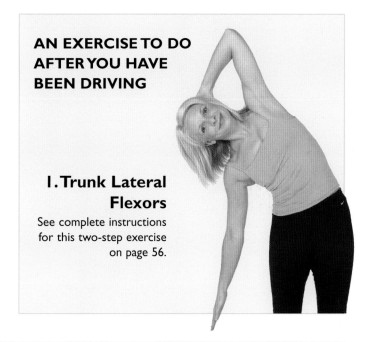

AN EXERCISE TO DO AFTER YOU HAVE BEEN DRIVING

1. Trunk Lateral Flexors
See complete instructions for this two-step exercise on page 56.

Choosing the Back-friendly Car

Protecting your back against travel-related back pain should begin before you even set foot in your car. Next time you're in the market for a new vehicle, keep these tips in mind – they could help you prevent pain well into the future.

- **Make sure you can get in and out easily –** if the car is too low to the ground, you might have trouble.
- **A tilt steering wheel** can make getting in and out easier on your back. Consider this feature.
- **The driver's seat should feel firm,** contoured and comfortable. Look for several features: easy forward and backward adjustment, adjustable lumbar support, lateral bolstering to 'cuddle' your buttocks and thighs, tilting seats, and headrests that can be adjusted to make contact with the middle of your head.
- **Electronic adjustments for the seats** will save wear and tear on your back and keep you from having to wrench and work to get things right. Consider automatic buttons and toggles.
- **Take a test drive** to make sure the suspension is firm to assure you of a smooth ride that will not vibrate or jar your back on long-distance trips. You want the car to absorb shock, not your back.
- **Try to find a car with a shallow boot –** deep boots force you to bend over and reach for items you are lifting in and out. This strains your back.
- **Take your favourite passenger along** and make sure he or she is as comfortable as you are in the car. Try to focus on the more practical features like lumbar support.

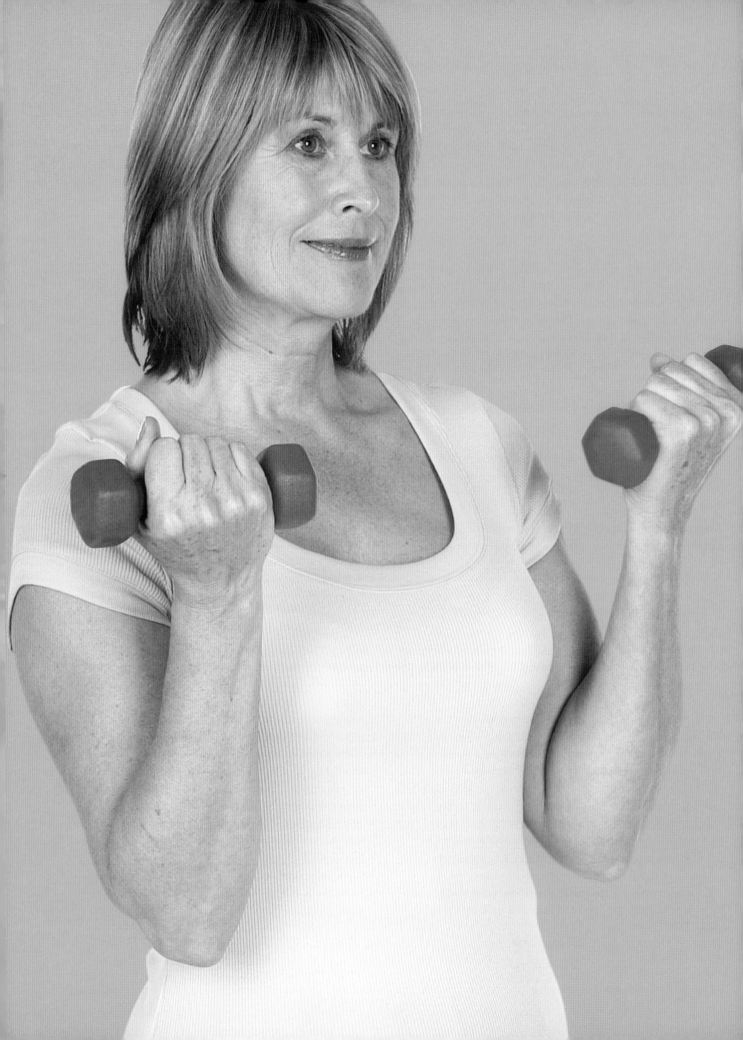

CHAPTER 16

YOUR HEALTHY BACK AT PLAY

Once you're in good shape and your back feels *great, it's time to return to play. Perhaps you'll resume a long-forgotten pleasure, or even find a new sport. The better you feel, the more you can play. The more you can play, the better you'll feel. It's a wonderful cycle of fitness and well-being. We've selected a few activities that are popular among our clients from which you might choose. Get out there and have fun.*

To get you off on the right foot, we've included brief discussions on a number of sports and activities with advice very similar to that which we deliver to our new athletes. We've also suggested a secret-weapon stretch or two, which you can do before you begin an activity, which will make all the difference in your performance.

BASKETBALL

We have worked with a number of basketball players in our career, including the New York Knicks team, and we can tell you one thing: flexibility is critical – for us! We are relatively short, so when we're talking to a 7-foot-tall (2.1m) basketball player, our necks and backs are in serious flexion from looking up. Good thing we're strong and flexible, or we would be in traction simply from talking to them.

The fact is, the bigger they are, the harder they fall. Although regulations are aimed at keeping body contact to a minimum, collisions send these players to the floor or somersaulting over camera crews and presenters on a regular basis. And the impact can be hard. Because players don't wear protective gear, a moving body meeting an immovable object can provide some fairly spectacular falls – most are pretty minor, but unfortunately some do result in serious injuries.

Basketball is a rigorous, fast-moving sport that keeps the players in perpetual motion. As a result, most players are in good shape. Repetitive movements, like running, jumping, pivoting, rapidly changing direction, rotating and shooting characterise the sport. These skills, sharpened by drills and honed by long games, put an athlete's body at risk of physical injury, particularly to tendons, ligaments and muscles that stabilise joints. Landing after a running-jump shot, for example, produces forces up to seven times your body weight.

The good news is that back injuries are rare and most commonly the result of trauma, particularly among young or inexperienced players. Girls and women are injured more frequently than their male counterparts, and their injuries tend to be more serious. Here are a couple of ways you can help prevent injuries on the court.

Know your weak spots. Most injuries take place in practice, and most often afflict the feet and ankles, where supersized feet can become stress-fractured by supersized workouts on a hard floor, or fractured by collision or stomping. In addition, strains and sprains are common. Trainers keep vast stores of tape in the locker room for just such occasions.

In order of greatest vulnerability, your body's weak points when playing basketball are the knee, ankle, lower back, shin, hip, shoulder, neck, wrist, foot, groin and fingers.

Proper stretching and conditioning. Using the Active-Isolated method can help prevent most of the overuse or traumatic injuries in these problem areas.

Shop for good shoes. Perhaps the best precaution you can take is to be very selective about your shoes. Basketball shoes are specifically designed to provide a little cushion between your foot and the floor and give support to the ankle. By virtue of special engineering in the sole, particularly at the ball of your foot, they are also constructed to pivot, where you'll bear the weight of that move.

Inspect that surface. If you're playing on an outside court, check it first to make sure that it's completely free from debris. You want a surface that is smooth, without holes or buckles in the paving.

Children, take precautions. Experts advise that children wear knee and elbow pads, mouth guards and eye protection. (Frankly, adults could learn a lesson here.)

Hydrate – carefully. Remember to drink frequently, so you're always hydrated, but be sure to keep your water off the court. A wet, slick spot could send you or one of your team-mates skidding.

Know your secret-weapon stretch: tibialis anteriors. The floor of a basketball court is hard and the cushioning in basketball shoes is minimal. Because you'll be running, stopping, turning, pivoting and jumping, you need to make sure that your heels can strike the floor without damaging the fronts of your shins. When the heel is down and the forefoot is up, your shin strains. It's exacerbated by the speed at which you thunder up and down the court. Don't hide this stretch from your team-mates, because you'll want them all to benefit from it, but don't ever do it in front of your opponents and give away one of the best-kept secrets in injury prevention and flexibility in movement.

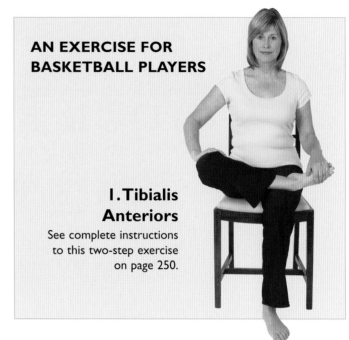

AN EXERCISE FOR BASKETBALL PLAYERS

1. Tibialis Anteriors
See complete instructions to this two-step exercise on page 250.

CRICKET

Cricket appears to be an innocuous, highly civilised game played by well-mannered people who follow polite rules that have governed the game since antiquity. So if it's so civilised and well-mannered and polite, why is it necessary for a cricket player to wear a helmet fitted with a shatter-proof face visor, a high-impact-resistant chest protector, forearm guard, gloves, box (genital protector), thigh pads and shin pads? What could eclipse a thousand years of gentility? A little 5.5-ounce (150g) ball rocketing towards you at a scorching 90 miles per hour (145kph) – so much for manners.

Of course, getting hit by a ball that moves faster than you can duck is not your only concern. Protective gear and a dead-eye bowler will assure you a hit-free day. Injuries in cricket are specific to the aspects of the game.

Bowling is much like throwing the javelin. Injuries to the bowler are nearly identical: lower-spine strain is common as the bowler runs into position, arches his back, rotates his hips, and then swings into and through the bowl, javelin-style. The mandatory straight elbow that distinguishes the 'bowl' from a 'throw' strains the shoulder, specifically the rotator cuff. Nerve impingement and overuse injuries of the shoulder are the most common problems in the sport.

In fielding, injuries occur when a quietly waiting player springs into action. From standing, alert and waiting, muscles are not prepared to move. When the ball rockets into the field, the player reacts quickly and dynamically. It's not uncommon for something to strain or tear.

Most batting injuries are caused because the back foot must remain on the ground when a player bats, so the Achilles tendon can suffer irritation and run the risk of rupture.

The wicket keeper's knees may strain and suffer fatigue from squatting for long periods of time. And we'll tell you something else. An extensive Australian study of injury in cricket suggests that fatigue contributes to injury as much as anything else.

Although cricket is generally considered to be a low-injury sport, it has its risks. You'll prevent injury and play better if you are strong, flexible and in shape. Preventing injuries, maximising performance and winning are matters of training and preparation; here are a few tips to keep you fit on the pitch.

Focus on your back and shoulders. The back needs to be strong and flexible in order to avoid straining, particularly for batting or bowling. The shoulder also requires special attention because it's the most commonly injured joint in cricket – throwing is the main culprit here. Strengthening the primary muscles such as your shoulders (deltoids), the top of your upper back (trapezius), and your chest (pectoralis) is necessary.

Don't forget to stretch. Equally critical are flexibility and generous ranges of motion in all joints. When you're loose and warmed up, you will find you can move more quickly and without irritation. Also, the greater your ranges of motion, the greater your reach, the longer your stride and the more torque and power you can put into rotation and wind-up.

Train hard. Being fit goes a long way in championship play. The good news is that cricket players are in better shape today than at any other time in the sport's history, because training methods have improved, along with our understanding of the complexity of the game's demands on the body. Also contributing to high-level athletics is the popularity of one-day cricket, which has put increasing demands on the players to survive the rigours of the accelerated game.

Know your secret-weapon stretch: rotator cuff 2. With ballistic throwing and catching, your shoulders need all the help they can get. The shoulder is the most mobile of all our joints. And yet, it's the most delicate, held together not by interlocking bone, but by muscles and connective tissue. It's highly susceptible to injury. To stay in the game and win, you have to keep your shoulders in great shape.

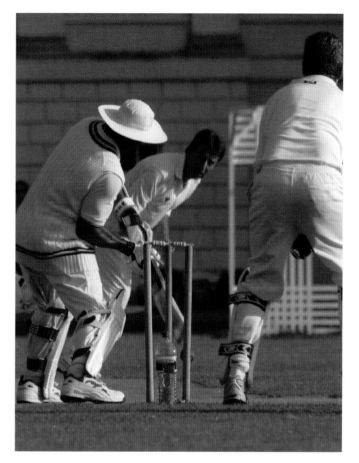

▲ Going batty
Although at first glance a 'safe' game, cricketers get their fair share of injuries – and not just from a hurtling ball. Bowling and batting are exertions that can easily strain muscles.

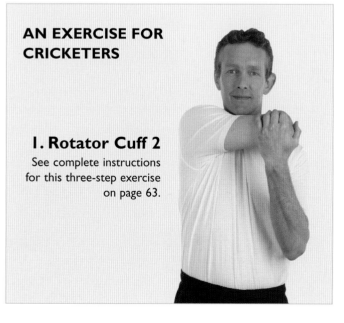

AN EXERCISE FOR CRICKETERS

1. Rotator Cuff 2
See complete instructions for this three-step exercise on page 63.

Cycling

Cycling started out as basic transport and remains so for many people around the world, but the complex partnership between an athlete and a bicycle can be thrilling. For some, it's a proper sport; for others, it's a joyful ride with the wind in their hair and a passing countryside. For everyone, cycling can be a great workout.

Many years ago, we started our practice in Gainesville, Florida, one of the best-kept secrets in training meccas. This wonderland of fantastic weather, landscape loaded with good trails, and plenty of sports-medicine professionals overflows with sports teams who come to train in privacy. When we worked with one of the major cycling teams, we noticed that their hamstrings were tight, their quads had blown up and their backs were damaged from hundreds of miles of training a week.

Their hamstrings and quads recovered quite easily, but this wasn't the case with their backs. In a rider, the back is always in flexion, bent over and stabilising to hold the cyclist in a perfect aerodynamic position. This position does not promote circulation, relaxation or recovery at all. Also, some of the younger, less-experienced riders tightened their hands around the handlebar grips and translated that tension up through their arms and shoulders and straight into their backs. Even short periods of time holding the grips too tightly would do it. We had to teach everyone to relax. And almost all the work we did with them was to unlock tortured backs.

Because cycling is primarily pedalling, the legs are the drivers in rotation. When pressing down and out on the pedal, you use hip and knee extensors (quads) and ankle flexors (tibialis anterior). When bringing the pedal up in rotation, you use your hip and knee flexors (hamstrings) and ankle extensors (gastrocnemius muscles). These rotations and the forces that drive them are consistent side to side, particularly with the use of toe clips that lock the feet into position on the pedals. Arm extensors help you turn the bike and support some of the weight of your body as you lean into the grips in that signature aerodynamic position. But the weight isn't fully supported by your hands on the grips; your flexed back and contracted abdominals stabilise your torso – transmitting the support work of your arms to your legs. Your upper back and neck are holding your head up, face forwards and made heavier by a helmet. As you pedal, you are getting a no-impact aerobic workout.

But cycling is not a perfect exercise. Pedalling around and around in a tight concentric circle shortens the muscles when they work, particularly the hamstrings. In order to be healthy and balanced, a muscle needs to be elongated as well as contracted and shortened, but cycling can produce imbalanced, inflexible muscles. Sports medicine experts also rank cycling high in injury statistics. In fact, injury

▼ Road racing
The backs of serious cyclists are always bent over, but correct posture and a relaxed grip will help to ensure an effective aerobic workout.

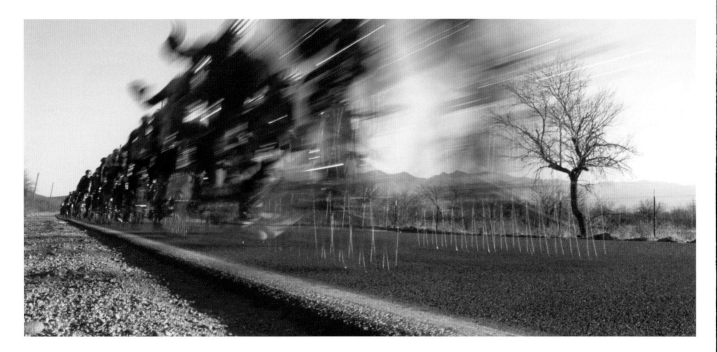

is an inherent part of cycling. Most common injuries are traumatic and the direct result of impact and skidding on pavement; these include grazes, cuts, bruises and broken bones. We also see repetitive stress injuries and overuse injuries that we can help you avoid with these tips.

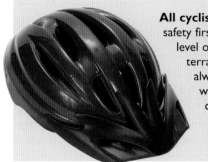

All cyclists should remember: safety first. Irrespective of your level of competence or the terrain you are riding on, always make sure you wear a helmet – it could save your life if you have a collision or a fall.

Take steps to combat nerve compression. Among the most common overuse injuries we see are nerve compressions of the hand (ulnar nerve) and forearm (radial distal nerve) from pressure on the handlebar grip – holding on too tightly for too long or resting one's weight too completely on the palm of the hand. Contracted muscles tighten up and put the nerves into compression, causing pain, numbness, fatigue, weakness and irritation. Wear padded gloves and remove your hands from the grips one at a time, shake them out and wiggle your fingers to get blood flowing.

We also see some nerve compression in the foot from wearing tight shoes, keeping too short a distance between the seat and the pedals, putting too much force down on the pedal for extended periods of time, and having weak muscles of the lower leg. Flexibility training will probably get you out of nerve compression, but it may take some time before you are 100 per cent.

Stretch and strengthen to avoid inflammation. We see inflammation of the tendons at their attachments at the hip, knee and ankle; overly tight quadriceps compressing the kneecap against the joint (major discomfort); pressure on the nerves of the cervical spine at the back of the neck from hyperextending and fatiguing the neck in holding the head up; lower-back pain as we explained earlier; and pain deep in the buttocks (sciatica or piriformis syndrome). Flexibility and strength will prevent all of these problems.

Select your seat carefully. Another injury we see is nerve compression between a rider's legs from sitting too long on a seat so hard that circulation is eventually cut off. Avoiding nerve compression between the legs is a matter of lifting your rear once in a while – make sure you periodically stand up on the pedals to help get the pressure off your backside. Another option is to get a better seat, one that is cushioned by padding or diffuses pressure with gel. Try as many as you can until you get a perfect fit for your physiology and comfort level. There are even seats that support your 'cheeks' but have a gap where more-sensitive body parts can be free. Unfortunately, this is one area where an exercise strap or rope just won't do.

Vary your posture. Sit straight upright from time to time and take the pressure off your back and neck. Move your head from side to side, but carefully. You don't want to throw off your equilibrium.

Be prepared for problems. Keep a repair kit and a spare inner tube with you in the event of a flat tyre, and always carry a mobile phone with you.

Don't forget the water. Remember to drink plenty of fluids while you are cycling. When you're flying along, it's so easy to get fooled into thinking that you're not really sweating, because at high speeds, sweat quickly dries to cool you.

Know your secret-weapon stretch: quadriceps. The correct rotation of the pedal limits range of motion in your joints and builds muscles that can easily become out of balance. Strong and flexible quads are essential for powering the cycle.

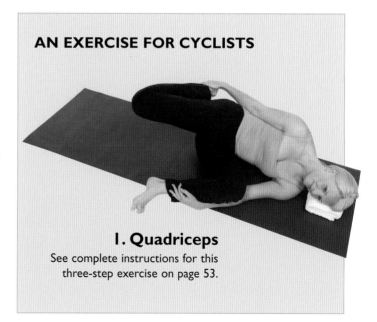

AN EXERCISE FOR CYCLISTS

1. Quadriceps
See complete instructions for this three-step exercise on page 53.

DOWNHILL SKIING

In skiing, control is a matter of simple physics – a breathless lift into weightlessness followed by digging in or side-slipping that causes a change in direction or speed.

Skiing is also a matter of shock absorption. Your hip extensors, knee extensors and plantar flexors carry your lead leg forwards. Your rear leg is held forwards by your hip flexors. Your abdominals and back support your torso, providing stability for your leg extensors. The metatarsal arch in your foot bears your weight when you plant your foot, providing stability during any balance of weight shifts from side to side.

Speaking of shock absorption, the design of today's ski closely mirrors the shock-absorbing properties of the human foot: there's a slight arch in the centre of the ski, which takes a pounding but then quickly dissipates those forces outwards. You swing, lift, plant and manoeuvre around your poles using your back, shoulders, arms,

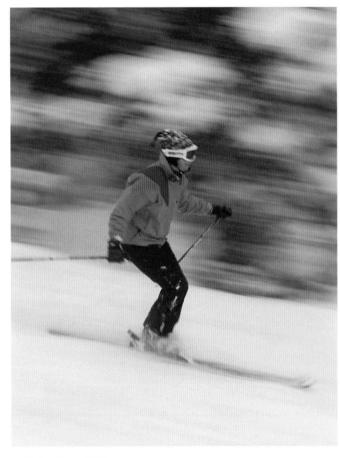

▲ Going downhill fast
The most common injury experienced by skiers is in the knees – a problem made worse by rigid skiing boots.

hands and wrists. With exercise like this, it's easy to fatigue everything, especially your back.

Millions of people go skiing each year, and the number is rising. Skiing can be wonderful fun and great exercise, but it can also be risky. The good news is that injuries are fewer than they were in the early days, because of better equipment, better slope development and maintenance, and better training. Lower-limb fractures used to top the list of maladies, but the high-tech, impact-resistant boots have provided a measure of protection that has lowered the statistic significantly.

Unfortunately, although ankles and shins are safer, the knees are still taking a pounding – particularly the anterior cruciate ligaments. This is the most common of all injuries. The boots allow limited movement of your ankles, so when you decide to change the angles of your feet and skis, you must effect that change from your knees and hips, exerting force on the front and sides of your shin to translate your decision down through the boot to the ski to the snow. The tibialis anterior and the triceps surae in your lower legs are also involved.

When you first begin skiing, you'll notice that the smallest moves make big differences, especially at high speeds. Good skiers make it look easy with very subtle, controlled adjustments in position. A beginner who is not quite as strong has to throw the whole body into a manoeuvre, which can be awkward and exhausting. As a skier improves, all movements are stronger, more subtle and more quickly performed – all of which is helped incredibly by overall fitness.

As we researched back injuries among skiers, we discovered that although back injuries don't top the list, no body part is immune from getting hurt when you're hurtling down a mountain at top speed and something goes wrong. The best defence is experience and training. In fact, inexperienced skiers hold the record for all accidents: four to one over the experts. Here are a few ways you can better those odds.

Stay in shape throughout the year. Strength and flexibility will give you some of the skills you require. You need good reflexes, coordination and balance. And all of these qualities can come from working out.

Don't forget your cardio. At some less-advanced levels, skiing is not a complete exercise, so you'll want to supplement your training with some cardio workouts. Running, cycling or inline skating at altitude all yield superior cardiovascular benefits. At altitude, the air isn't as dense in oxygen, so your body adjusts to it by increasing red blood cells to carry the little oxygen they can get as you cycle air through your lungs. This increase in red blood cells – and that little extra boost – is amazing when you return to sea level.

Eat and drink for fuel and warmth. Remember that being cold causes your body to shiver to keep you warm, which will burn extra calories. Eat small amounts often so that you can keep your blood sugar levels up for maximum, consistent energy.

Additionally, we encourage you to drink lots of water, since dehydration can creep up on you without warning.

Beware the weather. The blinding sun reflecting off the snow can be beautiful – but very dangerous to your eyes and skin. Wear goggles to protect you from glare and use high-SPF sunscreen. Also, dress in layers that will keep you warm and wick sweat away from your body.

Don't take unnecessary risks. Stay on marked slopes and trails. Please stay on slopes that are at your level. Mistakes in skiing can be dangerous – for you and others. Be sensible.

Know your secret-weapon stretch: hip abductors. Everyone will think you're making a snow angel, but the stretch shown below will keep you loose on the slopes and make manoeuvring and shock absorption easier on your legs. Take your boots off, then lie down on your back on hard-packed flat snow with both legs extended straight out.

AN EXERCISE FOR SKIERS

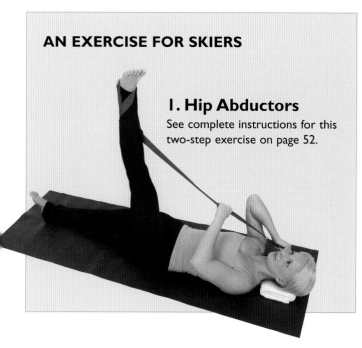

1. Hip Abductors
See complete instructions for this two-step exercise on page 52.

FOOTBALL

In 2001, we worked in Naples, Italy, preparing their football team for competition. In Italy, football is as competitive as it gets. The players are recruited worldwide and are elevated to celebrity status previously afforded only to Roman gods, especially when they're performing at the top of their game. Although we worked with the whole team, we were especially touched by Francesco Baldini. He had lost some of his speed because of constant back pain, and his status was in danger of fading in the eyes of the fickle fans. Baldini was more concerned about his team than the fans.

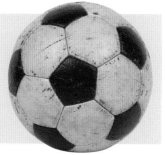

We love football. It's the world's most popular game, played in nearly every country in the world. Estimates place the number of amateur players at 40 million worldwide.

When we worked with Francesco, his injury responded so well that he brought in his whole team. Seventeen of the 30 team-mates were injured. Their title was on the line. We got 16 of the 17 back on the field. (The one player who was still unfit had a broken collarbone. We're good, but we're not that good.) It was incredible.

When we are in Africa working with marathon runners in Kenya, we see boys and men of all ages travel by foot for five hours from a neighbouring village to play football on a Saturday in Eldoret, where the marathon camp is located. At the end of a joyful day, they spend another five hours going home. You have to admit that there's something pretty compelling about a game for which people will go to that much effort. We heartily endorse football as a sport for nearly everyone without regard for age or gender.

Football is a great workout. The demands of play put most players into excellent physical condition with unusually refined coordination, power, speed and control. Repetitive, explosive movements define the sport: running, jumping, changing direction, rotating, pivoting, diving, heading and throwing. Unfortunately, they're also the explosive movements that cause injury, particularly to the connective tissues: tendons, ligaments and muscles that stabilise and mobilise joints.

While you're going to be running the equivalent of six or seven miles (10 km) during every game, you'll also be developing the skills of a sprinter: ballistic and high-speed. On the field, you're constantly on the move (aerobic exercise), then, frequently, you kick into warp drive (anaerobic). In fact, the workout provided by football is so intense that studies of top professional players reveal that, similar to what marathoners experience, football players can completely deplete their glycogen stores during the course of a game. (Glycogen is the energy fuel source your body stores and uses to fire muscles.)

At the same time you're running hard enough to exhaust glycogen, your arms and shoulders are pumping to help you stay in balance and rhythm, to amplify the force of your running, and to balance and counterbalance you as you quickly change direction and change the distribution of your weight. Your back and chest are holding you in an erect position. Your hands are relaxed. Your head is up. All your senses are on alert, primed to make that run or intercept that ball.

In football, most injuries occur in the lower extremities of the body. Bruises, ligament sprains (particularly of the ankle), and muscle strains of the ankles and legs account for 75 per cent of all injuries. Other injuries we see are iliotibial band (ITB) syndrome, an irritation of the outside of the knee; tendinitis; and other similar overuse problems caused by ballistic changes in direction. The constant hard charging sometimes leads to stress fractures of the tibia (shin). Collisions between players can also lead to bone breaks and fractures. Chronic groin pain seems to be an occupational hazard and is caused by forceful kicking when a player isn't flexible and strains connective tissue, such as tendons and ligaments. Goal keepers get injured by impacting with the ball, the ground or another player. In fact, goalies suffer 18 per cent of all injuries in soccer but comprise only six per cent of the total players. Statistically, that's a significantly increased risk. Here are a few ways to make football safer.

Watch your head. Football also claims an unusual injury found only in one other sport – boxing. A cyst may form in the centre of the forehead just over the bridge of the nose. This is caused by repeated blows to the head. Boxers get it from being struck with a fist in a boxing glove. Football players cause it themselves by heading the ball with their foreheads. Studies of players who said they headed the ball more than 10 times per game also scored lower than average on tests for attention, concentration and overall mental functioning, compared to other players. But that's not the only risk: when you get whacked on the head, your neck suffers a horrific jolt.

There is no support or padding worn around the neck to protect it from serious injury, so it's up to you to protect your cervical spine by being careful.

Do extra work on your upper body. Because football is strictly a 'hands-off' sport (unless you are the goal keeper), relying mainly on your legs, you are deficient in work on your shoulders, upper back, arms, wrists and hands. We would like to see you work overtime on developing a strong back and neck if you want to excel at twisting, turning and heading. Being strong, flexible, and well-trained through practice will help you.

Guard against the elements. Because football is almost always played outside, you need to protect yourself from the effects of the sun and the heat. Stay hydrated with plenty of fluids before, during and after the match. And don't forget the sunscreen.

Use protection. Also, if you are offered safety equipment, such as shin pads, which protect the lower front leg, seize the opportunity. Remember that football is a contact sport played at top speed. A lot can go wrong very quickly. Give yourself every advantage.

Know your secret-weapon stretch: hip adductors. In addition to your regular workout, here's a stretch you can do in the changing room to warm up your hips for a longer, more controlled gait – this will really help when it comes to running and kicking.

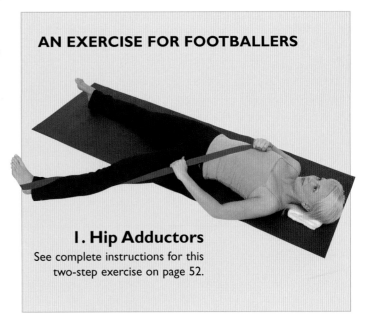

AN EXERCISE FOR FOOTBALLERS

I. Hip Adductors
See complete instructions for this
two-step exercise on page 52.

GOLF

A golf swing is one of the most complex of all athletic endeavours. The swing demands a full range of motion from nearly every joint in the body, so full flexibility is absolutely essential. The areas of your body that most affect a swing are your abdominals for stabilisation and rotation; your hip, trunk, arm and shoulder for the golf swing; and your wrist for grip, control and stability.

The forces that propel the swing actually start low, in your ankles and feet, travel up your legs as you begin your torque, go through your knees up your thighs to your hips, accelerate through your trunk, and drive up through your chest and shoulder as you tightly coil to draw back and lift into position your arms, wrists and hands. From this position, you're in full rotation with your eye on the ball. At this moment, you're gauging forces, speed, direction, finesse and power necessary to strike that ball perfectly to put it where you want it. You experience a moment of complete stillness, and then – pow! – you unwind explosively, sweeping your arms, wrists and hands down in that controlled, graceful arc that forms your swing.

Power and momentum drive your follow-through into a reverse 'C' finish. And here is a simple lesson in physics for you: the more flexible you are, the further you can bring the club away from the ball as you wind up; increasing this range creates more swing speed, which gives you more distance and accuracy on your drive; and being able to sweep into your follow-through means that you have smoother control of your shot. Flexibility means more power, control, distance, accuracy and fewer overuse injuries.

In professional golfers, the most common injuries are to the wrist, back, hand, shoulder and knee.

In amateur golfers, the situation is different. Amateur injuries line up as the lower back, elbow, wrist, shoulder and knee.

We want you out there on the links, so do your best to avoid injury by trying some of these strategies.

Work on that swing. With both professional and amateur players, most injuries are caused by ineffective swing mechanics and inefficient or incomplete warm-up techniques. The difference between amateur and professional lower-back pain is that amateurs, often less well trained, load the spine more. And they lack the organised muscle-firing patterns that develop only with time and experience.

Emphasise flexibility. Professional golfers have the highest incidence of back injury of any professional athlete. The culprit is usually torsional stress on a back that is too inflexible to absorb the rotation in the hips, knees and shoulders, and is unable to spread the stresses over the entire spine, which is where they should be. Lower-back pain can be caused by a poor swing. And a poor swing can be caused by lower-back pain. Get strong and flexible, and your swing will improve.

Prepare your body. Take the time to warm up and cool down. Preparing your body for exercise is always important, but Dr Mark McLaughlin, from the department of neurosurgery at Tufts University School of Medicine in Massachusetts, says it's especially important when your back is hurting or weak.

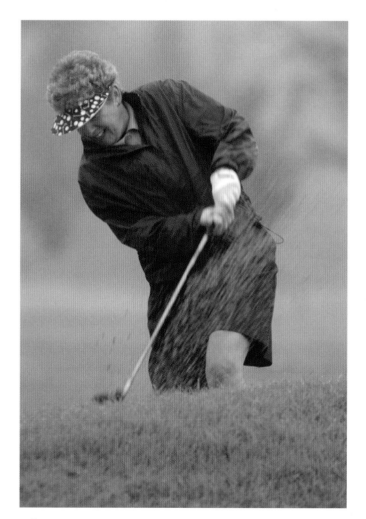

▲ Swingers

A surprising number of muscles are called upon when playing golf, and injuries can occur almost anywhere in the body.

Get in some cardio. If you can, leave the golf buggy and walk. If you can carry or pull your own clubs, all the better. Still, remember that golf will not give you a well-rounded workout. You'll need to augment your fitness programme with other cardio, strength and flexibility training.

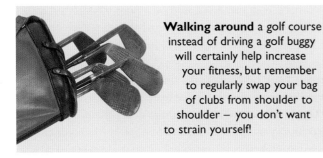

Walking around a golf course instead of driving a golf buggy will certainly help increase your fitness, but remember to regularly swap your bag of clubs from shoulder to shoulder — you don't want to strain yourself!

Don't be proud. If your back is in pain, move your ball out of angled lies, thick rough and pot bunkers rather than take the shot. If you're not up to playing, take some time off. A little rest now can preserve your game for the long term.

Take a water bottle. You're going to be out for a good few hours (usually in the sun), so stay hydrated.

Know your secret-weapon stretch: trunk lateral flexors. Here's a stretch that you can use in the changing room right before you step out on to the course. It gets your circulation going and loosens up the muscles in your back and along the sides of your trunk. The result? More dynamic torque in the wind-up and release of your swing.

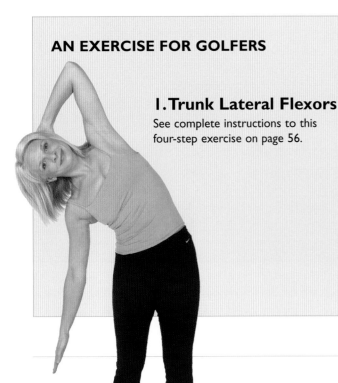

AN EXERCISE FOR GOLFERS

1. Trunk Lateral Flexors

See complete instructions to this four-step exercise on page 56.

INLINE SKATING

Inline skating was developed by Scott and Brennan Olson of Minnesota as an off-season training tool for skiers and ice hockey players. Done downhill, this skating closely approximates the physics of skiing, complete with weight transfer, edging and turns. Some ski resorts even have inline skating trails for training in the summer. On the flats – the way most of us will do it – inline skating closely approximates the physics of ice hockey.

Skating is a good, inexpensive, low-impact aerobic exercise that's great fun. Although it is enjoyed by people of all ages, it's now officially designated as an 'extreme' sport, a reputation earned by daring young skaters who defy gravity with impressive acrobatics.

For most of us, inline skating is uncomplicated. All you need is one inexpensive pair of skates, as much protective equipment as you can put on, and a vast expanse of pavement. Although the first thing you must learn to do is brake, skating begins with balance and coordination. You learn to roll forwards, then add pushing off, with each foot in a stabilising diagonal, from which pressure can be exerted to move the other foot forwards.

To stabilise, you use the abductors in your hips, buttocks (gluteals), thighs (quads) and calves (soleus). Your trunk flexes forwards from your hips with your back straight, engaging and contracting your abdominals, lower back and hip flexors and extensors to create that signature forward thrust. For turns and changing direction, you use hip abductors and adductors. For spins and rotations, you fire your hip and trunk rotators. For jumps, you lift off with your gluteals and abdominals and absorb shock with your hips. For backward movement, you turn your head with your neck rotators, hyperextend your hip for direction changes and abduct and adduct your hips for propulsion. Arm and torso swinging (rhythmic side-to-side motion) is controlled by your hip rotators, abductors and adductors, with your back and abdominals providing stabilisation. In other words, you get nearly a full-body workout.

Most injuries from inline skating are the results of trauma. Skaters fall down, crash into or fall off things, or slam into each other. But skaters have a high incidence of lower-back pain related to the repetitive movement and the extreme forward flexed position of the skater's trunk. This pain can be easily bypassed with stretching and adequate warm-up. Also, it's a good idea to stand up straight and take some of the tension out of your back with a few quick releases. Here are a few tips to make your inline skating injuries a little less 'extreme'.

Spare no precaution. Wear every bit of protection you can. Padding and bracing are critical for protecting knees, elbows and wrists. Also, we insist that you wear a helmet. Head injuries are very serious and totally avoidable.

Compensate the upper body. Inline skating, when you're really pumping, is a wonderful aerobic workout that lets you work your lower extremities, but your upper body can be neglected. You'll want to supplement your training with general strength and flexibility and with attention to upper body work.

Don't forget your lower half. Even though you're working your lower body pretty hard, don't forget that the skate boot restricts your foot and ankle movement and prevents your legs from getting a complete, well-balanced workout. Also make sure that you work legs, ankles and feet in your Stretching and Strengthening programme.

Boost your cardio. Again, it's a great cardio workout – but you can make it even better by buying yourself a set of ski poles with rubber tips and using the poles as you skate. Or join in a hockey game and swing a stick.

Know your secret-weapon stretch: ankle evertors. Because your ankles are going to be strapped into your boots and held rigidly, you have to introduce some flexibility for quick turning and shock absorption when you jump. Your skating will be smoother, and you'll feel better when you change from skates to your normal shoes.

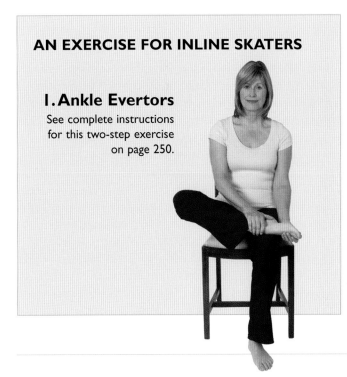

AN EXERCISE FOR INLINE SKATERS

1. Ankle Evertors

See complete instructions for this two-step exercise on page 250.

RUGBY

Rugby is a contact sport, and one of the features of the game is the scrum, where the two opposing packs of forwards group together with heads down and arms interlocked and push to gain ground. It's a tangle of pushing, pulling and kicking. It's not uncommon for a scrum to collapse and afford even more opportunity for physical contact, only this time everyone's off balance and on the ground head first. Stamping is common. Considering the studs on the bottom of everyone's boots, it can get pretty ugly.

Surprisingly, injuries are fairly infrequent. The most common variety are cuts – mainly to the head and face – half of which will require stitches. Second most common are joint injuries, usually incurred as one player defends the ball against another player – or the entire opposing team. After joint injuries are the following: neck strain, cervical spine injury, shoulder and arm injuries, and trunk trauma. Follow these tips to prevent injury on the pitch.

Fifteen per cent of all injuries suffered while playing rugby are the result of illegal moves, so somebody's not playing fair... but few players seem to mind. Like many Olympic sports, rugby has its roots in battle, one on one, and it's easy to get carried away in the passion of the moment.

Drop the beer, pick up the exercise strap. As with all sports, strength, flexibility and cardio fitness will help you stay alert and give you an advantage in defeating the opposing team. Warming up before a game is critical to get all muscles ready for contact.

Know your secret-weapon stretches: neck extensors and neck lateral flexors. Rugby is a sport where the back and neck are at risk, and there's little to be done about that, except to be highly conditioned and to stay out of the way of the thundering herd. Because tackling and scrummaging can get out of hand, the neck is particularly at risk. Make sure you're strong. Your mouth guard won't save you from an injury in the cervical spine. (See overleaf for exercises.)

TWO EXERCISES FOR RUGBY PLAYERS

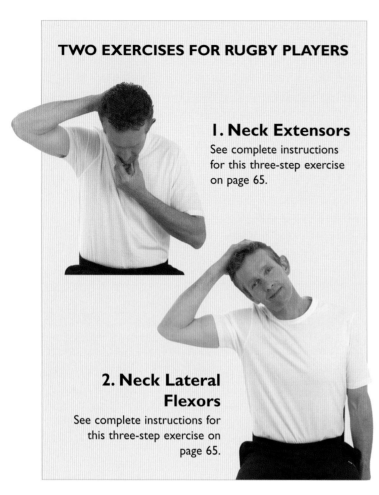

1. Neck Extensors

See complete instructions for this three-step exercise on page 65.

2. Neck Lateral Flexors

See complete instructions for this three-step exercise on page 65.

RUNNING

Running is a rewarding exercise and a passion shared by millions of people all over the world. It's inexpensive – all you need are a good pair of running shoes and some comfortable, loose clothing – and can be done almost anywhere. Perhaps the most beautiful thing about running is the basic biomechanics. Your running gait has three simple phases: the foot plant (this is when one foot is planted on the ground and your body literally rides over the top of it); the push-off (this is when that foot leaves the ground behind you in a thrust from your glutes and swings forwards to receive your weight in front of you, literally when the back leg becomes the front leg); and airborne (this is when both feet are off the ground before the front foot plants again and right after the back foot pushes off).

The third phase, airborne, is what distinguishes running from walking or racewalking. In the foot-plant phase, your ankle is the power generator, outworking your knee by 150 per cent and your hip by 300 per cent. (In fact, the ankle is responsible for 60 per cent of the total power, followed by

40 per cent from the knee, and 20 per cent from the hip.) Power for your push-off phase comes primarily from your gluteus maximus. Literally, you thrust, rather than lift, your knee and reach out with your leg for the next step. Your arms pump, amplifying forward momentum and counterbalancing your body.

As you run, your arms are pumping to help you stay in balance and rhythm and to amplify the energy of forward momentum. Your abs and back are holding you in an erect position. Your hands are relaxed. Your head is up. Your chest is open. And you are breathing.

Running is a superior cardiovascular workout, but because runners hold a specific form, the body ends up getting very little variety. Weakness and imbalance can set in. Because of this, runners hold the record for overuse injuries among all athletes in all fields – a massive 70 per cent. Of all runners, 37 to 56 per cent get hurt every year, although the injuries might be only minor. Injuries of the knee are most common, followed, in order of frequency, by feet, hips, upper legs and thighs, and lower back. Follow these tips to avoid injury.

Get strong and flexible. While running is great for your cardiovascular system and gives a good workout to many muscles, it's not a perfect exercise. You need to supplement it with Active-Isolated Stretching and Strengthening. Not only is variety good for complete fitness, it will improve your running.

General Active-Isolated Strengthening will help you hold your form and maintain efficiency, and it also will give your muscles some variety so that you can avoid imbalance and weakness. Flexibility training will allow you to lengthen your stride.

Don't forget to drink. Running is strenuous, sweating work. Hydrate before, during and after your run. Staying hydrated can help keep your blood volumes up, which helps your heart more efficiently pump blood and oxygen to the muscles. The muscles need the increased blood and oxygen to fire and, then, carry metabolic waste away.

Invest in good running shoes. It's an astonishing fact, but with every footstrike in running, you put between 1.5 and 5 times your body weight down through your legs to your feet. This works out at more than 110 footstrikes per mile (68 for each kilometre) or 5,000 footstrikes per hour. If you weigh 125lb (56kg), this can be as much as 625lb (280kg) of force 5,000 times an hour. That is an enormous amount of impact! Running places great demands on your body,

but your foot is remarkable in its shock-absorbing ability –
especially with the right footwear. Go to a reputable sports
outlet and ask them to fit you for the best shoes you can
afford. You'll feel the difference immediately. Once you
have a decent pair of shoes, you'll never go back.

Rest. And remember to make sure you get some rest.
One of the greatest secrets to top-level training is that a
day off between hard workouts allows the body to recover
and rebuild more effectively. You'll get stronger and faster
if you integrate easy workouts or complete rest between
sessions of tough training.

Know your secret-weapon stretch: standing quadriceps.
The stretch shown below is the best, but, unless you are
blessed with excellent balance and coordination, you might
want to stand facing something against which you can
steady yourself. There's nothing more heartening to your
opponents than to see you topple over on the starting line.

▶ Staying on track
Running is great exercise but injuries are common – particularly
in the knees and feet. Stretching can help prevent these.

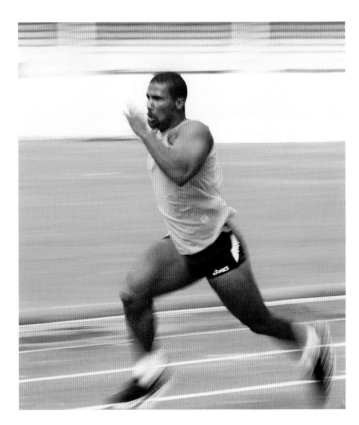

1 Standing Quadriceps

Active Muscles You Contract: Muscles in your buttocks and backs of your thighs
Isolated Muscles You Stretch: Muscles in the fronts of your thighs
Hold Each Stretch: 2 seconds **Reps:** 10 to the left, 10 to the right

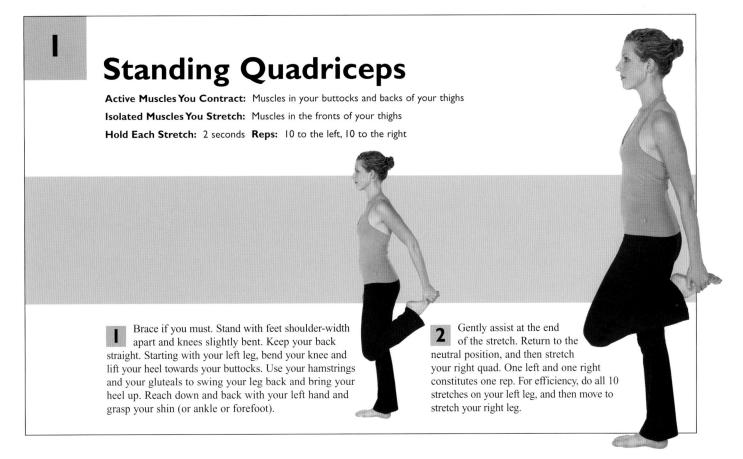

1 Brace if you must. Stand with feet shoulder-width
apart and knees slightly bent. Keep your back
straight. Starting with your left leg, bend your knee and
lift your heel towards your buttocks. Use your hamstrings
and your gluteals to swing your leg back and bring your
heel up. Reach down and back with your left hand and
grasp your shin (or ankle or forefoot).

2 Gently assist at the end
of the stretch. Return to the
neutral position, and then stretch
your right quad. One left and one right
constitutes one rep. For efficiency, do all 10
stretches on your left leg, and then move to
stretch your right leg.

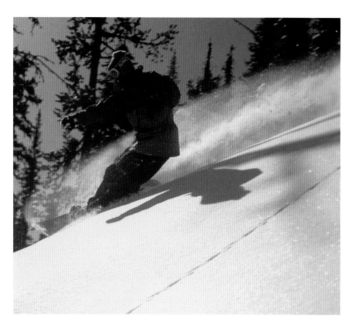

▲ Snowboarding
The backs of experienced snowboarders are loose and relaxed, with most injuries only being caused by wiping out (falling over).

SNOWBOARDING

Snowboarding actually made its debut in the 1920s, but today it is not only the fastest-growing winter sport in the world but also the fastest, no question. It has graduated from the exclusive domain of hotdoggers with their hell-bent downhill runs to choreographed, aerobatic, balletic international competitions. Snowboarding has been designated as an 'extreme' sport.

When you snowboard, you use your legs for stabilising and your ankle flexors and extensors, knee flexors and extensors, and hip abductors and adductors for balancing and turning. Your trunk is generally flexed forwards. Your abdominals provide support.

Your arms and wrists are extended for balance and counterbalance or for gripping the board to guide it. You are loose and relaxed, guiding the board by shifting your centre of gravity and putting pressure on one edge of the board. The physics are nearly identical to surfing, in which digging in on one side propels you in the opposite direction.

The most common snowboarding injuries are strains, sprains, fractures and bruises – and most of those, especially those above the waist, are caused by wiping out (falling over). Interestingly, since most boarders strap themselves in with the left foot in front, leg and foot injuries generally occur on the left side. It's no surprise that beginners are more at risk than veterans, but prevention is very logical. Use your common sense!

Stretch and strengthen before you hit the trails. Strength and flexibility are crucial for manoeuvring your board quickly and accurately. Because snowboarding is not a complete exercise, you'll want to supplement your training with some lifting and stretching.

Being fit means having more fun. Running, cycling or inline skating at altitude yields superior cardiovascular benefits. In fact, athletes in other endurance sports often retreat to high-altitude areas before major competitions. When they work out at altitude, their bodies adjust to the thin air by increasing oxygen-carrying capabilities. When they return to sea level, their performance levels improve measurably. We encourage you to take advantage of your location. Increased cardiovascular health translates to stamina: more fun for longer periods of time.

Respect the weather. Being out in the elements demands that you pay attention to them. Make an effort to stay warm, wear eye protection (from sun, glare and impact), and use sunscreen on your face and lips. Drink water to keep yourself hydrated.

Know your secret-weapon stretch: thoracic-lumbar rotators. Here's one stretch that you can do before you hit the slopes (see below). It will warm up your back for maximum manoeuvring and control.

AN EXERCISE FOR SNOWBOARDERS

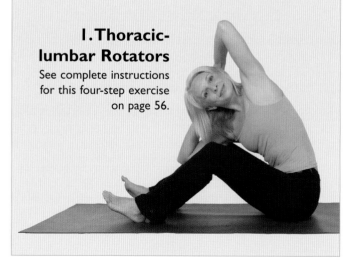

1. Thoracic-lumbar Rotators
See complete instructions for this four-step exercise on page 56.

SQUASH AND RACQUETBALL

Squash has been called the fastest of all racket sports. That's a good thing. Generally, the faster the sport, the better the workout. On the downside, however, being the fastest also means there's greater opportunity for getting hurt. In fact, it has the highest rate of injury in all racket sports – 59 per cent.

There's no way to identify individual muscles involved with the biomechanics of a squash player, because when you play, you work nearly everything, combining gymnastics, acrobatics, aerobatics and racket skills.

Squash requires enormous control, endurance, strength, finesse, eye-hand coordination and visual acuity. It all sounds wonderful, except that a falter in any one of these talents and skills can result in an injury to yourself or your opponent. Compared to other sports, injuries are generally quite low, but the majority of them are traumatic: slamming into the wall, getting whacked with a racket, tripping and falling.

Very few injuries are from overuse, and those that are often occur when the player is competing above his or her skill level or is on the court too long and is tired. Overhead strokes can cause shoulder problems such as rotator-cuff strains and nerve impingement, leading to pain and numbness. Because the racket is lightweight and the player snaps or slaps a stroke, the elbow and wrist may suffer fatigue and strain. Ballistically changing directions from side to side or from front to back and pivoting to catch a shot can result in sprains and strains of the ankles and feet. But, by far the most dangerous injuries in racket sports involve the eye and the head. It's easy to get into the line of fire of a rocketing ball or a racket badly swung.

Do what you can to stay out of that line of fire, and stay healthy with these tips.

Focus on balance. Squash is decidedly one-sided – unless you're ambidextrous and you switch the racket from side to side, only one arm, shoulder and side of your back are going to be worked out during a game. The other side will end up being weaker unless you plan your training to make certain that both sides of your body are strong, flexible and balanced all the way up and down the line.

Get fit first. Squash is a wonderful way to work off the tensions of the day and get a good workout, but it's not recommended as a way to get fit. Instead, think of it as a game to play *after* you're conditioned. We hate to tell you this, but sports medicine experts cite squash as having the potential for heart attack in players who play too hard without proper conditioning. Stamina and endurance will not only give you the edge over your exhausted competitors, it might also save your life. Put a high-level cardiovascular workout into your programme.

Wear eye protection. Choose shatterproof glasses made especially for racket sports. Make sure they fit properly and are secure on your face.

Don't skimp on stretching. Warm up properly so that the sudden, ballistic movements required in squash will not damage unprepared, cold muscles.

Choose court shoes. Leave your running shoes in your workout bag; they're made for moving forwards only. Wear shoes that will support your feet as you pivot and move side to side. Make sure they fit properly and are tightly fastened at all times.

Safety first. Never enter a court while a game is in play. Make sure your door is closed so that someone will not haplessly wander onto your court. And stay alert on the court. We don't want to hear the sickening sound of 'squash' coming from your court.

Know your secret-weapon stretch: hip abductors. This quick stretch is perfect for the locker room, right before the match. It will prepare your back, hips and upper legs for the demands of lunging, pivoting and jumping.

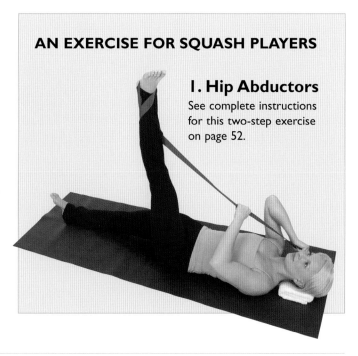

AN EXERCISE FOR SQUASH PLAYERS

1. Hip Abductors
See complete instructions for this two-step exercise on page 52.

SWIMMING

Swimming is the ultimate repetitive-movement sport, from kicking with legs to stroking with arms. Each movement takes place over and over and over and over… until something in the body becomes fatigued and strains.

Repetitive stress manifests itself most often in the shoulder. Tendinitis of the supraspinatus or biceps tendon – swimmer's shoulder – is found in about half of all competitive swimmers at some time in their careers.

No wonder the shoulder is so susceptible to overuse injury. As the most mobile of all the joints in the body, it is the most fragile with very little skeletal support. Strokes that are powered by the shoulder have to rely on complicated stabilising and mobilising relationships among the rotator-cuff muscles, the shoulder capsule, tendons, bones, ligaments and muscles of the chest and back. These balances are easily upset and can set off a cascade of injuries – many in the upper back. Other overuse injuries in the swimmer's body include strains, sprains, irritation and tendinitis in the feet, ankles, knees, elbows and back.

Although back injuries in swimming are few, the cervical spine and lumbar spine are at risk when you dive, with rapid extension and flexion changes and the arching of the back after entering the water. The butterfly stroke can also be hard on the lumbar spine, because of the extension and flexion of the back and legs against the resistance of the water. Younger swimmers are especially at risk.

Although the water in swimming pools is increasingly treated using more eye-friendly chemicals – instead of chlorine – it's still a good idea to wear goggles when swimming if your eyes are sensitive.

The good news is that swimming is great for treating back injuries. The pool provides a spectacular workout without any jarring or pounding. The weightlessness of a body in water tends to take a lot of pressure off the back, so that some measure of fitness can be maintained or even enhanced without irritating the back further. Make your swimming even safer with these tips.

Don't forget your bones. Although swimming is a wonderful exercise, it doesn't provide a full workout, so you'll want to supplement your training with strength and flexibility. Remember that swimming isn't a load-bearing exercise – that is, swimming does not put any impact on the bones. Women who rely on exercise for osteoporosis

▼ Keeping afloat
Swimming is a terrific sport – whether done seriously or just for pleasure. Injuries are rare and occur mainly in the shoulder.

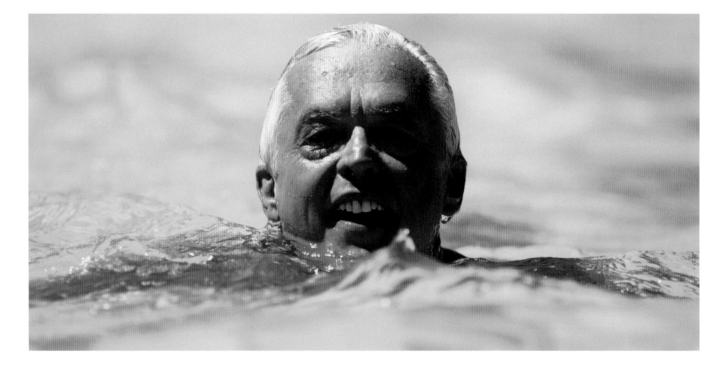

prevention need load-bearing work and should consider adding some more appropriate fitness components to their training, such as strength training and walking.

Drink plenty of water. When you swim, it's easy to forget that you need to hydrate adequately. When you're already wet, you might forget that swimming is hard work and you're sweating. Drink plenty of fluids. Keep a bottle of water by the side of the pool and stop by for a drink at regular intervals.

Know your secret-weapon stretch: shoulder external rotators. Swimming is extra tough on your shoulders because you have to move powerfully – but you have to do it against the resistance of the water. Certainly, it's a superior workout, but it's also hard on your shoulders and upper back. Let's warm you up with a stretch that will give you an advantage.

AN EXERCISE FOR SWIMMMERS

1. Shoulder External Rotators

See complete instructions for this three-step exercise on page 62.

Case Study:

Top-level athletes often suffer from muscle injuries, and swimming the butterfly with spasming back muscles is a sure-fire recipe for disaster.

We met Brian, a champion junior Olympian, at a workshop we were conducting at his swimming club on Long Island. He was a junior in high school at the time. He had a frozen shoulder and severe upper-back pain.

An examination showed that the infraspinatus muscle in his rotator cuff had become shortened. He had only about five degrees range of motion in the joint, radiating pain into his forearm and hand. Back muscles that cross over the cuff spasmed to protect it. It wasn't long before they were overloaded from compensation and shorting out. Because his forearm and hand were losing function, his shoulder was frozen, and his back was aching. He was miserable.

Brian's injuries were serious, so we started his therapy with minimal movements – in millimeters – so that we could get things moving and get neural control back for him. We started by unlocking his body with Active-Isolated Stretching.

Eventually, we were able to unlock Brian's cervical spine, but there was a lot of scar tissue within his muscles that had to be broken up. Swimming powerfully and rotating his neck and lifting his head against water resistance had taken a mighty toll. We had to repattern his muscles and restore neural drive so they would react to commands from his brain.

Once we released his cervical spine, his frozen shoulder started to give.

When we could get him through a stretch routine, we moved into strengthening. Again, we had to go very slowly and recognise that all these little improvements were adding up fast.

Even though he was a big kid, we started with 1lb (455g) weights. Eventually, we got him up to 25lb (11.3kg). It took time, but Brian learned the work and did it. He was back in the pool at competition level – and without pain – within a couple of months.

By the end of his senior year, he earned a swimming scholarship to the US Naval Academy. He's now a Navy Seal. And he gets other Seals to work out with exercise straps.

TENNIS

We have worked with tennis players for many years and find them to be among the fittest of all our athletes. Tennis is a spectacular workout, which also seems to be a lot of fun. After all, the equipment is fairly inexpensive, there are indoor courts and outdoor courts almost everywhere, and partners and coaches are plentiful.

Tennis is a game that keeps you on high alert at all times. You have to be ready for anything, from diving to the ground to leaping into the air. These high-speed manoeuvres are both the blessing and the bane of the sport. Although they help develop a powerful athlete, they also put a great deal of stress on the body.

The most common injuries of tennis players, in order of frequency, are the shoulder, back, elbow, knee and ankle.

Notice that we start at the top and move south? Most injuries are the result of overuse – repetitive movements that simply cause fatigue and then damage. In tennis, repetitive movements are also traumatic. Players hit hard, and even the smallest little injuries can become problematic after the 100th time they're irritated. Eventually, these small traumas will result in tendinitis, strain and stress fractures. A good example of a tennis injury made worse by repetition is tennis elbow – lateral epicondylitis.

Not all injuries result from repetition and hammering. A little over a third of all tennis injuries are simply accidents: turning an ankle, wrenching a knee or fracturing a bone in the foot.

As for the back, it's involved 110 per cent. Tennis is second only to squash in back injuries, and nearly 40 per cent of professional players have missed tournaments because of back pain. The back takes massive force to haul back at the shoulder, go into rotation, and then unwind in an explosion that gets the ball over the net. Small imbalances can create big problems. Follow this advice to make sure you play only when you're strong and flexible and have the endurance to beat your opponent.

Look for a mentor. Your form is very important, so you'll need time to perfect it. One great way to avoid injury is to study with an experienced coach who will make sure your moves are perfect.

Go at your own pace. Also, be sure to advance slowly from one level to the next. Too much, too soon guarantees fatigue, discouragement and injury. Build a solid foundation every step of the way, and your game will be much stronger.

Cross-train. To play tennis well, you have to be light on your feet. Active-Isolated Stretching and Strengthening are the perfect programmes to achieve this because you need flexibility for quick moves and strength, not bulk, for driving the ball. You also need a good cardio workout to supplement your training and playing. Tennis is far too much 'stop and start' for you to get your heart rate up and keep it there long enough for a good cardio programme, but you do need to have stamina and endurance. We recommend running, cycling, swimming, cross-country skiing or inline skating.

Protect yourself from the sun. As a side note, remember that there is no shade on a tennis court, so wear sunscreen with a high SPF, a hat and sunglasses that are shatter-proof. Also, drink plenty of water before, during and after play. Put a large bottle of water at the edge of your court and use every opportunity to swing by for a sip – like when your opponent is busy trying to locate the ball you just rocketed straight out of the court.

Make the most of pauses in play. As you are strolling to the side or swapping ends in between games, use the time to stretch out your shoulders and shake off some tension. If anything hurts, stop the game.

Know your secret-weapon stretch: hip abductors. Before you hit the court, try the stretch below to warm up your back, hips and legs and put speed and power into your ability to run, pivot, jump and back up.

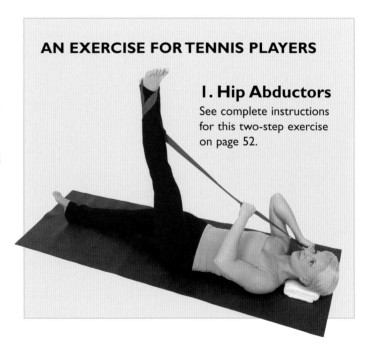

AN EXERCISE FOR TENNIS PLAYERS

1. Hip Abductors
See complete instructions for this two-step exercise on page 52.

WALKING

Humans, by all accounts, have been walking for at least three million years. Almost everyone can do it, from toddlers right on up to the eldest among us. It's an inexpensive, low-impact, tension-busting, cardiovascular exercise that gets your heart rate up and burns off excess calories. In 30 minutes of walking at a fast pace up hills, you can burn up to 300 calories. We believe in it so much that we made it a large part of our programme. (See 'Your Cardio Programme' on page 88.)

We describe the biomechanics of walking in chapter 2, but we want to point out that another fascinating aspect of walking is the action of your arms. The opposite arm will swing in perfect cadence with the swinging leg: right arm with left leg and left arm with right leg. Nature has designed it this way to counterbalance you as your weight shifts from foot to foot and to amplify the momentum of your gait. The faster you go, the more energetic and higher the arm swing. If you have never noticed it, try swinging your left arm forwards when you swing your left leg forwards: it's nearly impossible.

Injuries in walking are few and far between. To make it even safer, just take it easy, increase your distance and difficulty slowly, and keep these pointers in mind.

Don't forget to stretch and strengthen. Much as we extol the virtues of walking, we must admit that it is not the perfect exercise. You still need Active-Isolated Stretching and Strengthening to keep your muscles strong and flexible. Follow all three facets of the programme for total fitness.

Walk unencumbered. We want to caution you about carrying handheld weights or strapping on shot-filled ankle and wrist weights as you walk. They change the dynamics of your stride and add stress to the arm muscle attachments at the shoulder joints.

Know your secret-weapon stretch: tibialis anteriors. Walking plants your heel flat on the ground over and over. If you're not used to it, it can strain the front of your shin, maybe even causing the dreaded shin splints. Try the above exercise to help ensure that your shin can support the lift of your forefoot and the strike of your heel.

▶ Take a hike
Walking is a brilliant cardiovascular exercise that forms the basis of many enjoyable pursuits. Backpacking, in particular, is a great way to work out while enjoying the outdoors.

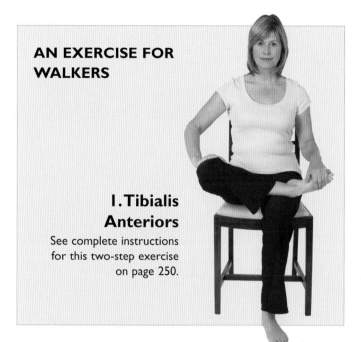

AN EXERCISE FOR WALKERS

1. Tibialis Anteriors
See complete instructions for this two-step exercise on page 250.

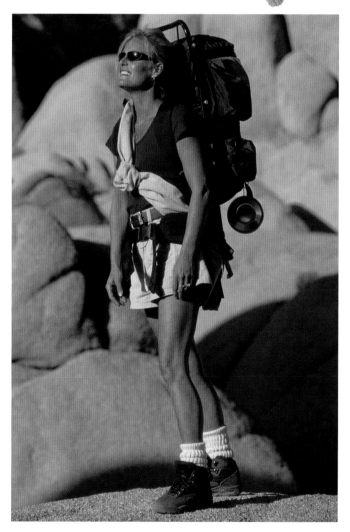

THE PRINCIPAL MUSCLE SETS OF THE BODY

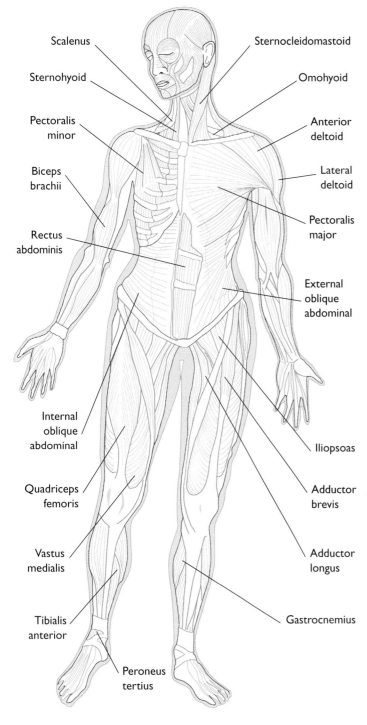

Scalenus

Sternohyoid

Pectoralis minor

Biceps brachii

Rectus abdominis

Internal oblique abdominal

Quadriceps femoris

Vastus medialis

Tibialis anterior

Peroneus tertius

Sternocleidomastoid

Omohyoid

Anterior deltoid

Lateral deltoid

Pectoralis major

External oblique abdominal

Iliopsoas

Adductor brevis

Adductor longus

Gastrocnemius

Abdominals: Including the rectus abdominis, the internal oblique abdominal and the external oblique abdominal. These are also referred to as the abs.

Ankle evertors: Including the peroneus longus, the peroneus brevis, the peroneous tertius and the extensor digitorum longus.

Ankle invertors: Including the tibialis anterior and the tibialis posterior.

Biceps: The biceps brachii.

Deltoids: Including the anterior deltoid, lateral deltoid and posterior deltoid.

Gastrocnemius: Also referred to as the gasrocs.

Gluteals: Including the gluteus maximus, the gluteus medius and the gluteus minimus. Also referred to as the glutes.

Hamstrings: Including the semimembranous, biceps femoris and semitendinous.

Hip abductors: Including the gluteus medius and the gluteus minimus.

Hip adductors: Including the adductor brevis, the adductor longus and the adductor magnus.

Hip extensors: Including the hamstrings and the gluteus maximus.

Hip external rotators: Including the gluteus maximus and the piriformis.

Hip flexors: Including the iliopsoas (psoas and iliacus), the quadriceps femoris and the tensor fascia latae.

Hip internal rotators: Including the gluteus minimus and the tensor fascia latae.

Knee extensors: Including the quadriceps femoris and the vastus medialis.

Neck extensors: Including the sternocleidomastoid, scalenus, levator scapulae, trapezius, rectus capitis posterior major, rectus capitis posterior minor.

Neck flexors: Including the scalenus, the sternocleidomastoid, the sternohyoid and the omohyoid.

Neck rotators: Including the splenius capitis and the levator scapulae.

Pectoralis: The pectoralis major and the pectoralis minor.

Pronators: See evertors.

Quadriceps: Including the quadriceps femoris.

Sacrospinalis: Beneath the erector spinae.

Shoulder internal rotators: Including the subscapularis (beneath the deltoids).

Shoulder external rotators: Including the infraspinatus.

Supinators: See invertors.

Thoracic (lumber) rotators: Including the longissimus thoracis and the spinalis thoracis.

Tibialis: The tibialis anterior and the tibialis posterior. These are ankle invertors.

Trapezius: Also referred to as rotator cuff 2.

Trunk lateral flexors: Including the rectus abdominis and the internal oblique abdominal.

Trunk extensors: Including the erector spinae and the splenius capitis.

Rhomboid: The rhomboideus major and the rhomboideus minor. Also referred to as rotator cuff 1.

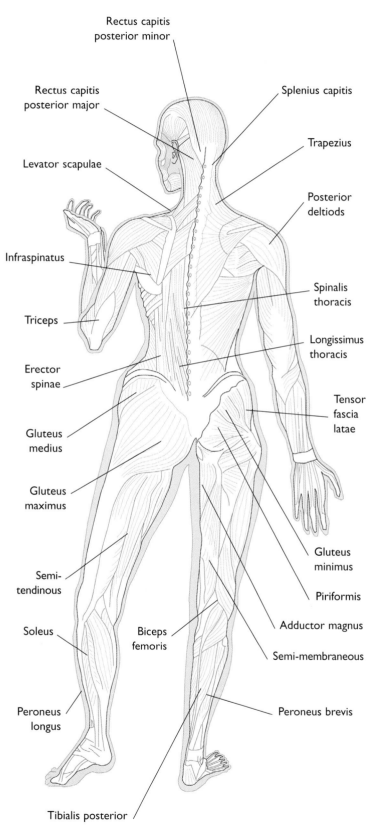

Rectus capitis posterior minor

Rectus capitis posterior major

Levator scapulae

Splenius capitis

Trapezius

Posterior deltiods

Infraspinatus

Triceps

Spinalis thoracis

Longissimus thoracis

Erector spinae

Tensor fascia latae

Gluteus medius

Gluteus maximus

Gluteus minimus

Piriformis

Semi-tendinous

Adductor magnus

Soleus

Biceps femoris

Semi-membraneous

Peroneus longus

Peroneus brevis

Tibialis posterior

FURTHER RESOURCES

■ ANKYLOSING SPONDYLITIS

**National Ankylosing Spondylitis
Society**
PO Box 179
Mayfield
East Sussex, TN20 6ZL, UK
www.nass.co.uk

■ ARTHRITIS

Arthritis Foundation of Western Australia
17 Lemnos Street
Shenton Park, WA 6008, Australia
www.arthritiswa.org.au

Arthritis Research Campaign
Copeman House
St Mary's Court
St Mary's Gate
Chesterfield
Derbyshire, S41 7TD, UK
www.arc.org.uk

■ CHIROPRACTORS

British Chiropractic Association
17 Blagrave Street
Berkshire, RG1 1QB, UK
www.chiropractic-uk.co.uk

**Chiropractors Association
of Australia**
Suite 7
Castlereagh Street
Penrith, NSW 2750, Australia
www.chiropractors.asn.au

New Zealand Chiropractors Association
PO Box 46 7144
Herne Bay
Auckland, New Zealand
www.chiropractic.org.nz

**Chiropractic Association
of South Africa**
www.chiropractic.co.za

■ COMPLEMENTARY AND ALTERNATIVE THERAPY

**Association of Massage
Therapists (AMTA)**
Level 2
85 Queen Street, VIC 3000, Australia
www.amta.asn.au

**Association of Specialised
Kinesiologists (KZN branch)**
Kwa-Zulu Natal Branch
Gudrun Lauterbach
PO Box 277
Warburg 3233, South Africa
www.kinesiology.co.za

**Australian Acupuncture &
Chinese Medicine Association Ltd**
PO Box 5142
West End, QLD 4101, Australia
www.acupuncture.org.au

**Australasian College
of Natural Therapies**
57 Foveaux Street
Surry Hills
NSW 2010, Australia
www.acnt.edu.au

Australian Kinesiology Association
AKA Inc.
PO Box 233
Kerrimuir, VIC 3129, Australia
www.aka-oz.org

**Australian Naturopathic
Practitioners Association (ANPA)**
PO Box 1190

Hartwell, VIC 3125, Australia
www.anpa.asn.au

**The Australian Society of
Hypnosis (ASH)**
Publications Office, ASH
PO Box 5114
Alphington, VIC 3078, Australia
www.ozhypnosis.com.au

**The Ayurvedic Company
of Great Britain Ltd**
81 Wimpole Street
London, W1G 9RF, UK
www.ayurvedagb.com

British Acupuncture Council
63 Jeddo Road
London, W12 9HQ, UK
www.acupuncture.org.uk

**British Homeopathic
Association**
Hahnemann House
29 Park Street West
Luton
Bedfordshire, LU1 3BE, UK
www.trusthomeopathy.org

**The British Medical
Acupuncture Society**
www.medical-acupuncture.co.uk

British Society of Clinical Hypnosis
www.bsch.org.uk

**The Confederation of Complementary
Health Associates of Southern Africa
(COCHASA)**
COCHASA National Office
PO Box 2471
Clareinch 7740, South Africa
www.cochasa.org.za

**Complementary Medicine
Association (CMA)**
CMA Federal Administration Office
PO Box 6412
Baulkham Hills, NSW 2153, Australia
www.cma.asn.au

**The General Council and
Register of Naturopaths**
Goswell House
2 Goswell Road
Street
Somerset, BA16 0JG, UK
www.naturopathy.org.uk

**Institute for Complementary
Medicine**
PO Box 194
London, SE16 7QZ, UK
www.icmedicine.co.uk

Kinesiology Federation
PO Box 28908
Edinburgh, EH22 2YQ, UK
www.kinesiologyfederation.org

**Massage Therapy Association
South Africa (MTA)**
PO Box 53320
Kenilworth 7745, South Africa
www.mtasa.co.za

**National Herbalists Association
of Australia (NHAA)**
NHAA Office
13 Breillat Street
Annandale, NSW 2038, Australia
www.nhaa.org.au

**New Zealand Association
of Medical Herbalists**
nzamh.org.nz/index.htm

**New Zealand Association of
Professional Hypnotherapists**
PO Box 90-314
AMSC
Auckland 1030, New Zealand
www.nzaph.co.nz

**Therapeutic Massage
Association (TMA)**
PO Box 19005
Courtney Place
Wellington, New Zealand
www.tmanz.org.nz

**New Zealand Council
of Homeopaths**
New Zealand Council of Homeopaths
PO Box 51-195
Tawa, Wellington, New Zealand
www.homeopathy.co.nz

**New Zealand Register
of Acupuncturists**
PO Box 9950
Wellington 6001, New Zealand
www.acupuncture.org.nz

**New Zealand Register of
Complementary Health
Professionals**
c/o New Zealand Health Network
PO Box 337
Christchurch, New Zealand
www.nzhealth.net.nz

**New Zealand Society
of Naturopaths**
PO Box 90-170
Auckland Central Post Office
Auckland, New Zealand
www.naturopath.org.nz

The Reiki Association
Cornbrook Bridge House
Clee Hill
Ludlow
Shropshire, SY8 3QQ, UK
www.reikiassociation.org.uk

Reiki New Zealand
PO Box 39 416
Howick, Auckland, New Zealand
www.reiki.org.nz

**The South African Society
of Physiotherapy**

PO Box 92125
Norwood 2117, South Africa
www.physiosa.org.za

**TFH Kinesiology Association
of New Zealand (Inc)**
PO Box 10343
Hamilton, New Zealand
www.kinesiology.gen.nz

■ GENERAL HEALTH

**Australian Traditional
Medicine Society Ltd**
Suite 3
Fisrt Floor
120 Blaxland Road
Ryde NSW 2112, Australia
www.atms.com.au

**BBC Online Health
and Fitness**
www.bbc.co.uk/health

**Health Development Agency
(HDA)**
7th Floor
Holborn Gate
330 High Holborn
London, WC1V 7BA, UK
www.hda.nhs.uk

■ HEALTHY NUTRITION

**British Nutrition
Foundation (BNF)**
High Holborn House
52–54 High Holborn
London, WC1V 6RQ, UK
www.nutrition.org.uk

**Exercise Science and
Rehabilitation Centre**
University of Wollongong
Northfields Avenue
Wollongong, NSW 2522, Australia
www.nutritionaustalia.org

**The Institute for
Optimum Nutrition**
13 Blades Court
Deodar Road, Putney
London, SW15 2NU, UK
www.ion.ac.uk

**New Zealand Nutrition
Foundation**
Private Bag 25 905
St Heliers
Auckland, New Zealand
www.foodworks.co.nz/nutritionfoundation

**NICUS
Department of
Human Nutrition**
PO Box 19063
Tygerberg 7505, South Africa
webhost.sun.ac.za/nicus

■ **HOME SAFETY**

**Accident Compensation
Corporation (ACC)**
www.acc.co.nz

**Department of Trade
and Industry – Home
Safety Network**
www.dti.gov.uk/homesafetynetwork

**National Occupational Safety
Association (NOSA)**
Johannesburg, South Africa
www.nosa.co.za

**National Safety Council
of Australia**
322 Glenferrie Road
Malvern, VIC 3144, Australia
www.safetynews.com

**Royal Society for the
Prevention of Accidents**
353 Bristol Road
Edgbaston
Birmingham, B5 7ST, UK
www.rospa.co.uk

■ **OSTEOPATHY**

**Australian Osteopathic
Association**
PO Box 5044
Chatswood, NSW 1515, Australia
www.osteopathic.com.au

**General Osteopathic Council and
Osteopathic Information Service**
176 Tower Bridge Road
London, SE1 3LU, UK
wwww.osteopathy.org.uk

■ **OSTEOPOROSIS**

**National Osteoporosis
Foundation (NOF)**
www.nof.org

**National Oesteoporosis
Foundation of South
Africa (NOF)**
PO Box 481
Bellville
7535
South Africa
www.osteoporosis.org.za

National Osteoporosis Society
Camerton
Bath, BA2 0PJ, UK
www.nos.org.uk

Oesteoporosis Australia
PO Box 121
Sydney, NSW 2001, Australia
www.osteoporosis.org.au

Osteoporosis New Zealand
PO Box 688
Wellington, New Zealand
www.bones.org.nz

■ **PAIN**

**The Australian
Pain Society**
PO Box 571

Crows Nest
NSW 1585, Australia
www.apsoc.org.au

**New Zealand Pain
Society Inc**
PO Box 5303
Wellington, New Zealand
www.nzps.org.nz

**Pain Management Society
of South Africa (PMSSA)**
PO Box 12800
Amalinda
East London, 5252
South Africa
www.pain-management.co.za

Pain Relief Foundation
Clinical Sciences Centre
University Hospital Aintree
Lower Lane
Liverpool, L9 7AL, UK
www.painrelieffoundation.org.uk

■ **PREGNANCY**

Babyassist
www.babyassist.co.za

Babytimes
www.babytimes.co.nz

**Pregnancy, Birth
and Beyond**
27 Hart Street
Dundas, NSW 2117, Australia
www.pregnancy.com.au

Wellbeing
www.wellbeing.org.uk

■ **PHYSIOTHERAPY**

**Australian Physiotherapy
Association (APA)**
Level 3
201 Fitzroy Street
St. Kilda

Melbourne
Victoria 3182, Australia
www.physiotherapy.asn.au

**Chartered Society
of Physiotherapy**
14 Bedford Row
London, WC1R 4ED, UK
www.csp.org.uk

**New Zealand Society
of Physiotherapists Inc**
PO Box 27386
Wellington, New Zealand
www.nzsp.org.nz

South African Society of Physiotherapy
PO Box 92125
Norwood 2117, South Africa
www.physiosa.org.za

■ PRIMARY CARE DOCTORS

**National Association of
Patient Participation**
PO Box 999
Nuneaton
Warwickshire, CU11 5ZD, UK
www.napp.org.uk

Private Healthcare UK
Intuition Communication Ltd
Concept House
271 High Street
Berkhamsted
Hertfordshire, HP4 1AA, UK
www.privatehealth.co.uk

**Royal College of
General Practitioners**
14 Princess Gate
Hyde Park
London, SW7 1PU, UK
www.rcgp.org.uk

■ SCOLIOSIS

Scoliosis Research Society (SRS)
www.srs.org

■ SENIOR HEALTH

Age Concern
1268 London Road
London, SW16 4ER, UK
www.ace.org.uk

**Centre for Policy
on Ageing**
25–31 Ironmonger Row
London, EC1V 3QP, UK
www.cpa.org.uk

■ SPINES AND BACKS

BackCare
16 Elmtree Road
Teddington
Middlesex, TW11 8ST, UK
www.backpain.org

Spine-health.com
www.spine-health.com

SpineUniverse.com
www.spineuniverse.com

■ SPORTS MEDICINE

**Osteopathic Sports
Care Association**
PO Box 221
Sunbury-on-Thames
Middlesex, TW16 5AD, UK
www.osca.org.uk

**The Physician and
Sportsmedicine Online**
www.physsportsmed.com

SportsMedicine.com
www.sportsmedicine.com

■ WORKPLACE SAFETY

**The Information Network
of the European Agency for
Safety and Health at Work**
europe.osha.eu.int

**Institute for Occupational
Safety and Health**
The Grange
Highfield Drive
Wigston
Leicestershire, LE18 1NN, UK
www.iosh.co.uk

■ YOGA

**BKS Iyengar Yoga Association
of Australia Ltd**
www.iyengaryoga.asn.au

**BKS Iyengar Yoga Association
of New Zealand (IYANZ)**
www.iyengar-yoga.org.nz

British Wheel of Yoga
25 Jermyn Street
Sleaford
Lincolnshire, NG34 7ES, UK
bwy.org.uk

Iyengar Yoga Institute (London)
www.iyi.org.uk

Calories to Kilojoules (kj)

These equivalents have been slightly
rounded to make measuring easier.

Calories x 4.186 = Kilojoules

Calories	Kilojoules (kJ)
1	4.186
10	41.86
25	104.65
50	209.3
75	313.95
100	418.6
200	837.2
300	1,255.8
400	1,674.4
500	2,093
600	2,511.6
700	2,930.2
800	3,348.8
900	3,767.4
1,000	4,186

INDEX

Underlined page references indicate boxed text and tables. **Boldface** references indicate illustrations and photographs.

ACKNOWLEDGEMENTS

To the people from all walks of life and ends of the world, thank you for honouring us to help you help yourselves out of pain, for giving us the gift of witnessing the extension of the healing spirit; and to the doctors, health-care professionals and flexibility technicians who carry the torch in our mission of healing.

No book of ours can go to print without heartfelt thanks to the greatest agent and friend, Reid Boates. As he always says, "Onwards!" And many, many thanks to Mariska van Aalst, our talented and tireless editor at Rodale Inc. She's truly amazing.

Jim and Phil Wharton

Rodale Books International and Studio Cactus would like to thank the following people for their assistance in creating this book:

Aaron Brown, Phil Carré, Lorna Hankin, Kate Hawkins and Will Jones
for editorial and design assistance, Ann Marangos for proofreading,
and Lynda Swindells for indexing.

Thanks also go to all the models:

Nadia Anne, Charles Craven, Will Hall, Binny Lee Smith (BMA Model Agency),
Lynne Shillitto (MOT Model Agency),
Jacqueline Shaw (International Model Management),
Kate Hawkins.

Picture Credits

(b = bottom, bl = bottom left, br = bottom right, cl = centre left, cr = centre right, tl = top left, tr = top right)

Commissioned exercise photography: Gary Ombler

All other photography by Photos.com except for the following: Alamy 28; PhotoDisc 13, 14, 15, 20, 33, 43, br44, 45, 47, 66, tr88, tr101, 106, 107, 116, 117, 129, 142, 155, bl166, cr166, tl171, bl188, 193, 199, 220, b225, b270, br273; Studio Cactus bl98, tr98, br100, cl234, br248, tr270.